Migraine

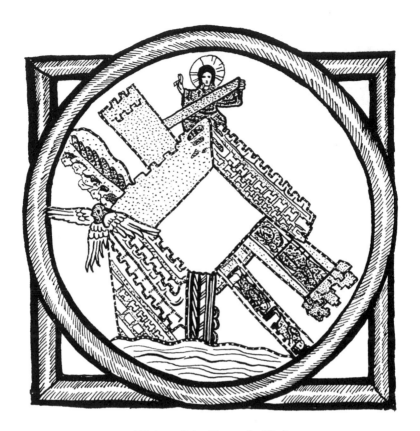

'Vision of the Heavenly City'

From a MS of Hildegard's *Scivias*, written at Bingen about 1180. This figure is a reconstruction from several visions of migrainous origin (see Appendix I).

Migraine

Revised and Expanded

Oliver Sacks

UNIVERSITY OF CALIFORNIA PRESS
Berkeley · *Los Angeles* · *London*

The publisher is grateful to Basic Books and Tavistock Publications for permission to reproduce two diagrams from *Higher Cortical Functions in Man* by A. R. Luria; to Constable and Co. for permission to reproduce five diagrams from C. Singer's *From Magic to Science*; and to the American Medical Association for permission to reproduce two diagrams from an article by K. Lashley published in the *Archives of Neurology and Psychiatry* of 1941. These, and other diagrams from original sources, have been redrawn and somewhat modified. The publisher is also grateful to the British Migraine Association and Boehringer Ingelheim Ltd. for permission to reproduce paintings from their collection of migraine art; and to Dr. Ronald K. Siegel for permission to reproduce Figure 10.

University of California Press
Berkeley and Los Angeles, California

University of California Press
London, England

Library of Congress Cataloging-in-Publication Data

Sacks, Oliver W.
    Migraine/Oliver Sacks.—Rev. and expanded ed.
        p.   cm.
    Includes bibliographical references and index.
    ISBN 0–520–08101–3 (cloth : alk. paper)
    ISBN 0–520–08223–0 (pbk. : alk. paper)
    1. Migraine.   I. Title.
    [DNLM: 1. Migraine.   WL 344 S 121ma]
RC392.S33   1992
616.8′57—dc20
DNLM/DLC
for Library of Congress   92–407
                                  CIP

Printed in the United States of America

3 4 5 6 7 8 9

To my parents

Socrates, in Plato, would prescribe no Physick for Charmides' headache till first he had eased his troublesome mind; body and soul must be cured together, as head and eyes. . . .

—*Robert Burton*

Whoever . . . sees in illness a vital expression of the organism, will no longer see it as an enemy. In the moment that I realise that the disease is a creation of the patient, it becomes for me the same sort of thing as his manner of walking, his mode of speech, his facial expression, the movements of his hands, the drawings he has made, the house he has built, the business he has settled, or the way his thoughts go: a significant symbol of the powers that rule him, and that I try to influence when I deem it right.

—*George Groddeck*

Contents

PART II The Occurrence of Migraine

Response to Flickering Light, Patterned Stimuli, and Visualisation of Scotomata · Miscellaneous Determinants: Food, Constipation, Menstrual Cycles, Hormones, Allergies, etc. · Self-Perpetuation of Migraines · Provocation of Attacks in Relation to "Tuning" and Homeostatic Limits Within Nervous System

Migraine in Relation to Intolerable Emotional Stress · Preliminary Comments on "Migraine Personality" and Relation of Attacks to Repressed Hostility · Case-Histories Illustrating Wide Range of Situations and Character-Types in which Repeated Migraines May Occur

PART III The Basis of Migraine

Clarification of the Term "Cause" in Relation to Migraine · Necessity to View Migraine in Three Ways: as a Process in the Nervous System, as a Reaction to Certain Stimuli, and as a Particular Form of Experience

Historical Introduction: Classical Theories (Humoral and Sympathetic), Vascular and Vasomotor Theories of the Nineteenth Century · Critiques of These · Liveing's Theory of "Nerve Storms" · Current Theories of Migraine Mechanisms and their Supporting Data · Vasomotor Theories (Latham-Wolff) Considered and Disputed · Chemical Theories of Migraine, with Particular Reference to Acetylcholine, Histamine, and Serotonin: Critique of These · Electroencephalographic Findings in Migraine: Notion of "Dysrhythmic Migraine," and of "Spreading Depression" in Relation to Migraine · Limitations of Current Theory and Data

Introductory Comments · Migraines as Polymorphous Parasympathetic or Trophotropic Events · Migraine as a Slow Form of Centrencephalic Seizure · Consideration of Visual Hallucinations in Migraine and Their Cortical Basis · Hierarchical Organisation of Migraines, and

Part v Migraine as a Universal

Illustrations

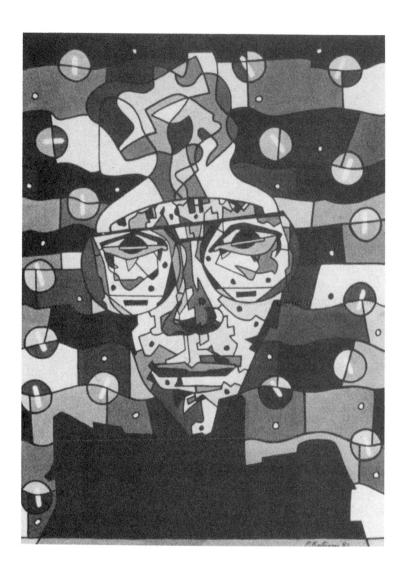

Many perceptual alterations may occur in migraine. The strangest and profoundest is *mosaic vision*, here shown in a painting done by a migraine sufferer asked to paint what he experienced during his attacks. (Courtesy British Migraine Association and Boehringer Ingelheim Limited.)

Preface to the Revised (1992) Edition

The chief features of migraine—its phenomena, and how these are experienced by the patient, its mode of occurrence, the triggers that may provoke it, the general ways in which one may live with it or combat it—none of these has changed in 2,000 years. Thus a vivid and detailed description of these matters is always relevant, and cannot become obsolete.

Many patients with migraine—especially young patients who experience a migraine aura, or an attack of classical migraine for the first time—have no idea what is happening to them, and may be terrified that they have a stroke, a brain tumour, or whatever—or conversely, that they are going mad, or suffering from some bizarre hysteria. It is an immense reassurance for such patients to learn that what they have is neither grave nor factitious, but a morally neutral, recurrent yet essentially benign condition which they share with countless others, and which is well understood. "Fear of this disease," wrote Montaigne, "used to terrify you, when it was unknown to you." A patient who has read *Migraine* will not be cured, but at least he will know what he has, and what it means, and will no longer be terrified.

Migraine, of course, is not just a description, but a meditation on the nature of health and illness, and how, occasionally, human beings may *need*, for a brief time, to be ill; a meditation on the unity of mind and body, on migraine as an exemplar of our psychophysical transparency; and a meditation, finally, on migraine as a *biological* reaction, analogous to that which many animals show. I think that these wider considerations, of migraine as part and parcel of the human condition, also retain their relevance—they constitute the unchanging *taxonomy* of migraine.

There have been reissues of *Migraine* over the years, but all of these, to my mind, have suffered from abridgement—from omitting some of the detail or discussion of the original, or watering it down, or trying to make the book more "popular" or "practical." Such attenuations, I have come to think, are wrong—the book is strongest in its original form, without ceasing to be accessible to the general reader.

And yet, clearly, there have been important advances in the last twenty years, relating to our new understanding of the mechanism of migraine, and to the development of new drugs and other techniques which can aid in its management. A patient who suffers severe and frequent migraines has a much better chance of dealing with this than he had in 1970. I am therefore making various additions to the book, including a new chapter (16) dealing with the exciting physiological and pharmacological discoveries of the last two decades, and the new modes of treatment for migraine which these now make available. I have added postscripts to three chapters, exploring migraine in relation to chaos and consciousness theory. I have also added a number of further case histories, a historical appendix, and numerous footnotes throughout the book. With these additions, the current edition becomes the fullest, as well as the most current, edition of *Migraine*.

In the original manuscript of *Migraine* (1967–68) there was a Part V, which consisted of a re-examination of the most complex geometric forms of the aura, and an attempt to provide a deep explanation of these. I came to feel that I had not succeeded in this, and that any such attempt, indeed, was premature at the time. So I omitted that part from the published book. It has been an especial pleasure, now, to be able to return to this project, and, with my colleague Ralph Siegel, to suggest a general theory or explanation of these aura phenomena of a sort which would not have been possible 25 years ago. Thus, in this 1992 edition, there is, finally, a Part V.

O. W. S.
New York
February 1992

Preface to the Original (1970) Edition

When I saw my first migraine patient, I thought of migraine as a peculiar type of headache, no more and no less. As I saw more patients, it became apparent to me that headache was never the sole feature of a migraine, and, later still, that it was not even a necessary feature of all migraines. I was moved, therefore, to enquire further into a subject which appeared to retreat before me, growing more complex, less capable of circumscription, and less intelligible, the more I learned of it. I delved into the literature of the subject, submerged, and then re-emerged, more knowledgeable in some ways but more confused in others. I returned to my patients whom I found more instructive than any book. And after I had seen a thousand migraine patients, I saw that the subject made *sense*.

I was at first disconcerted, but later delighted, at the complexity of the histories I received. Here was something which could pass, in a few minutes, from the subtlest disorders of perception, speech, emotion and thought, to every conceivable vegetative symptom. Every patient with classical migraine opened out, as it were, into an entire encyclopaedia of neurology.

I was recalled from my neurological preoccupation by the suffering of my patients and their appeals for help. Some patients I could help with drugs, and some with the magic of attention and interest. The most severely-afflicted patients defeated my therapeutic endeavours until I started to enquire minutely and persistently into their emotional lives. It now became apparent to me that many migraine attacks were drenched in emotional significance, and could not be usefully considered, let alone treated, unless their emotional antecedents and effects were exposed in detail.

I thus found it necessary to employ a sort of continuous double-vision, simultaneously envisaging migraine as a *structure* whose forms were implicit in the repertoire of the nervous system, and as a *strategy* which might be employed to any emotional, or indeed biological, end.

I have endeavoured, in the composition of this book, to keep these two perspectives constantly in view, portraying migraines as both physical and symbolic events. Part I is devoted to describing the forms of migraine attacks as experienced by the patient and observed by the physician. Part II is concerned with the many circumstances—physical, physiological, and psychological—which may provoke isolated or repeated migraine attacks. Part III is divided between a consideration of the physiological mechanisms of the migraine attack, and a discussion of the biological and psychological roles which migraines, and certain allied disorders, may fill. Part IV is concerned with the therapeutic approach to migraine, and forms both a corollary and a supplement to the preceding portions of the book.

I have used simple language wherever possible, and technical language wherever necessary. Although the first two parts of this work are primarily descriptive, in contrast to the third part which is explanatory and speculative, I have at all times moved freely, perhaps too freely, between the statement of facts and the questioning of their meaning. If the frame of reference is steadily broadened, its expansion is demanded by the many, various, and sometimes very strange facts we are forced to consider.

I entertain the hope that three groups of readers may find something of interest in this book. First sufferers from migraine, and their physicians, who seek an intelligible account of what migraine is, and how to treat it. Secondly, students and investigators of migraine who may be assured of finding a detailed, if somewhat discursive, reference-book on the subject. Lastly, general readers of a speculative turn of mind (not necessarily medical men!), who are invited to see in migraine something which has countless familiar analogies in human and animal functioning, a model which illuminates the entire range of psychophysiological reactions, by reminding us, again and again, of the absolute continuity of mind and body.

Acknowledgments

My first debt is to my many and long-suffering migraine patients, to whom I owe the possibility of this book. They have provided me with the clinical reality from which all observations were derived, and against which every idea has had to be tested. In a very real sense, therefore, this is *their* book.

A special visual reality has been provided by patients who have made paintings of their own visual experiences during migraine auras, so enabling all of us to see what is scarcely imaginable, and usually seen only by sufferers of migraine.

I am particularly indebted to Dr. William Gooddy, who read the original manuscript of *Migraine* in 1968, suggested many valuable additions and emendations, and with great generosity provided a foreword to it.

I am grateful to a succession of editors who have seen the book through various editions—above all, Miss Jean Cunningham, who edited the original edition, Hettie Thistlethwaite, Stan Holwitz, and Kate Edgar. The original drawings for the original edition were done by Audrey Besterman, and the photographic illustrations have been provided through the courtesy of Derek Robinson of Boehringer Ingelheim Limited.

Since publishing the original edition, I have enjoyed contact with the work of many colleagues eminent for their contributions to our understanding of migraine—in particular, Walter Alvarez, J. N. Blau, G. W. Bruyn, Donald Dalessio, Seymour Diamond, Arthur Elkind, the late A. P. Friedman, Vladimir Hachinski, Neil Raskin, Clifford Rose, Clifford

Saper, Seymour Solomon, J. C. Steele, Marcia Wilkinson, and most especially James W. Lance. I am deeply grateful to these for the stimulation they have afforded, though my opinions, and errors, are wholly my own. Finally, I must express my deep indebtedness to my friend and colleague Ralph Siegel, who has been my collaborator in composing the final chapter of the book, and has provided the computer graphics with which it is illustrated.

Foreword

The affliction of migraine has been described for at least the past 2,000 years; and no doubt every generation of modem man, with his history of perhaps 250,000 years, has its experience of this constellation of disorders. Yet it is a very common opinion of the public and the medical profession that little is known about migraine and even less to be done about it. Only in 1970 have arrangements been made for a clinic to deal with migraine to be set up in the City of London.

It is true that migraine is listed in textbooks of medicine and especially of neurology, but usually rather briefly among other intermittent disorders such as epilepsy and neuralgia. The common attitude is that migraine is merely a form of mainly non-disabling headache which occupies far more of a busy doctor's time than its importance warrants. Some of the accompaniments, such as vomiting and visual disturbances, are well recognised; sometimes to the extent that a diagnosis of migraine will be made only when a set pattern of visual upset, headache and vomiting occur in regular order. Some tablets and the current inelegant cliché of "learning to live with it" are advised by the physician, who hopes that he will not be on duty the next time the patient comes for advice. Because of the lack of full comprehension of the complexities and variabilities of a condition which is in every way fascinating in its phenomenology, many doctors are only too pleased when a patient, in desperation, takes himself off to the practitioners of "fringe medicine," almost hoping that the results will be both disastrous and very costly.

Is the medical profession entirely at fault? Does the name of an authoritative or "definitive" textbook spring to mind? Are there numerous
well-equipped and properly organised centres where the condition may
be studied? Are there extensive statistics about the whole problem, such
as there are for, say, industrial accidents, bronchial carcinoma or mea-
sles? Did we have as students a single lecture on migraine, and did anyone
tell us that migraine is not just a tiresome form of occasional headache
which someone else rather boringly suffers from? Almost certainly not;
and the awareness that migraine is an expression of the genetics, personality, way of life of an individual is only very recently being pro-
claimed.

Another remarkably neglected aspect of the migrainous process is the
disorder of physiology which it expresses. In no other condition may we
find the complete physiological experiment in a human being which the
migrainous attack provides. We see, we may feel ourselves, the gradual
disintegration of function of the normal person, exactly as we do in a
case of stroke or of brain tumour; but without the disaster of the permanent disability. Within a few minutes or an hour or so the attack is
past; the symptoms and signs, which may include those of dysphasia and
hemiplegia, double vision, vertigo, vomiting, bowel disturbance, water
balance changes, personality disorders, have vanished. However, few
studies have been carried out under these circumstances; and research,
such as it is, is more likely to have been carried out on more or less
anaesthetised animals, who probably do not have migraine as we know
of it.

To redress this imbalance of interest, experience, physiological knowledge and therapeutic enterprise, we need a synoptic work which sets out
for us all the whole scope of the migrainous space-time continuum, the
lifelong pattern of ever-changing features and factors which the patient
with migraine both suffers and creates. His social circle, his work asso-
ciates, and especially his physicians are inseparable elements in this continuum.

Dr. Oliver Sacks has undertaken the task of providing the general
view which has for so long been lacking. In an immensely energetic act
of clinical scholarship, he has brought together virtually all the features
of modern knowledge on the subject of migraine. It is an interesting
academic exercise for the neurologist to try and detect the omission of
some minor point which he believes that he, almost alone, may have
noted. It is extremely hard to find any such omission.

Let us hope that this work will achieve full success from its determination to illumine the grand scheme of migraine. Any such success must have immense benefits to individual patients, and also to both medical practitioners and society in general.

WILLIAM GOODDY

Historical Introduction

Migraine affects a substantial minority of the population, occurs in all civilisations, and has been recognised since the dawn of recorded history. If it was a scourge, or an encouragement, to Caesar, Paul, Kant, and Freud, it is also a daily fact of life to anonymous millions who suffer in secrecy and silence. Its forms and symptoms, as Burton remarked of melancholy, are "irregular, obscure, various, so infinite, Proteus himself is not so diverse." Its nature and causes puzzled Hippocrates, and have been the subject of argument for two thousand years.

The major clinical characteristics of migraine—its periodicity, its relation to character and circumstance, its physical and emotional symptoms—had all been clearly recognised by the second century of our era. Thus Aretaeus describes it, under the name of Heterocrania:

> And in certain cases the whole head is pained, and the pain is sometimes on the right, and sometimes on the left side, or the forehead, or the fontanelle; and such attacks shift their place during the same day . . . This is called Heterocrania, an illness by no means mild . . . It occasions unseemly and dreadful symptoms . . . nausea; vomiting of bilious matters; collapse of the patient . . . there is much torpor, heaviness of the head, anxiety; and life becomes a burden. For they flee the light; the darkness soothes their disease; nor can they bear readily to look upon or hear anything pleasant . . . The patients are weary of life and wish to die.

While his contemporary Pelops described and named the sensory symptoms which might precede an epilepsy (the aura), Aretaeus observed the analogous symptoms which inaugurated certain migraines:

1

. . . flashes of purple or black colours before the sight, or all mixed together, so as to exhibit the appearance of a rainbow expanded in the heavens.

Four hundred years elapsed between the observations of Aretaeus and the treatises of Alexander Trallianus. Throughout this period repeated observations confirmed and elaborated the terse description of Aretaeus, while reiterating, unquestioned, the theories of antiquity concerning its nature. The terms *heterocrania*, *holocrania*, and *hemicrania* struggled with each other for many centuries; hemicrania (ἡ μικρανία) ousted its rivals, and has finally evolved, through an immense number of transliterations, to the migraine or megrim we speak of today. The terms sick-headache, bilious-headache (cephalgia biliosa) and blind-headache have been in popular use for many centuries.[1]

Two categories of theory have dominated medical thinking on the nature of migraine since the time of Hippocrates; both were still a matter of serious dispute at the end of the eighteenth century, and both, variously transformed, command wide popular assent today. It is, therefore, no work of supererogation, but one of the greatest relevance to trace the evolution of these two classical theories; we will speak of the humoral theory and the sympathetic theory.

An excess of yellow or black bile, it was supposed, could occasion not only a liverish feeling, a black humour, or a jaundiced view of life, but the bilious vomiting and gastric upset of a sick-headache.[2] The essence of this theory, and of the form of treatment which it implies, is precisely expressed by Alexander Trallianus:

[1]The *Oxford English Dictionary* provides an exhaustive list of these transliterations and their usages. A mile fraction of these may be cited:

Mygrane, Megryne, Migrane, Mygrame, Migrym, Myegrym, Midgrame, Midgramme, Mygrim, Magryme, Maigram, Meigryme, Megrym, Megrome, Meagrim . . .

The first use of any of these terms in English was apparently in the fourteenth century: "the mygrame and other euyll passyons of the head." The French term "Migraine" was in use a century earlier.

The visual auras of migraine were generally denoted (as were other elementary visual hallucinations) by the term *suffusio*, and qualified by specific descriptive terms: Suffusio dimidans, Suffusio scintillans, Suffusio scotoma, Suffusio objecta emarginans, etc.

[2]A variant of the humoral theory attributed migraines to the spleen and splenetic humours. Pope (himself an inveterate migraineur) has preserved this concept in his description of the Cave of Spleen

There screen'd in shades from day's detested glare,
Spleen sighs for ever on her pensive bed,
Pain at her side, and *megrim* at her head.

If therefore headache frequently arises on account of a superfluity of bilious humour, the cure of it must be affected by means of remedies which purge and draw away the bilious humour.

Purging and drawing away the bilious humour—in this lies the historical justification of innumerable derivative theories and treatments, many of them practised at the present day. The stomach and bowel may become laden with bilious humours: hence the immemorial use of emetics, laxatives, cathartics, purgatives, etc. Fatty foods draw bilious humours to the stomach, therefore the diet of the migraineur must be sparse and ascetic. Thus, the puritanical Fothergill, a lifelong sufferer from migraine, considered the following especially dangerous:

Melted butter, fat meats, spices, meat-pies, hot buttered toast, and malt liquors when strong and hoppy . . .

Similarly, it has always been considered, and is still so held, that constipation (i.e. retention of bilious humours in the bowel) may provoke or prelude an attack of migraine. Similarly, bilious humours might be reduced at their source (a variety of "liver pills" is still recommended for migraine), or diminished if their concentration in the blood became too high (blood-letting was particularly recommended in the sixteenth and seventeenth centuries as a cure for migraine). It is not, perhaps, unduly far-fetched to regard current chemical theories of the origin of migraine as intellectual descendants of the ancient humoral doctrines.

Contemporary in origin with the humoral theories, and evolving concurrently with them, have been a variety of "sympathetic" theories. These hold that migraine has a peripheral origin in one or more of the viscera (the stomach, the bowel, the uterus, etc.), from which it is propagated about the body by a special form of internal, visceral communication; this occult form of communication, hidden from and below the transactions of consciousness, was termed "sympathy" by the Greeks, and "consensus" by the Romans, and was conceived to be of particular importance in connecting the head and the viscera ("mirum inter caput et viscera commercium").

The classical notions of sympathy were revived, and given a more exact form by Thomas Willis. Willis had come to reject the Hippocratic notions of hysteria as arising from the physical trajectory of the womb about the body, and instead came to visualise the uterus as *radiating* the phenomena of hysteria through an infinitude of minute pathways about the body. He extended this concept to the transmission of a migraine throughout the body and of many other paroxysmal disorders.

Willis set out, three centuries ago, to review the entire domain of nervous disorders (*De Anima Brutorum*), and in the course of this work included a section ("De Cephalalgia") which must be considered as the first modern treatise on migraine, and the first decisive advance since the time of Aretaeus. He organised a vast mass of medieval observations and speculations on the subjects of migraine, epilepsy and other paroxysmal reactions, and added to these clinical observations which were extraordinary in their accuracy and sobriety.[3] Consulted on one occasion by a lady with a headache, he has passed down to us the following incomparable description of migraine:

> Some years since, I was sent for to visit a most noble Lady, for above twenty years sick with almost a continual Headach, at first intermitting . . . she was extremely punished with this Disease. Growing well of a Feavour before she was twelve years old, she became obnoxious to pains in the Head, which were wont to arise, sometimes of their own accord, and more often upon very light occasion. This sickness being limited to no one place of the Head, troubled her sometimes on one side, sometimes on the other, and often thorow the whole compass of the Head. During the fit (which rarely ended under a day and a night's space, and often held for two, three, or four days) she was impatient of light, speaking, noise, or of any motion, sitting upright in her Bed, the Chamber made dark, she would talk to nobody, nor take any sleep, or sustenance. At length about the declination of the fit, she was wont to lye down with an heavy and disturbed sleep, from which awakening she found herself better . . . Formerly, the fits came not but occasionally, and seldom under twenty days of a month, but afterwards they came more often; and lately she was seldom free.

Willis, discussing this case, shows himself fully aware of the many predisposing, exciting and accessory causes of such attacks: ". . . An evil or weak constitution of the parts . . . sometimes innate and hereditary . . . an irritation in some distant member or viscera . . . changes of season, atmospheric states, the great aspects of the sun and moon, violent passions, and errors in diet." He was well aware, also, that migraine, though frequently intolerable, is benign:

---

[3] A rare prodrome of migraine is bulimia, and this Willis observed with another patient:

On the day before the coming of the spontaneous fit of this disease, growing very hungry in the evening, she eat a most plentiful supper, with an hungry, I may say a greedy appetite; presaging by this sign, that the pain of the head would most certainly follow the next morning; and the event never failed this augury.

... But although this Distemper most grievously afflicting this noble Lady, above twenty years ... having pitched its tents near the confines of the Brain, had so long besieged its regal tower, yet it had not taken it; for the sick Lady, being free from a Vertigo, swimming in the Head, Convulsive Distempers, and any Soporiferous symptoms, found the chief faculties of her soul sound enough.

The other classical concept revived by Willis was that of *idiopathy*, a tendency to periodic and sudden explosions in the nervous system.[4] Thus the migrainous nervous system, or the epileptic nervous system, could be detonated at any time, by a variety of influences—physical or emotional—and the remotest effects of the explosion were conveyed throughout the body by sympathy, by presumed sympathetic nerves whose existence Willis himself could only infer.

Sympathetic theories were particularly favoured and elaborated in the eighteenth century. Tissot, observing that stomach disorders might precede and apparently inaugurate a migraine headache, and that vomiting could rapidly bring the entire attack to a close, suggests:

It is then most probable that a focus of irritation is formed little by little in the stomach, and that when it has reached a certain point, the irritation is sufficient to give rise to acute pains in all the ramifications of the supraorbital nerve ...

Contemporary with Tissot, and also lending the weight of his authority to such sympathetic theories, was Robert Whytt; observing "... the vomiting that generally accompanies inflammation of the womb; the nausea, the disordered appetite, that follows conception ... the headache, the heat and pains in the back, the intestinal colic suffered when the time of the menstrual flow approaches ... etc.," Whytt pictures the human body (in Foucault's eloquent paraphrase) as riddled, from one extremity to another, by obscure but strangely direct paths of sympathy: paths which could transmit the phenomena of a migraine, or a hysteria, from their visceral origins.

It is important to note that the finest clinical observers of the eighteenth century—Tissot (who wrote voluminously on migraine, and whose 1790 treatise was the true successor of Willis's "De Cephalalgia"),

[4]Willis writes elsewhere (*De Morb. Convuls*, 1670): Quod si *explosionis* vocabulum, in Philosophia ac Medicina insolitum, cuipiam minus arrideat; proinde ut pathologia σπασ-μῶδης huic basi innitens, tantum *ignoti per ignotius explicatio* videatur; facile erat istiusmodi effectus, circa res tum naturales, tum artificiales, instantias et exempla quamplurima proffere; ex quorum analogia in corpore motuum in corpore animato, tum regulariter, tum ἀνώμαλος peractorum, rationes aptissimae desumuntur.

Whytt, Cheyne, Cullen, Sydenham, etc.—made no arbitrary distinctions between physical and emotional symptoms: all had to be considered together, as integral parts of "nervous disorders." Thus Robert Whytt brings together, as intimate and interrelated symptoms,

> . . . An extraordinary sensation of cold and heat, of pains in several parts of the body; syncopes and vaporous convulsions; catalepsy and tetanus; gas in the stomach and intestines . . . vomiting of black matter; a sudden and abundant flow of clear pale urine . . . palpitations of the heart; variations in the pulse; *periodic headaches*; vertigo and nervous spells . . . depression, despair . . . madness, nightmares or incubi.

This central belief, this concept of the inseparable unity of psychophysiological reactions, was fractured at the start of the nineteenth century. The "nervous disorders" of Willis and Whytt were rigidly divided into "organic" versus "functional," and as rigidly partitioned between neurologists and alienists; Liveing and Jackson, it is true, did portray migraine as an indivisible psychophysiological entity without internal divisions, but their views were exceptional and against the bias of their century.

Superb descriptions of migraine appeared in great numbers with the opening of the nineteenth century, almost all of which had a vividness which seems to have vanished from the medical literature. Looking back on the riches of this older literature one is tempted to imagine that every physician of note either had migraine or made it his business to describe the phenomenon: included in this galaxy of names are those of Heberden and Wollaston, in the first decade of the century, Abercrombie, Piorry and Parry in its second and third decades, Romberg, Symonds, Hall, and Möllendorff around the middle of the century; brilliant descriptions were also provided by a number of non-medical men, among whom the astronomers Herschel and the Airies (father and son) were pre-eminent.

Almost all of these descriptions, however, dwelt on the *physical* aspects of migraine attacks, while neglecting their emotional components, antecedents, and uses. The theories of the nineteenth century, likewise, lacked the generality of the earlier doctrines, and were usually concerned with very specific mechanical aetiologies of one type or another. Vascular theories were very popular, whether these envisaged general plethora, cerebral congestion, or specific dilatations and constrictions of the cranial vessels. Local factors were given great weight: swelling of the pituitary gland, inflammation in the eyes, etc. Hereditary "taint" and masturbation were also inculpated towards the middle of the century (they had also been summoned to explain epilepsy and insanity), and in such theories—as in later theories of auto-intoxication, infective foci, etc.—an anachronistic quality is apparent, for the mode of action was ostensibly physical, but covertly and implicitly moral.

Homage must be singled out for a remarkable Victorian masterpiece, Edward Liveing's treatise *On Megrim, Sick-Headache, and Some Allied Disorders*, which was composed between 1863 and 1865, but only published in 1873. Bringing to his subject the acumen and learning of a Gowers, and the imaginative depth and range of a Hughlings Jackson, Liveing encompassed and ordered the entire range of migrainous experience, and its place amid an immense surrounding field of "allied and metamorphotic disorders." As Hughlings Jackson utilised the phenomena of epilepsy to visualise the evolution and dissolution of hierarchically-organised functions in the nervous system, so Liveing performed a comparable task using the data of migraine. Historical depth and generality of approach must be the justifications of any medical essay, and in these respects Liveing's masterpiece has never been equalled.

An essential part of Liveing's vision (and in this he was more related to Willis and Whytt than to his contemporaries) was the realisation that the varieties of migraine were endless in number, and that they coalesced with many other paroxysmal reactions. His own theory of "nerve-storms," of great generality and power, explained, as no other theory could, the sudden or gradual metamorphoses so characteristic of migraine attacks. The same thesis was expanded by Gowers, who portrayed migraine, faints, vagal attacks, vertigo, sleep-disorders, etc. as related to each other and to epilepsy—all such nerve-storms being mutually if mysteriously transformable amongst themselves.

The present century has been characterised both by advances and retrogressions in its approach to migraine. The advances reflect sophistications of technique and quantitation, and the retrogressions represent the splitting and fracturing of the subject which appears inseparable from the specialisation of knowledge. By a historical irony, a real gain of knowledge and technical skill has been coupled with a real loss in general understanding.

A migraine is a physical event which may also be from the start, or later become, an emotional or symbolic event. A migraine expresses both physiological and emotional needs: it is the prototype of a psychophysiological reaction. Thus the convergence of thinking which its understanding demands must be based, simultaneously, both on neurology and on psychiatry (the convergence envisaged and brought nearer by Cannon, the physiologist, and Groddeck, the analyst); finally, migraine cannot be conceived as an exclusively human reaction, but must be considered as a form of biological reaction specifically tailored to human needs and human nervous systems.

The fragments of migraine must be gathered together and presented, once more, as a coherent whole. There have been innumerable technical papers and monographs which have extended and crystallised our knowledge of specific aspects of the subject. But there has not been a general essay since the time of Liveing.

The Experience of Migraine

Introduction

Our first problem arises from the word *migraine*, which implies the existence of a (hemicranial) headache as a defining characteristic. It is necessary to state, at the very outset, that headache is *never* the sole symptom of a migraine, nor indeed is it a necessary feature of migraine attacks. We shall have occasion to consider many types of attack which exhibit every characteristic of migraines—clinically, physiologically, pharmacologically, and otherwise—but lack a headache component. We must retain the word *migraine* in view of its long and customary usage, but allow its extension far beyond the limits of any dictionary definition.

A variety of different syndromes may be recognised within the migraine-complex, and these may overlap, merge, and metamorphose into one another. The most frequently-occurring of these is the *Common Migraine* in which we find an assortment of migrainous symptoms grouped around the cardinal symptom of migraine headache (Chapter 1). When components other than headache come to dominate an otherwise similar clinical picture, we may speak of *Migraine Equivalents*, and under this head we will consider periodic and recurrent attacks dominated by nausea and vomiting, abdominal pain, diarrhoea, fever, drowsiness, mood-changes, etc. (Chapter 2). We must also discuss, in conjunction with these, certain other forms of attack and reaction which bear a clear if more remote relation to migraine: motion-sickness, fainting, vagal attacks, etc.

Separate consideration must be given to a peculiarly acute and dramatic type of attack—the *Migraine Aura*. Such auras may occur as isolated events, or they may be followed by headache, nausea, and other features of the migraine-complex. The entire syndrome, in the latter event, is termed a *Classical Migraine* (Chapter 3).

Somewhat isolated from the above syndromes is a highly distinctive variant of migraine which has been described under a variety of names, and is best termed *Migrainous Neuralgia*. Very rarely, a common or classical migraine may be followed by long-lasting neurological deficits: these are termed *Hemiplegic* or *Ophthalmoplegic Migraines*. In conjunction with these rare variants we will allude to *Pseudo-Migraines*, the mimicking of true migraines by organic lesions (Chapter 4).

Part I concludes with an attempt to define, in the terms already employed, some formal characteristics common to all types of migraine attack, i.e. the general structure of migraine.

ONE

Common Migraine

Since about my twentieth year, though otherwise in good
health, I have suffered from migraine. Every three or four
weeks I am liable to an attack . . . I wake with a general feeling of disorder, and a slight pain in the region of the right
temple which, without overstepping the mid-line, reaches its
greatest intensity at midday; towards evening it usually
passes off. While at rest the pain is bearable, but it is
increased by motion to a high degree of violence . . . It
responds to each beat of the temporal artery. The latter
feels, on the affected side, like a hard cord, while the left is
in its normal condition. The countenance is pale and sunken,
the right eye small and reddened. At the height of the attack,
when it is a violent one, there is nausea . . . There may be left
behind a slight gastric disorder; frequently, also, the scalp
remains tender at one spot the following morning . . . For a
certain period after the attack I can expose myself with impunity to influences which before would have infallibly caused
an attack.

du Bois Reymond, 1860

The cardinal symptoms of common migraine are headache and nausea.
Complementing these may be a remarkable variety of other major symptoms, in addition to minor disorders and physiological changes of which
the patient may not be aware. Presiding over the entire attack there will
be, in du Bois Reymond's words, "a general feeling of disorder," which
may be experienced in either physical or emotional terms, and tax or
elude the patient's powers of description. Great variability of symptoms
is characteristic, not only of attacks in different patients, but between
successive attacks in the same patient.

These, then, are the *ingredients* of a common migraine. We will list
and describe them one by one, while understanding that migrainous
symptoms never occur in such schematic isolation, but are linked to one

another in various ways. Some symptoms are conjoined to form characteristic *constellations*, while others present themselves in a definite and
often dramatic order, so that we may recognise a basic *sequence* to the
attacks.

HEADACHE

The *character* of the pains varied very much; most frequently they were of a hammering, throbbing or push-
ing nature . . . [in other cases] pressing and dull . . .
boring with sense of bursting . . . pricking . . . rending
. . . stretching . . . piercing . . . and radiating . . . in a
few cases it felt as if a wedge was pressed into the
head, or like an ulcer, or as if the brain was torn, or
pressed outwards.

Peters, 1853

Migraine headache is traditionally described as a violent throbbing
pain in one temple, and not infrequently takes this form. It is impossible,
however, to specify a constant site, quality, or intensity for in the course
of a specialised practice one will encounter all conceivable varieties of
head-pain in the context of migraine. Wolff, whose experience is un-
matched in this area, has stated (1963):

> The sites of the migraine headache are notably temporal, supra-orbital, fron-
> tal, retrobulbar, parietal, postauricular, and occipital . . . They may occur as
> well in the malar region, in the upper and the lower teeth, at the base of the
> nose, in the median wall of the orbit, in the neck and in the region of the
> common carotid arteries, and down as far as the tip of the shoulder.

One may say, however, that migraine headache is unilateral in *onset*
more frequently than not, although it tends to become diffuse in distribution later in the attack. One side is generally attacked by preference,
and in a few patients there may be an invariable left- or right-sided
involvement throughout life. More commonly there is only a relative
preference, often associated with the severity of pain: severe frequent
hemicrania on one side with mild occasional hemicrania on the opposite
side. A number of patients complain of an alternation of hemicrania
from one side to the other in successive attacks, or even in the same
attack. At least a third of all patients experience a bilateral or diffuse
headache (holocrania) from the outset of the attack.

The *quality* of migraine headache is similarly variable. Throbbing occurs in less than half of all cases, and in these may characterise the headache only at its inception, soon giving way to a steady aching. Continued throbbing throughout the attack is uncommon, and occurs chiefly in those who drive themselves to continued physical activity despite a migraine. Throbbing, when it occurs, is synchronised with arterial pulsation, and may be accompanied by visible pulsation of extracranial arteries.

Its intensity is proportional to the increased amplitude of such arterial pulses (Wolff), and the pain may be interrupted by pressure on the affected artery, or the common carotid artery, or sometimes the eyeball, on the affected side. Such occlusion is immediately followed, when the finger is released, by a violent resurgence of the arterial pulse and the head-pain. Throbbing is not, however, a *sine qua non* of vascular headache, and its absence does not have the significance of its occurrence. One may say, however, that almost all vascular headaches are aggravated by active or passive head-movement, or by the transmitted impulse of coughing, sneezing or vomiting. The pain is therefore minimised by rest, or by splinting of the head in one position. It may also be mollified by counter-pressure; many migraine sufferers will press the affected temple into their pillows, or hold the affected side with their hand.

The *duration* of migraine headache is very variable. In extremely acute attacks ("migrainous neuralgia") the pain may last only a matter of minutes. In a common migraine, the duration is rarely less than three hours, is commonly of eight to twenty-four hours' duration, and on occasion may last several days, or in excess of a week. Tissue changes may become manifest in very extended attacks. The superficial temporal artery (or arteries) may become exquisitely tender to the touch and visibly indurated. The surrounding skin may also become tender, and remain in this state for more than a day following the subsidence of the headache. Very rarely a spontaneous hygroma or haematoma may form about the affected vessel.

The *intensity* of migrainous headache is extremely variable. It may be of incapacitating violence, or so faint that its presence is only detected by the transient pain consequent upon jolting of the head or coughing.[5]

---

[5]The earlier literature provides some remarkable examples of "splitting" headaches. Thus Tissot (1790) records in his treatise: "C. Pison (a physician) experienced on himself such violent attacks of migraine that he believed his skull's sutures were splitting . . . Stalpart Van der Viel *saw* the sutures of the skull actually splitting in an attack of migraine, the object of which was the gardener's wife . . . "

Nor need the intensity remain constant throughout the attack; a slow waxing and waning with a period of a few minutes is commonly described, and much longer remissions and exacerbations may also occur, particularly in protracted menstrual migraines.

Migrainous headache is frequently complicated by the simultaneous or antecedent occurrence of other types of head-pain. Characteristic "tension-headache," localised especially in the cervical and posterior occipital regions, may inaugurate a migraine headache, or accompany it, particularly if the attack is marked by irritability, anxiety, or continued activity throughout its duration. Such tension-headache must not be construed as an integral portion of the migraine, but as a secondary reaction to it.

NAUSEA AND ASSOCIATED SYMPTOMS

Eructations occur, either inodorous and without taste,
or of an insupportable mawkishness; abundant
mucosities and salivary fluid flow into the mouth,
intermixed at times with those of a bitter, bilious taste;
there is extreme disgust for food; general malaise
. . . paroxysmal distensions of the stomach with gas,
followed by belchings, with transient relief; or vomiting may occur . . .

Peters, 1853

Nausea is invariable in the course of a common migraine, whether it is trifling and intermittent, or continuous and overwhelming. The term "nausea" is used, and has always been used, in both literal and figurative senses, as denoting not only a specific (if unlocalisable) sensation, but a state of mind and pattern of behaviour—a turning-away, from food, from everything, and a turning-inwards. Even if there is no overt nausea, a vast majority of migraine patients will be averse to eating during the attack, knowing that the act of eating, the sight, the smell, or even the very thought of food may bring on overwhelming nausea. We might almost speak of *latent* nausea in this connection.

A variety of other symptoms, local and systemic, are likely to be associated with nausea. Increased salivation and reflux of bitter stomach-contents ("waterbrash"), with the necessity of swallowing or spitting, may not only accompany the sensation of nausea, but precede it by several minutes. Not uncommonly patients are alerted to the imminence of a severe sick-headache by finding their mouths filled with saliva or water-brash, and may be enabled, by this timely signal, to take appropriate medication and ward off further oncoming symptoms.

Established nausea provokes various forms of visceral ejaculation: hiccup, belching, retching, and vomiting. If the patient is fortunate, vomiting may terminate not only his nausea but the entire migraine attack; more commonly, he will fail to secure relief from vomiting, and suffer instead an excruciating aggravation of concurrent vascular headache. When florid, nausea is far less tolerable than headache or other forms of pain, and in many patients, especially youthful ones, nausea and vomiting dominate the clinical picture and constitute the crowning misery of a common migraine.

Repeated vomiting first empties the existing stomach-contents, is followed by vomiting of regurgitated bile, and finally by repeated "dry" heaving or retching. It is the chief cause (in company with profuse sweating and diarrhoea) of the severe fluid and electrolyte depletion which can prostrate patients suffering protracted attacks.

FACIAL APPEARANCE

The picturesque terms "red migraine" and "white migraine" were introduced by du Bois Reymond, and retain a certain descriptive value. In a red migraine, the face is dusky and flushed: in the words of an old account

> congested, with rushing and roaring in the head, bloating, glowing, and shining of the face, with protrusion of the eyes . . . great heat of the head and face . . . throbbing of the carotid and temporal arteries . . . (Peters, 1853)

A full-blown, plethoric appearance, as Peters describes, is distinctly uncommon, occurring in less than a tenth of cases of common migraine. Patients predisposed to red migraines often have a marked propensity to flush with anger or blush with embarrassment: facial erythema, we may say, is their "style":

Case 40   A 60-year-old man of irascible temperament subject to common migraines since the age of 18, and bilious attacks and severe motion-sickness in childhood. He has a beef-red face, with tiny dilated arterioles in the nose and eyes. He flushes in his frequent rages, and indeed his face always seems to glow with a red smouldering fire which is the precise physiological counterpart of his chronic smouldering irritability. His face becomes crimson a few minutes before the onset of migraine headache, and remains flushed throughout the attack.

Much more familiar is the picture of white migraine, in which the face is pale, or even ashen, thin, drawn and haggard, while the eyes appear small, sunken, and ringed. These changes may be so marked as to suggest the picture of surgical shock. Intense pallor is always seen if there is severe nausea. On occasion, the face becomes flushed in the first few minutes of an attack, and then abruptly pale, as if, in Peters's words, "all the blood passed suddenly from the head to the legs."

Oedema of the face and scalp may occur, either as isolated features or in the context of a very general fluid-retention and oedema (see p. 22). Facial, lingual and labial swelling, reminiscent of an angioneurotic oedema, may occur at the inception of the attack in some patients. In one such patient whom I was able to observe at the inauguration of an attack, a massive periorbital oedema developed on one side a few minutes before the onset of headache. More commonly, facial and scalp oedema develop *after* prolonged dilatation of extracranial vessels, and are associated, as Wolff and others have shown, with fluid transudation and sterile inflammation about the involved vessels. The oedematous skin is always tender and has a lowered pain-threshold.

OCULAR SYMPTOMS

It is almost always possible to detect changes in the appearance of the *eyes* during or before an attack of migraine headache, even though the patient himself may not volunteer any visual or ocular symptoms. There is usually some suffusion of small vessels in the globe, and in particularly severe attacks the eyes may become grossly bloodshot (this feature is characteristic in attacks of migrainous neuralgia). The eyes may appear moist (chemotic) from an increase in lacrimation—analogous to, and often synchronised with, the increased salivation—or bleary from an exudative inflammation of the vascular bed. Alternatively, the eyes may appear lustreless and sunken: a true enophthalmos may occur.

These changes in the eyeball, when severe, may be associated with a variety of symptoms: itching and burning in the affected eye(s), a painful sensitivity to light, and blurring of vision. Blurring of vision may be of incapacitating severity ("blind-headache") and one may find it impossible to visualise the retinal vessels with any clarity at such times, due to the exudative thickening of the cornea.

NASAL SYMPTOMS

Descriptions of migraine rarely pay much attention to nasal symptoms, although careful questioning of patients will reveal that at least a quarter of them develop some "stuffiness" of the nose in the course of an attack. Examination at this time will show engorged and purple turbinates. Such symptoms and findings, when they are present, may mislead both patient and physician into making a diagnosis of "sinus" or "allergic" headache.

Another nasal symptom, which may come either towards the beginning or at the resolution of the attack, is a profuse catarrhal secretion. It will be readily understandable that the combination of a running nose with a sense of malaise and headache may mimic a "cold" or other viral infection, and there can be no doubt but that a number of such migraines are misdiagnosed as such. When, however, the "cold" shows some propensity to occur every weekend, or after acute emotional disturbances, the true diagnosis may become apparent.

The following case-history will illustrate how conspicuous a part may be played by nasal and other secretions in the course of a migraine, as well as certain other premonitory symptoms to be discussed later:

Case 20   A 53-year-old lady who has had common migraines of unusually elaborate format for nearly thirty years. At one time she used to have "a feeling of extreme well-being" the night before her attacks. More recently, she has tended to have feelings of intense drowsiness during the preceding evening, accompanied by repeated and uncontrollable yawning. She lays stress on the "unnatural . . . irresistible . . . ominous" qualities of this drowsiness. She will go to bed early, and her sleep will be of unusual length and density.

She will awake the next morning with what she terms "a feeling of unrest . . . My whole system is set off in some way, and everything starts to move inside me . . . " This feeling of unrest and internal motion resolves itself into a diffuse secretory activity, with profuse catarrh, salivation, lacrimation, sweating, watery diuresis, vomiting and diarrhoea. After two or three hours of this massive internal activity she develops an intense throbbing headache on the left side.

ABDOMINAL SYMPTOMS AND ABNORMAL BOWEL-ACTION

About one-tenth of adults who suffer from common migraine complain of abdominal pain or abnormal bowel-action during the course of the attack. The proportion is notably higher in younger patients, and the abdominal symptoms described here as a minor component of a common migraine may constitute the predominant or only symptoms in so-called "abdominal migraines" (see Chapter 2).

Two types of abdominal pain are described with some frequency: the first is an intense, steady, boring, "neuralgic" type of pain, usually felt in the upper abdomen and sometimes radiating to the back—it may mimic the pain of a perforated ulcer, cholecystitis or pancreatitis. Somewhat more commonly, the patient describes a colicky abdominal pain, often referred to the right lower quadrant, and not infrequently taken for appendicitis.

Abdominal distension, visceral silence, and constipation tend to occur in the prodromal or earlier portions of a migraine, and contrast-studies performed at this stage have confirmed that there is stasis and dilatation throughout the entire gastro-intestinal tract. This is succeeded in the later or closing portions of the attack by increased peristaltic activity throughout the gut, clinically manifest as colicky pain, diarrhoea, and gastric regurgitation.

LETHARGY AND DROWSINESS

Although many patients, especially indomitable and obsessional ones, make no concessions to a migraine and insist on driving themselves through the usual round of work and play, a degree of listlessness and a desire for rest are characteristic of all severe common migraines. A vascular headache exquisitely sensitive to motion of the head may in itself enforce inactivity, but we cannot accept this as the only, or even the chief, mechanism at work. Many patients feel weak during an attack and exhibit diminished tone of skeletal muscles. Many are dejected, and seek seclusion and passivity. Many are drowsy.

The relation of sleep to migraine is a complex and fundamental one, and we will have occasion to touch upon it in many different contexts: the incidence of syncope and stupor in the acutest forms of migraine (migraine aura and classical migraine), the tendency for migraines of all types to occur during sleep, and their putative relation to dream and nightmare states. At this point we must pay attention to three aspects of a complex relationship: the occurrence of intense drowsiness or stupor before or during a common migraine, the occasional abortion of attacks by a short sleep of unusual density, and the typical protracted sleep in which many attacks find their natural termination.

Nowhere in the literature can we find more vivid and accurate descriptions of migrainous stupor than in Liveing's monograph.

It is important [he writes] to distinguish this drowsiness from the comparatively natural and graceful sleep which, in a large proportion of cases, terminates, and sometimes shortens the paroxysm. It is, on the contrary, of a most uncomfortable and oppressive character, sometimes verging on coma.

Liveing compares this drowsiness with the altered states of consciousness which may sometimes precede an asthmatic attack, citing the following introspective description of the latter:

> Symptoms of an approaching fit began to appear at 4 p.m. The principal were fullness in the head, dullness and heaviness of the eyes, and disagreeable drowsiness. The drowsiness increased so much that I spent a great part of the evening in a succession of "trances," as I call them. This horrid drowsiness generally prevents one from being sensible of the approach of a fit till it has commenced.

I have already cited a case from my own experience (Case 20, p. 19) in which the patient describes a very similar state of irresistible and unpleasantly-toned drowsiness as a prodromal feature of her attacks, and such descriptions may be multiplied manifold. Sometimes the drowsiness may precede other symptoms by minutes or hours, while at other times it presents itself *pari passu* with the headache and other symptoms. Repeated yawning is a characteristic feature of these lethargic states, presumably an attempted arousal mechanism to stave off the torpor. Migrainous drowsiness is not only "irresistible," glutinous and unpleasantly toned, but tends to be charged with peculiarly vivid, atrocious and incoherent dreams, a state verging on delirium. It is best, therefore, not to yield to it.[6]

Some patients do, however, discover that a brief deep sleep near the commencement of a migraine may prevent its subsequent evolution.

Case 18   A 24-year-old man who suffers both from classical and common migraines, and has experienced, on other occasions, both nocturnal asthmas and somnambulistic episodes. He finds that he may fall into "a very deep sleep . . . they can hardly wake me" shortly after the onset of a migraine, and that if circumstances permit him to do this, he will awake within an hour with a sense of great refreshment, and the complete dispersal of all his symptoms. If he is prevented from sleeping in this fashion, the attack runs its course for the remainder of the day.

The duration of such curative sleeps may be very brief. Liveing cites the case of a gardener with typical abdominal migraines; this patient

---

[6]The "nightmare" song in *Iolanthe* provides a splendid description, not of a nightmare, but of a migraine delirium (the song mentions eleven other symptoms of migraine). As Gilbert and Sullivan observe: "Your slumbering teems with such horrible dreams that you'd very much better be waking."

was able to abort the development of a full-blown attack if he could lie down under a tree and secure ten minutes' sleep at its inception.

DIZZINESS, VERTIGO, FAINTNESS AND SYNCOPE

True vertigo must be considered quite exceptional in the course of a common migraine, although it is often experienced in a migraine aura or classical migraine. Milder states of "lightheadedness" occur with notable frequency. Selby and Lance (1960), in a clinical study of 500 patients with migraine of all types, found that "some 72 per cent complained of a sensation of dizziness, lightheadedness and unsteadiness . . . " They further observed that "sixty patients of 396 had lost consciousness in association with attacks of headache."

The possible causes of such symptoms may, of course, be multiple, and will include autonomic reactions to pain and nausea, vasomotor collapse, prostration due to fluid loss or exhaustion, muscular weakness and adynamia, etc., in addition to the action of direct central mechanisms inhibiting the level of consciousness.

ALTERATIONS OF FLUID BALANCE

A number of migraine patients complain of increased weight, or tightness of clothes, rings, belts, shoes, etc. in association with their attacks. These symptoms have been submitted to precise experimental investigation by Wolff. Some weight-gain preceded the headache stage in more than a third of the patients he studied; since however the headache could not be influenced either by experimental diuresis or hydration, Wolff concluded that "weight gain and widespread fluid retention are concomitant but not causally related to headache," an important conclusion which we shall have occasion to refer to, when we come to discuss the interrelationship of different symptoms in the migraine-complex.

During the period of water-retention urine is diminished in output and highly concentrated.[7] The retained fluid is discharged through a profuse diuresis, sometimes associated with other secretory activities, as the migraine attack resolves.

---

[7] I have had one patient, an intelligent woman whose testimony I am inclined to trust, who affirms that she develops a peculiar fruity odour in the periods of water-retention which inaugurate her occasional migraines. Unfortunately, however, she had no attacks during the six-month period that I saw her, so that no opportunity presented itself of identifying the nature or cause of this odour.

Case 35   This 24-year-old woman has invariable menstrual migraines and one or two further attacks in the course of an average month. Both menstrual and extra-menstrual attacks are preceded by a weight-gain which may be as much as 10 lb.; the fluid is distributed in the trunk, feet, hands, and face, and takes about two days to accumulate. Coincident with the fluid-retention is "a great increase in nervous energy," as the patient terms it, characterised by restlessness, hyperactivity, loquacity, and insomnia. This is followed by a 24- to 36-hour period of intestinal cramps and vascular headache. The detumescence of these attacks occurs, very literally, with a massive diuresis and an involuntary epiphora.

FEVER

Many patients may complain that they *feel* feverish during the course of a common migraine, and they may indeed demonstrate flushing of the face, coldness and cyanosis of the extremities, shivering, sweating, and alternating feelings of heat and cold preceding or accompanying the onset of headache. These symptoms are not necessarily accompanied by fever, although the latter *may* be present, and are of considerable severity, especially in youthful patients.

Case 60   A 20-year-old man with a history of common migraines going back to his eighth year. The headaches are accompanied by intense nausea, pallor and gastro-intestinal disturbances, chills, cold sweats, and occasional rigors. I had the opportunity of examining him while he was in the throes of a severe attack, and found an oral temperature of 103.5°F.

MINOR SYMPTOMS AND SIGNS

Contraction of one pupil, ptosis, and enophthalmos (Horner's syndrome) may produce a striking asymmetry in cases of unilateral migraine. There is no consistency, however, concerning pupillary size. In the earlier stages of an attack, or if pain is very intense, the pupils may be enlarged; later in an attack, or if nausea, lethargy, collapse, etc., dominate the picture, small pupils will be seen. The same considerations apply to pulse-rate: an initial tachycardia is likely to be followed by a protracted bradycardia, the latter sometimes associated with significant hypotension and postural faintness or syncope. Observant patients may comment on such changes of pulse and pupil during their worst attacks.

Case 51   A 48-year-old man has had migraines since childhood, and also suffers from chronic tachycardia. He has been struck, therefore, by the slowing of his pulse during the attacks, and has also observed that his pupils, normally large, become minute. I was able to confirm these observations while seeing him in the course of an attack: there was striking pallor and diaphoresis, congested chemotic eyes, pinpoint pupils, and a bradycardia of 45.

There is no end to the number of odd, miscellaneous alterations of physiological function which *may* occur as a result of migraine; a complete listing of these would provide a fascinating catalogue of *curiosa*. It will suffice, however, to make brief reference to the occurrence of widespread vascular changes and occasional trophic changes associated with migraines. We have already noted that a spontaneous effusion or ecchymosis may develop about an involved scalp artery. I have had the opportunity of seeing one patient whose "red" migraines were associated with flushing of the entire body, followed, in the later portions of the attack, by the development of many spontaneous ecchymoses on the trunk and limbs. Another patient, a woman of 25, suffered pain in the palms of both hands with her migraine headaches; during the painful period the hands appeared flushed and congested: this syndrome is very similar to the "palmar migraine" described by Wolff.

The literature makes many references to whitening and loss of scalp hair following repeated migraines. The only case suggestive of this, in my own experience, was that of a middle-aged woman who had had very severe, frequent attacks of invariably left-sided hemicrania, and in her mid-twenties developed a startling streak of white hair on this side, the remainder of her hair remaining jet-black until many years later.

ORGANIC IRRITABILITY

... the patient could not bear anything to touch his
head, and the least sight or sound, even the ticking of
his watch, was insupportable.

Tissot, 1778

Irritability and photophobia are exceedingly common in the course of migraine attacks, and have been adopted, by Wolff and others, as pathognomonic features aiding the diagnosis.

We are concerned with two types of irritability as accompaniments of the migraine state. The first is an aspect of the mood-change and defensive seclusion which may be so prominent in the behaviour and social posture of many migraine patients. The second type of irritability arises from a diffuse sensory excitation and excitability, so great that it may render all sensory stimuli intolerable, as the old words of Tissot remind us. In particular, migraine patients are prone to photophobia, an intense discomfort, both local and general, provoked by light, and an avoidance of light which may become the most obvious external characteristic of the entire attack. Some of this photophobia is on the basis of conjunctival hyperaemia and inflammation, as described earlier, and is associated with burning and smarting of the eyes. But a major component of photophobia is a central irritability and sensory arousal, which may be accompanied by very vivid and protracted visual after-images and turbulent visual imagery. Alvarez has provided a graphic description of such symptoms in himself; during the early part of his own migraines, he sees such brilliant after-images on his television-screen that he is unable to watch the picture. Observant patients frequently note, if they close their eyes at such a time, that they are submitted to an involuntary visual barrage, a kaleidoscopic presentation of rapidly-changing colours and images, the latter either crude or as highly-organised as dream images.

An exaggeration and intolerance of sounds—phonophobia—is equally characteristic of the severe attack; distant sounds, the noise of traffic, or the dripping of a tap, may appear unbearably loud and provoke the patient to fury.

Very characteristic of this state is an exaggeration, and often a perversion of the sense of smell; delicate perfumes appear to stink, and may elicit an overwhelming reaction of nausea. Similarly with the sense of taste, the blandest foods acquiring intense and often disgusting flavours.

It is important to note that sensory excitability of this type may precede the onset of headache, and, in general, is characteristic of the *early* portions of the migraine attack. It is often followed by a state of sensory inhibition or indifference for the remainder of the attack: in Peters's words, "by a general hebetude of sensorial power . . . " The alterations of sensation and sensory threshold which occur in common migraine, however distressing to the patient, are very mild in comparison to the intense hallucinations and perversions of sensation which are characteristic of migraine aura and classical migraine.

MOOD-CHANGES

The interrelationship of affective states and migraine is one of the greatest complexity, and as such will demand repeated exploration as we traverse the subject. Obvious difficulties present themselves, from the start, in distinguishing cause and effect, and very careful questioning, or observation over a prolonged period, may be needed to dissect out those affective changes which form an *integral* part of the migraine syndrome from antecedent moods and feelings which have played a part in precipitating the attack, and from the secondary, emotional consequences of the attack itself.

When these factors have been duly weighed, we will continue to be struck by the fact that profound affective changes may occur during, and only during, a migraine attack, changes which are particularly startling in patients of normally equable temperament. Moreover it will become clear that such mood-changes are not simply reactions to pain, nausea, etc., but are themselves primary symptoms proceeding *concurrently* with the many other symptoms of the attack. Very profound mood-changes may also occur *before* and *after* the bulk of the attack, and as such will be considered in the concluding section of this chapter. The most important emotional colourings during the clinically-recognised portion of a common migraine are states of anxious and irritable hyperactivity in the early portions of the attack, and states of apathy and depression in the bulk of the attack.

The common picture of anxious irritability has already been sketched in the preceding section. The patient is restless and agitated; if confined to his bed, he will move about constantly, rearranging the bedclothes, finding no position of comfort; he will tolerate neither sensory nor social intrusions. His irascibility may be extreme. Such states are exacerbated if the patient continues to drive himself through his habitual routine of work, and their exacerbation, by a vicious circle, is likely to provoke a further increase in other symptoms of the attack.

Very different is the picture presented in the fully-established or protracted attack. Here the physical and emotional posture is characterised by accepted suffering, dejection and passivity. Such patients, unless compelled to act otherwise by internal or external factors, *withdraw* or regress into illness, solitude and seclusion. The emotional depression at such times is very real, often serious, and occasionally suicidal. The following account is taken from an eighteenth-century description:

> From the first perception of uneasiness in the stomach the spirits begin to flag. They grow more and more depressed, until cheerful thoughts and feelings fly away, and the patient conceives himself the most wretched of human beings and feels as if he were never to be otherwise . . .

This old description brings out the true depressive quality—the sense of utter hopelessness and permanence of misery—a reaction which is clearly far in excess of a realistic response to a short-lived benign attack of which the patient has had innumerable experiences.

Feelings of depression will be associated with feelings of anger and resentment, and in the severest migraines there may exist a very ugly mixture of despair, fury and loathing of everything and everyone, not excluding the self. Such states of enraged helplessness may be intolerable both for the patient and his family, and their potential severity must never be underrated by the physician who undertakes to look after the severely incapacitated and depressed patient in the throes of an attack.

SYMPTOM-CONSTELLATIONS IN COMMON MIGRAINE

We have now listed the major symptoms of a common migraine *as if* they were unrelated to one another and occurred at random. Certain groups of symptoms tend, however, to occur with some consistency. Thus, severe vascular headache usually occurs in association with other evidences of dilatation in extracranial vessels: suffusion and chemosis of the eyes, vascular engorgement within the nose, facial flushing, etc. In other patients, gastro-intestinal symptoms form a coherent phalanx: gastric and intestinal distension, abdominal pains, followed by diarrhoea and vomiting. A "shock" picture is seen in severe "white" migraines, constituted by pallor, coldness of the extremities, profuse cold sweating, chilliness, shivering, slowness and feebleness of the pulse, and postural hypotension; this picture is frequently seen in association with very severe nausea, but may occur when nausea is not prominent. In such constellations, there is a fairly obvious physiological linkage of the symptoms, an expected concurrence. The type of conjunction is less readily explained in certain other constellations which tend to occur, in particular, in the earliest or prodromal stages of an attack, or during its resolution. Thus we may recognise, in the former case, a tendency for hunger, thirst, constipation, physical and emotional hyperactivity to be linked together; or, in the latter case, for a great number of secretory activities to proceed in unison.

THE SEQUENCE OF A COMMON MIGRAINE

A migraine attack is likely to be described by the patient in terms of a single symptom, or a mass of symptoms. Patient questioning and observation of repeated attacks may be necessary before it becomes clear that there is a preferred order or sequence of symptoms. The appreciation of such a sequence at once raises problems of terminology and definition: what constitutes the attack "proper"? Where does it begin and end?[8]

As generally understood and described, a common migraine is constituted by vascular headache, nausea, increased splanchnic activity (vomiting, diarrhoea, etc.), increased glandular activity (salivation, lacrimation, etc.), muscular weakness and atonia, drowsiness and depression. We will find, however, that migraine neither starts nor ends with these symptoms, but is both preceded and followed by symptoms and states which are clinically and physiologically the reverse of these.

We may speak of premonitory or *prodromal symptoms*, while recognising that these pass, insensibly, into the earlier phases of the attack proper. Some of these prodromal or early symptoms are local, some systemic; some are physical, and others are emotional. Among the commoner physical prodromes we must include states of water-retention and thirst, states of visceral dilatation and constipation, states of muscular tension and sometimes hypertension. Among the emotional or psychophysical prodromes we must recognise states of hunger, restless hyperactivity, insomnia, vigilance, and emotional arousal which may have either an anxious or euphoric colouring. Thus George Eliot, herself a sufferer from severe common migraines, would speak of feeling "dangerously well" the day before her attacks. Such states, when they are acute and extreme, may achieve an almost maniacal intensity.

Case 63   This middle-aged man was of normally phlegmatic nature, and presented a forbidding austerity of appearance and manner. He had experienced infrequent common migraines since childhood, and described the prodromal excitement of these attacks with some embarrassment. For two or three hours before the onset of his headaches he would be "transformed": he would feel thoughts rushing through his head, and would have an almost uncontrollable tendency to laugh or sing or whistle or dance.

[8]This point came up with great force—and a somewhat unexpected answer—when I had occasion to question one patient (Case 12), an eminent novelist, about the onset of his migraines. "You keep pressing me," he said, "to say that the attacks start with this symptom or that symptom, this phenomenon or that phenomenon, but this is not the way I experience them. It doesn't start with one symptom, it starts as a whole. You feel the whole thing, quite tiny at first, right from the start. . . . It's like glimpsing a point, a familiar point, on the horizon, and gradually getting nearer, seeing it get larger and larger; or glimpsing your destination from far off, in a plane, having it get clearer and clearer as you descend through the clouds." "The migraine *looms*," he added, "but it's just a change of scale—everything is already there from the start."

This business of "looming," of huge changes of scale, gives us a very different picture of what we might call the migraine landscape, makes us see it in dynamic, temporal terms —the terms of chaos theory—and not in the static, classical ones.

States of pre-migrainous excitement are more commonly of unpleasant tone, and take the form of irritable or agitated anxiety-states. Very
occasionally such states will reach panic or psychotic intensity. Affective
prodromes of this type are particularly common as part of a premenstrual syndrome.

Case 71   A 29-year-old woman with stormy menstrual syndromes of great
severity. The pre-menstrual phase would be marked by increasing water-
retention for two days, accompanied by a crescendo of diffuse anxiety and
irritability. Her sleep would be poor and punctuated by nightmares. The emotional disturbance would reach its maximum in the hours immediately preceding the menses, at which time the patient would become hysterical, violent,
and hallucinated. The emotional state would return to normal within a few
hours of the onset of menstruation, and be followed, the next day, by severe
vascular headache and intestinal colic.

The *resolution* of a common migraine, or indeed of any variety of
migraine attack, may proceed in three ways, as has been recognised since
the seventeenth century. It may, in its natural course, exhaust itself and
end in sleep; the post-migrainous sleep is long, deep, and refreshing, like
a post-epileptic sleep. Secondly, it may resolve by "lysis," a gradual
abatement of the suffering accompanied by one or more secretory activities. As Calmeil wrote, almost 150 years ago:

> Vomiting sometimes terminates a Migraine. An abundant flow of tears does
> the same, or an abundant secretion of urine. Sometimes hemicrania is termi-
> nated by an abundant perspiration from the feet, hands, half of the face, or
> by a nose-bleeding, a spontaneous arterial haemorrhage, or a mucous flux
> from the nose.

One must, of course, add to Calmeil's list that an abundant diarrhoea,
or menstrual flow, may similarly accompany the resolution of a migraine.
The hateful mood of a migraine—depressed and withdrawn, or furious
and irascible—tends to melt away in the stage of lysis, to melt away *with*
the physiological secretion. "Resolution by secretion" thus resembles a
catharsis on both physiological and psychological levels, like weeping
for grief. The following case-history illustrates a number of these points.

Case 68   This 32-year-old man was an ambitious and creative mathematician
whose life was geared to a weekly psychophysiological cycle. Towards the
end of the working week, he would become fretful, irritable and distractable,
"useless" at anything save the simplest routine tasks. He would have difficulty
sleeping on Friday nights, and on Saturdays would be unbearable. On Sunday

mornings he would awaken with a violent migraine, and would be forced to remain in bed for the greater part of the day. Towards evening he would break out in a gentle sweat and pass many pints of pale urine. The fury of his sufferings would melt away with the passage of these secretions. Following the attack he would feel a profound refreshment, a tranquillity, and a surge of creative energy which would carry him to the middle of the following week.

The third mode of resolution of a migraine is by *crisis*—a sudden accession of physical or mental activity, which brings the attack to an end within minutes.

Violent physical exercise may avert an attack, or truncate an existing attack. Many patients who lie abed late on Sunday and wake with a migraine find that early rising and hard physical work will prevent its occurrence. One patient of mine, a mesomorphic Italian of violent temperament, employs coitus to terminate his migraines if he is at home, or arm-wrestling if an attack comes on when he is at work, or drinking with his mates. Both are effective within five to ten minutes. Sudden fright, or rage, or other strong emotion may disperse and displace a migraine almost within seconds. One patient, asked how he terminated his attacks, said: "I have to get my adrenaline up . . . I have got to run around, or shout, or get in a fight, and the headache vanishes." Various forms of paroxysmal visceral activity may accomplish the same end. Violent vomiting is the classical example, but other activities may be equally effective.

Case 66   This patient, whose migraines were invariably terminated by paroxysmal vomiting, developed an ulcer in middle life, and was submitted to subtotal gastrectomy and vagotomy. When he had his first migraine after the operation he found himself unable to vomit, and felt disconsolate. Suddenly, however, he started sneezing with extraordinary violence and when the fit of sneezing had subsided his migraine was gone. Subsequently he adopted the use of snuff to facilitate the resolution of his attacks, and in so doing has unwittingly adopted an eighteenth-century prescription.

Other patients may hiccup, or belch repeatedly, with rapid resolution of their attacks. Even voracious eating may secure an early abortion of the attack, monstrous as such an activity would appear to most migraine patients. The relief comes *with the act* of eating.[9] Whichever method is utilised—violent physical, visceral, or emotional activity—the common

---

[9]Pavlov remarked on the frequency with which a hypnoidal state in a dog might be broken up by eating. The act of eating, often followed by scratching and sneezing, serves to arouse the dog from its trance-like state and was therefore termed by Pavlov an "autocurative" reflex.

factor is *arousal*. The patient is, as it were, awoken from his migraine as if from sleep. We shall further have occasion to see, when the specific drug therapies of migraine are under discussion, that the majority of these too serve to arouse the organism from a state of physiological depression.

We have already intimated an analogy between migraine and sleep, and this analogy is dramatised by the sense of extreme refreshment, and almost of rebirth, which may follow a severe but compact attack (see Case 68, p. 29). Such states do not represent a mere restoration to the pre-migraine condition, but a swing in the direction of arousal, a *rebound* after the migrainous trough. In the words of Liveing: ". . . [the patient] awakes a different being." Rebound euphoria and refreshment is particularly common after severe menstrual migraines. It is least in evidence after a protracted attack with vomiting, diarrhoea and fluid loss; such attacks fail to "recharge" the patient, and necessitate a period of convalescence.

One may describe an epilepsy simply in terms of the convulsion, while conceding that this may be preceded, in many patients, by a period of pre-ictal excitement and myoclonus, and followed by post-ictal stupor and exhaustion. But the violence and acuteness of the paroxysm justifies a restriction of the word "epilepsy" to cover this alone. In the case of a much more protracted paroxysmal reaction, like a migraine, it does not make sense—clinically, physiologically, or semantically—to limit the meaning of the word to the headache stage, or to any stage. The *entire sequence*—which we may then subdivide into prodromal stages, "attack proper," resolution, and rebound—must be denoted by the term "migraine." If this is not done, it becomes impossible to comprehend the nature of migraine.

POSTSCRIPT (1992)

Yet, when all this has been said, when one has set out tidy symptom constellations and sequences, one may have oversimplified and placed insufficient emphasis on the *unstable* quality of migraine, the difficulty of "fixing" it, of predicting its course, and the nature of that complex state that is best called "unsettled." Du Bois Reymond spoke of "a general feeling of disorder" at the very start of his attacks, and other patients speak, simply, of feeling "unsettled." In this unsettled state one may feel hot or cold, or both (see, for example, Case 9); bloated and tight, or

loose and queasy; a peculiar tension, or languor, or both; there are head
pains, or other pains, sundry strains and discomforts, which come and
go. *Everything* comes and goes, nothing is settled, and if one could take
a total thermogram, or scan, or inner photograph of the body, one would
see vascular beds opening and closing, peristalsis accelerating or stop-
ping, viscera squirming or tightening in spasms, secretions suddenly increasing or lessening—as if the nervous system itself was in a state of
indecision.

Intermittency, instability, fluctuation, oscillation are of the essence in
this unsettled state, this "general feeling of disorder," which runs before
a migraine. After minutes or hours this unsettledness starts to settle, very
rarely, alas!, into "health," much more commonly into the fixed and
settled forms of illness, those transfixed forms which are the textbook
symptoms and signs of migraine. Migraine starts as instability, disturbance, a far-from-equilibrium, unstable (or "metastable") state, which
sooner or later gravitates into either of two relatively stable positions,
that of "health" or that of "illness." There may, tantalizingly, be fluctuations between these—moments of stability, moments of health—as
this is happening, which tease with the promise that all is well; but the
overwhelming momentum is in the other direction.

McKenzie once called Parkinsonism "an organized chaos," and this
is equally true of migraine. First there is chaos, then organization, a sick
order; it is difficult to know which is worse! The nastiness of the first
lies in its uncertainty, its flux; the nastiness of the second in its sense of
immutable heavy permanence. Typically, indeed, treatment is only possible early, before migraine has "solidified" into immovable fixed forms.

The term "chaos," indeed, may be more than a figure of speech here,
for the sort of instability, of fluctuation, of sudden change, one sees here
is strongly reminiscent of what one may see in other complex systems—
the weather, for example—and may require for its understanding the
formal notion of "chaos" and a theory of complex, dynamical systems
(chaos theory). It may be important, then, to consider migraine in this
way, as a complex, dynamical disorder of neural behaviour and regula-
tion. The exquisite control (and, normally, latitude) of what we call
"health" may, paradoxically, be based on chaos. This is known to be
true of the nervous system as well (see Part V), especially perhaps with
the autonomic nervous system, with its fine tuning, its homeostasis, its
controls. Perhaps this is especially true in patients with migraine, in
whom, at certain "critical" times, the smallest stress will cause a physiological imbalance which, instead of being quietly corrected, leads rapidly

to further imbalances, overcompensations, playing on each other, rapidly amplifying, until it reaches that end-point we call "migraine." Perhaps migraine itself, to use a favorite term of chaos theorists, can itself act as a "strange attractor," pulling the nervous system, at certain times, into chaos.

TWO

Migraine Equivalents

Consideration of the many symptoms which may compose a common migraine has shown us that the term cannot be identified with any one symptom. A migraine is an aggregate of innumerable components, and its structure is composite. The emphasis of the components is extremely variable within the framework of a general pattern. Headache may be the cardinal symptom; it may constitute only a subsidiary symptom; it may even be entirely absent. We use the term "migraine equivalent" to denote symptom-complexes which possess the generic features of migraine, but lack a specific headache component.

This term is comparable to that of "epileptic equivalent," which denotes a form of epilepsy without convulsion. We justify the use of the term "migraine equivalent" if the following circumstances are fulfilled: the occurrence of discrete non-cephalgic attacks with a duration, a periodicity, and a clinical format similar to attacks of common migraine, and a tendency to be precipitated by the same type of emotional and physical antecedents. These clinical affinities will be matched, and confirmed, by physiological and pharmacological similarities.

Although earlier writers provided vivid case-histories of different types of migraine ("gastric megrim," "visual megrim," etc.), it remained for Liveing to trace the mutual convertibility of such attacks, and to speak of "transformations" and "metamorphoses" in this context. Thus, he would speak of asthmatic, epileptic, vertiginous, gastralgic, pectoralgic, laryngismal, and maniacal "transformations" of migraine.

The notion of migraine equivalents has not, for the most part, been sympathetically received. The physician who presumes to diagnose an "abdominal migraine" will be regarded, by many of his colleagues, as talking mumbo-jumbo or worse, and it may only be after endless diagnostic investigations and negative laparotomies, or the sudden replacement of attacks of abdominal pain by typical vascular headaches, that the old Victorian term is exhumed and reconsidered.

The concentrated experience of working with migraine patients must convince the physician, whatever his previous beliefs, that many patients *do* suffer repeated, discrete, paroxysmal attacks of abdominal pain, chest pain, fever, etc., which fulfil every clinical criterion of migraine save for the presence of headache. We will confine ourselves at this stage to a discussion of the following syndromes: cyclic vomiting and "bilious attacks," "abdominal migraines," "precordial migraines," and periodic, neurogenic disorders of body temperature, mood, and level of consciousness.

In addition to these acute, periodic, paroxysmal syndromes, there are a great variety of other states which bear *some* affinity to migraines, e.g. travel-sickness, "hangovers," reserpine reactions, etc. Consideration of these syndromes will be deferred to Part II.

CYCLIC VOMITING AND BILIOUS ATTACKS

We have observed the frequency and severity of nausea as a component of juvenile migraines. Frequently, it forms the cardinal symptom of a migraine reaction, and as such is often dignified with the term "bilious attack." Selby and Lance provide the following figures from their large series:

> . . . of 198 cases [of migraine] 31 per cent recalled frequently-occurring bilious attacks. Of a further 139 patients, 59 per cent have a history of some bilious attacks or severe motion-sickness during their early years.

I have not tabulated incidence-figures from my own practice, but would estimate—in accordance with Selby and Lance's figures—that nearly half the migraine patients one questions have suffered such symptoms at one time or another. Severe nausea is always accompanied by multiple autonomic symptoms—pallor, shivering, diaphoresis, etc. A majority of attacks are put down to dietary indiscretion in childhood, and in adult life ascribed to "gastric flu" or gall-bladder pathology, according to the persuasion of the physician.

Such attacks may persist throughout life, or may undergo a gradual or sudden transition to the "adult" form—common migraine. The following case-history, provided by Vahlquist and Hackzell (1949), illustrates the genesis and evolution of such attacks in a young patient:

> . . . When he was 10 months old he was badly frightened by an air-raid siren, and after this had abnormal fear-reactions and *pavor nocturnus* . . . The first typical attack occurred at the age of one year. He suddenly turned pale, and later had an attack of violent vomiting. During the next two years he had several attacks a week, always of the same type . . . When he was about three, he began to complain of a pain in his head during the attacks . . . They generally ended in a heavy sleep.

We may note, in passing, that cyclic vomiting of this type is also commonly associated with abnormal rage-reactions, and frequently coexists with temper tantrums.

ABDOMINAL MIGRAINE

The symptoms in any type of migraine are multiple, and the division between "bilious attacks" and "abdominal migraines" is an arbitrary one. The dominant feature in the latter is epigastric pain of continuous character and great severity, accompanied by a variety of further autonomic symptoms. The following incisive description is provided in Liveing's monograph:

> When about 16 years old, enjoying otherwise excellent health, I began to suffer from periodic attacks of severe pain in the stomach . . . The seizure would commence at any hour, and I was never able to discover any cause for it, for it was preceded by no dyspeptic symptoms or disordered bowels . . . The pain began with a deep, ill-defined uneasiness in the epigastrium. This steadily increased in intensity during the next two or three hours, and then declined. When at its height the pain was very intolerable and sickening—it had no griping quality whatever. It was always accompanied by chilliness, cold extremities, a remarkably slow pulse, and a sense of nausea . . . When the pain began to decline there was generally a feeling of movement in the bowels . . . The paroxysm left very considerable tenderness of the affected region, which took a day or two to clear off, but there was no tenderness at the time.

Some years later, this particular patient ceased to have his abdominal attacks, but developed instead attacks of classical migraine coming at similar intervals of three to four weeks.

I have notes of more than 40 patients (out of a total of 1,200) who consulted me with the presenting symptoms of common or classical migraine, but admitted to having had abdominal attacks similar to those described, for months or years in the past. Observant patients may comment on the slowness of the pulse and other autonomic symptoms accompanying the abdominal pain. Thus a patient cited earlier (Case 51, p. 23) had for a period of five years abdominal attacks in place of his common migraines, but had observed slowing of the pulse, smallness of the pupils, suffusion of the eyes and pallor in both types of attack. I have been given descriptions by three patients of what might be termed classical abdominal migraines.

Case 10   This 32-year-old man had suffered from classical migraines since the age of 10, the attacks coming with great regularity every four weeks. On some occasions, the migraine scotoma would be followed, not by headache, but by severe abdominal pain and nausea lasting 6 to 10 hours.

An excellent account of the presentations of abdominal migraine in children, and the problems of diagnosis to which they may give rise, has been provided by Farquhar (1956).

PERIODIC DIARRHOEA

We have observed the frequency of diarrhoea as a symptom in common migraine, especially in the later phases of the attack. Diarrhoea *per se*, often preceded by severe constipation, may be abstracted as an isolated symptom occurring in the same circumstances, or with the same periodicity, as attacks of common migraine—one of the commonest of such complaints is "weekend diarrhoea." Such neurogenic diarrhoeas tend to be ascribed to dietary indiscretion, or food-poisoning, or "intestinal 'flu,' " etc., until such explanations lose their acceptability, and it is borne in upon patient and physician that the attack represents a cyclical or circumstantial equivalent of migraine.

A certain number of such patients, especially those under severe chronic emotional stress, may proceed from a benign pattern of isolated migrainous diarrhoeas to a chronic mucous diarrhoea, or, rarely, a true ulcerative colitis. One suspects, in such patients, that the bowel has been a "target-organ" from the start (see Chapter 13).

PERIODIC FEVER

High fever may occur in the course of severe common migraines, particularly in children. It may also be abstracted as an isolated periodic symptom occurring in its own right, and sometimes alternating with common migraines.

I have seen half a dozen patients, currently suffering from common or classical migraines, who have had such attacks of periodic neurogenic fever in the past. The differential diagnosis may be laborious and tricky in such cases, for all possible causes of organic disease must be considered and excluded before one dare postulate a functional or neurogenic origin for such a symptom. The following case-history is summarised from Wolff:

> The patient, an engineer aged 43, began suffering from intermittent attacks of fever up to 104°F. in 1928, and he had continued to be afflicted with them . . . until 1940. It is of special interest that similar intermittent attacks of fever associated with "sick-headache," nausea and vomiting, had occurred in the patient's father . . .
>
> During late adolescence the patient himself began suffering from periodic headaches . . . especially frequent at times of emotional strain, and diagnosed as migraine . . . Before each [febrile] episode there were prodromal symptoms . . . a feeling of unrest and difficulty in concentration. The temperature rose rapidly to a peak and returned to normal within 12 hours. Leucocytosis (in the neighbourhood of 15,000 cells) occurred. After the fevers he had a "purged" feeling with a sense of especial well-being and mental efficiency.

The admirable case-history illustrates that attacks of febrile migraine equivalent may present a similar sequence to attacks of common migraine, with prodromal "arousal," and post-migrainous rebound and replenishment. It may also be noted that the patient's fevers ceased following therapeutic discussion of his emotional problems and general situation, and the presumed mechanism of his attacks.

PRECORDIAL MIGRAINE

The term "precordial migraine" (pectoralgic, or pseudo-anginal migraine) denotes the occurrence of chest-pain as a major constituent of a common or classical migraine, or its occurrence as a periodic, paroxysmal symptom with migrainous rather than anginal qualities and antecedents.

The symptom is a rare one, and I have encountered it only twice in my experience of over 1,000 migraine patients, once associated with common, and once with classical, migraines. The following case-history illustrates its occurrence during, and alternating with, classical attacks:

Case 58 A 61-year-old woman who had had attacks of classical migraine since adolescence. The majority of her attacks are ushered in by scintillation and paraesthesiae, bilaterally, followed by intense unilateral vascular headache, nausea and abdominal pain. A further symptom, during such severe attacks, is a feeling of painful tightness in the chest, accompanied by the radiation of pain to the left scapula, and down the left arm: it generally lasts for two to three hours.

The chest-pain is not aggravated by exercise, nor is it accompanied by cardiographic abnormalities; it is not alleviated by nitroglycerin, but is diminished, in company with its other accompanying symptoms, by ergotamine.

On occasion, this patient has had attacks of similar chest-pain occurring as an isolated symptom, and sometimes ushered in by migrainous scotomata and paraesthesiae.

The presentation and diagnosis of such attacks has been very fully considered by Fitz-Hugh (1940).

PERIODIC SLEEP AND TRANCE-STATES

The drowsiness which often accompanies or precedes a severe common migraine is occasionally abstracted as a symptom in its own right, and may then constitute the sole expression of the migrainous tendency. The following case illustrates the "transformation" of common migraine to a sleep equivalent.

Case 76 The patient was a nun who had been subject to common migraines of great severity at least twice weekly for some 20 years. Treatment was initially prophylactic and symptomatic in view of her wish to avoid discussion of personal matters. After three months of such treatment, her cephalgic attacks abruptly disappeared, but there occurred, in their stead, once or twice weekly sleeps of almost stuporous intensity. These attacks would last 10 to 15 hours, and constituted an unprecedented *addition* to her usual nocturnal sleep.

We have alluded to the frequency of torpor in post-prandial migraines. The following case-history, which we will have occasion to refer to in other contexts, illustrates the occurrence of post-prandial stupors as an isolated symptom.

Case 49 The patient, an obsessively hard-working engineer—in his own words, "I never stop—I wish I didn't have to sleep"—suffers from a remarkable variety of migrainous equivalents and analogues. Unless he forces himself to take a brisk walk after meals, he will fall into an irresistible torpor. He describes this as follows: "I go into a trance, where I am able to hear things around me, but can't move. I am soaked with a cold sweat. My pulse gets very slow." The state lasts between one and two hours, rarely less or more than this. He "wakes," if one may use the word, with a feeling of intense refreshment and bounding energy.

We may also note briefly, at this stage, that migrainous sleeps and stupors not infrequently alternate with other and briefer periodic trance-states, such as narcolepsies, "daymares," and somnambulistic episodes. Particular attention will be paid to such relationships in later chapters.

PERIODIC MOOD-CHANGES

We have already spoken of the affective concomitants of common migraines—elated and irritable prodromal states, states of dread and depression associated with the main phase of the attack, and states of euphoric rebound. Any or all of these may be abstracted as isolated periodic symptoms of relatively short duration—some hours, or at most two or three days, and as such may present themselves as primary emotional disorders. The most acute of these mood-changes, generally no more than an hour in duration, usually represents concomitants or equivalents of migraine aura. We may confine our attention at this stage to attacks of depression, or truncated manic-depressive cycles, occurring at intervals in patients who have previously suffered from attacks of undoubted (classical, common, abdominal, etc.) migraine. Alvarez, who is particularly alert to the occurrence of such migrainous equivalents, cites the following history:

> A woman aged 56 complained of spells of deep depression lasting for a day or two. Her home physician thought they were probably menopausal in origin, but I found they were migrainous, and associated with a slight unilateral headache. I learned that in her early girlhood she had had spells of typically migrainous vomiting . . . In her forties, she had had severe migrainous headaches with much retching.

An unusually clear-cut case from my own experience was provided by the following patient, part of whose history has already been cited in another context:

Case 10   This 32-year-old man had suffered both from classical cephalgic and classical abdominal migraines since childhood, the attacks coming with considerable regularity at monthly intervals. In his mid-twenties, he had been free of such attacks for more than a year, but suffered during this time from equally regular attacks of elation followed by severe depression, the entire episode lasting no more than two days.

Characteristic of such affective equivalents is their *brevity*—manic-depressive cycles, as generally understood, occupy several weeks, and frequently longer. Monthly affective equivalents of this type—or "lunacies" if we may venture the term—are most commonly seen in the context of menstrual syndromes.

MENSTRUAL SYNDROMES

A large minority of women experience marked affective and autonomic disturbances about the time of menstruation. Greene has estimated that "about 20 women in every 100 suffer sometimes from premenstrual migraine," and if we include under this heading autonomic and affective disturbances not accompanied by headache, the figure must be substantially higher than this. Indeed, we may say that the menstrual cycle is *always* associated with some degree of physiological disturbance, even though this may pass unobserved by the patient. The disturbance tends to be in the direction of psychophysiological arousal prior to the menses, and "let-down" followed by rebound after the menses.

The arousal period may be characterised by "tension," anxiety, hyperactivity, insomnia, fluid-retention, thirst, constipation, abdominal distension, etc. and, more rarely, asthma, psychosis, or epilepsy. The "let-down" period, or "de-rousal," may be manifest as lassitude, depression, vascular headache, visceral hyperactivity, pallor, sweating, etc. In short, virtually all the symptoms of migraine, as they have been described thus far, may be condensed into the biological turmoil surrounding menstruation.

Of particular relevance in the present context is the frequent alternation, during the life-history of a single patient, of differing formats of menstrual syndrome, with the emphasis on vascular headache at one time, at another on intestinal cramping, etc. The following case-history illustrates a sudden "transformation" between two types of menstrual migraine.

Case 32   A 37-year-old woman had experienced severe abdominal (probably intestinal) cramping at the menstrual period between the ages of 17 and 30. She suddenly ceased to experience these symptoms at that age, but suffered, in their place, typical premenstrual migraine headaches.

Other patients may suffer severe menstrual syndromes for several years, lose these to acquire frequent attacks of paroxysmal headache or abdominal pain unrelated to the menstrual periods, finally reverting to the original pattern of menstrual disturbance.

The precise timing of such menstrual syndromes, and their physiological and psychological relationship to menstruation, will be considered at length in Chapter 8.

ALTERNATIONS AND TRANSFORMATIONS

It is legitimate to speak of abdominal, precordial, febrile, affective, etc., "equivalents" of migraine, in that the general format and sequence of migraine, as pictured in Chapter 1, persists despite the varying emphasis of individual symptoms. There are, in addition to such acceptable equivalents, many other forms of paroxysmal illness or reaction which may insidiously or suddenly "replace" migraine attacks in the life-history of an individual; they occur, for the most part, with the same periodicity as the original migraines, or in response to much the same circumstances. It would be absurd, without doubt, to speak of paroxysmal asthma, angina, or laryngospasm as being migraine equivalents, yet clinical observation forces us to wonder whether they may not, on occasion, fill a biological role analogous to that of migraine attacks. Semantic argument is profitless in this context, and we may content ourselves, for the moment, with the non-committal term which Liveing uses: "allied disorders".

Heberden (1802) recorded the already established observation that "the hemicrania . . . has ceased upon the coming of an asthma," and it is impossible to doubt that there may be sudden transitions from one species of paroxysm to the other during the life-history of a patient. I have myself observed such alternations, generally abrupt, in at least 20 patients under my care. The following case-history, already presented in part, typifies such a transformation.

Case 18   This 24-year-old man had suffered from frequent nightmares and somnambulistic episodes until the age of 8, attacks of periodic, usually nocturnal, asthma until the age of 13, and classical and common migraines thereafter. The classical migraines would come, with considerable regularity, every Sunday afternoon. The use of ergot compounds effectively aborted these attacks, and after three months of therapeutic care, he suddenly ceased to experience even the premonitory migraine auras. Some weeks after this he returned to me angrily complaining that his long-defunct attacks of asthma had returned, and that they came, in particular, on Sunday afternoons. He regretted the change, finding his migraines preferable to, and altogether less frightening than, the asthmas.

We will have occasion to return to this particular and illuminating case-history in the following chapter. This was one of my first patients, and his experience, our joint experience, early persuaded me that merely symptomatic treatment in certain patients might do no more than drive them through an endless repertoire of "allied reactions."

Similar case-histories may be collected, and similar considerations adduced, with regard to the mutual transformations of migraine with attacks of neurogenic angina or laryngospasm, the former of these transformations also being well known to Heberden: "Instances are not wanting," he writes, ". . . where attacks of this complaint and now of headache have afflicted the patient by turns." Perplexing problems of differential diagnosis are presented by certain patients in whom attacks of *angina sine dolore*, neither precipitated by exercise nor accompanied by cardiographic changes alternate with migraines. The following description, taken from Beaumont (1952), shows the common clinical ground which may be shared by the two types of attack.

> . . . The patient is suddenly seized by a sensation of imminent death, becomes pale and motionless, and yet experiences no pain. During an attack salivation or vomiting may occur, the attack ceasing with eructation of wind, or a copious flow of urine.

Neurogenic laryngospasm (croup) provides another example of an exceptionally acute paroxysmal reaction which may show mutual transformations with attacks of migraine. An excellent example of this is provided by Liveing. We have already alluded to the abdominal migraines experienced by his patient "Mr. A" (periodic attacks between the ages of 16 and 19), and the attacks of classical migraine which succeeded these (between the ages of 19 and 37). Subsequently, this patient "lost" his classical migraines, but suffered from periodic attacks of paroxysmal croup:

> . . . after having been asleep an hour or so, he would suddenly wake to consciousness in the act of jumping out of bed, tearing open his collar-band and struggling violently for breath with loud stridulous breathing; after a few minutes of this, which appeared to him a prolonged and intolerable agony, the throat spasm would relax and respiration again become free. These attacks have occurred at very irregular intervals, sometimes several months apart, but generally two or three on successive or neighbouring nights.

BORDERLANDS OF MIGRAINE

Gowers (1907), in his preface to a series of lectures on "The Borderland of Epilepsy," announced his intention to speak of attacks which were *near* epilepsy, but not of it. He was concerned with the consideration of faints, vagal attacks, vertigo, sleep symptoms, and, above all, migraine. Epilepsies, in their most clearly recognisable form, are characterised by suddenness, brevity, loss of consciousness. But let us imagine, argues Gowers,

> . . . a minor epileptic attack that is extended, its elements protracted with no tendency to be terminated by loss of consciousness; its features would be so different that its nature would not be suspected.

It is indeed in these terms, as extended epilepsies, that Gowers would categorise many of the attacks he describes. He quotes, for example, the following case-history as exemplifying a *vagal attack* akin to epilepsy:

> The subject . . . was a man, an officer in the army, aged 20. The seizures were not frequent; they had occurred about once in 6 months for 12 years, ever since he was 18 years old. Earlier in the day he had been in especially good spirits—an antecedent often noted. Quite suddenly a dreamy mental state came on, a reminiscent state, the well-known feeling that whatever was happening had happened before. It was not momentary, as in epilepsy, but continued. With it, or just after its commencement, his hands and feet became cold . . . With the coldness his face became increasingly pale, and physical prostration set in, speedily reaching such a degree that he was scarcely able to move. If he tried to sit up, he fell back at once. His extremities became icily cold, even to an observer. So great was the prostration that he could only utter one or two words at a time . . . His pulse became smaller and smaller, until it was hardly perceptible. There was not a moment's loss of consciousness throughout. His own sensation was that he was dying, passing out of physical existence. The state lasted about half an hour, and then he became aware, simultaneously, that his mental state was improving and that his feet were a little less cold. The amelioration went on, but two or three minutes after its commencement a distinct rigor set in, with shivering and chattering of the teeth . . . A few minutes after the rigor an urgent need for micturition was felt and went on during the rest of the day, a large quantity of limpid urine being passed . . . He continued pale for the rest of the day.

The reader will recognise a large number of symptoms we have hitherto termed "migrainous" in this admirably detailed description. The antecedent feeling of well-being, the duration of the attack, its lysis with a protracted diuresis, are all features we have encountered in the sequence of common migraines. By what warrant, therefore, is such an attack to be termed an extended epilepsy rather than a quite brief and severe, let us say, a *condensed* migraine?

Virtually all the patterns of migraine equivalent we have considered in this chapter may present themselves in a more contracted format. Lennox and Lennox (1960) provide many instructive case-histories under the title of autonomic or diencephalic epilepsy. Sometimes such autonomic attacks may evolve from or into clear-cut epilepsies or migraines, and at other times they may alternate with such attacks.

An obvious and important type of attack which bears obvious clinical affinities to both migraines and epilepsies—in terms of its widespread autonomic features to the former, and in terms of its suddenness and loss of consciousness to the latter—is the *faint*. Fainting not uncommonly coexists with recurrent migraine, and may occur with much the same periodicity as, or in similar provocative circumstances to, the migraine attacks. One may observe, as with vagal attacks, a continuous transition in the clinical picture from a dramatic and sudden collapse to protracted autonomic reactions with haziness, but not loss, of consciousness. The still briefer attacks which Gowers considers—vertigos, narcolepsies, cataplexies, etc.—will be considered in the next chapter, for their affinities are to migraine aura rather than common migraine and the migraine equivalents we have so far discussed.

Acute attacks of this type which are near migraine, but not of it, we may term *migranoid attacks*, and like migraine they tend to be periodic, recurrent, and strongly familial. We may reserve the term *migranoid reactions* for certain types of response akin to migraine in their clinical aspects, but circumstantially provoked rather than spontaneous and periodic. Here we must place the hyperbolic reactions to *heat* (and fever), *exhaustion, passive motion*, and certain *drugs* which are both common and characteristic in migraine patients. The distinction of what is a migraine and what a migranoid reaction is purely one of convenience. Thus it is awkward to call *motion-sickness* a migraine attack, but we may very conveniently term it a migranoid reaction, and note, in support of its affinities, that a large minority (almost 50 per cent, according to Selby and Lance) of adult migraine sufferers experienced severe motion-sickness in childhood. Similarly a *hangover*—with its vascular headache, malaise, lethargy, nausea, and penitential depression—is usefully considered as a migranoid reaction; many migraine patients are highly intolerant of alcohol, and may suffer a spectrum of symptoms in its wake, from an acute nausea or headache reaction, to a full-blown hangover the following day. Feverish headaches and autonomic reactions may similarly be accounted migranoid in quality.

Similarly, there is a spectrum of drug-responses, acute and sub-acute, characterised by diffuse central and autonomic reactions, akin both to syncopal and to migraine attacks. Thus, the following description of a "nitritoid crisis" is cited by Goodman and Gilman (1955):

> Normal robust male, aged 28, given 0.18 gm of sodium nitrite by mouth . . . Yawning appeared and became progressively more prominent; the respirations deepened and assumed a sighing character; restlessness, belching and borborygmus were noted; and a cold perspiration broke out over the entire body-surface. In about 20 minutes the skin was ashen grey, the subject became drowsy . . . the blood-pressure reading became unobtainable . . . and unconsciousness ensued.

Reactions of a similar acuteness may occur following visceral dilatation or injury, reflex or haemorrhagic fall of blood-pressure, toxic and metabolic insults (e.g. hypoglycaemia), and in allergic and anaphylactoid responses.

We will have to concern ourselves later with the question of whether such responses afford useful "models" of the migraine reaction, and content ourselves, at this point, with noting their clinical affinity and place in the borderlands of migraine.

ALTERNATIONS AND CONCOMITANCES WITH OTHER DISORDERS

Even more complicated than these cases in which two allied symptoms alternate, are those patients who present with a *polymorphous* syndrome in which a large variety of symptoms—with clinical and physiological affinities to each other—occur simultaneously or cyclically in the history of the individual:

Case 49   This 31-year-old engineer has already been cited in connection with a tendency to post-prandial stupors. He suffers from a variety of further symptoms, as follows:

> (a) A continuous "latent" vascular headache, which becomes manifest on stooping, jolting, or coughing.
> (b) Attacks of common migraine.
> (c) Night sweats, for which no organic basis has been found.
> (d) Attacks of nocturnal salivation.

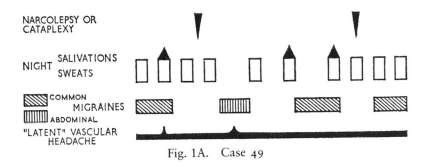

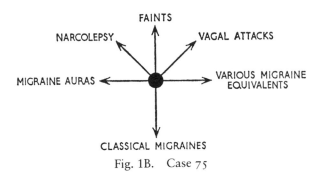

Fig. 1A.   Case 49

Fig. 1B.   Case 75

(e) Attacks of abdominal pain and diarrhoea—contrast studies of the bowel have always been negative.

(f) Orthostatic hypotension.

(g) Occasional sleep-paralysis, narcolepsy, and cataplexy.

He is otherwise in excellent health.

Case 75   A 35-year-old physician subject to migraine auras and classical migraine has also experienced, as alternative reactions, abdominal migraines, bilious attacks, stuporous migraine equivalents, "vagal attacks" (exceedingly similar in type to that described by Gowers), and, more rarely, fainting and narcolepsy. All of these reactions are circumstantially determined, either by exhaustion or acute emotional stress, especially if these factors are conjoined. He cannot predict *which* somatic response will occur: all of them seem equally available and equivalent to one another.

Case 64   A polysymptomatic woman of 45 with the following history: Intrinsic (usually nocturnal) asthma until the age of 20, recurrent duodenal ulceration between the ages of 20 and 37. At the age of 38 she had an initial episode of rheumatoid arthritis, and has had several episodes subsequently. Coincident with the inauguration of this symptom, she started to have frequent attacks of angioneurotic oedema and of common migraine. These two

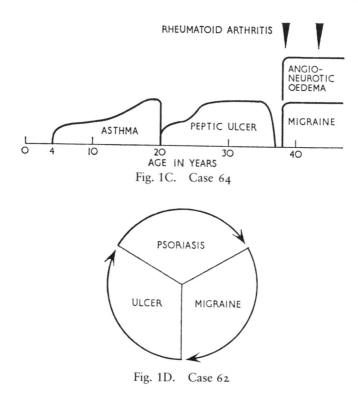

Fig. 1C.   Case 64

Fig. 1D.   Case 62

latter syndromes have coalesced, and since the age of 43 her attacks of migraine have been ushered in by facial and periocular oedema.

Case 62   A 51-year-old woman whose social and emotional history will be elaborated in Part II. She had suffered for more than twenty years with three somatic manifestations: common migraine, ulcerative colitis, and psoriasis. She would suffer for several months from one of these symptoms, before remitting and passing to another symptom. She was thus trapped within an endless malignant cycle.

Case 61   A 38-year-old woman who presented herself for treatment of common migraine although she also had disfiguring psoriasis. Her family background was one of polymorphous functional disease: migraine, hayfever, asthma, urticaria, Menière's disease, peptic ulcer, ulcerative colitis, and Crohn's disease. It was difficult to avoid the feeling that this stricken family was, in effect, committing physiological suicide.

Case 21   A highly intelligent 25-year-old woman who combines severe neurotic symptoms with a variety of somatic syndromes. She had had classical migraines since childhood, of which there is a prominent family history: the

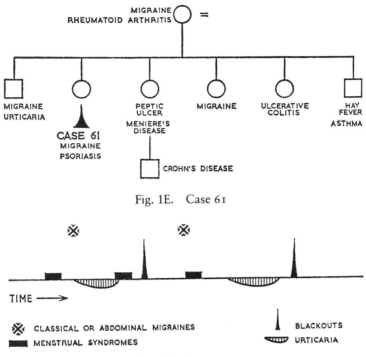

Fig. 1E. Case 61

Fig. 1F. Case 21

majority of these attacks arise at dawn with a nightmare or night-terror—the figments of nightmare and unmistakable scotomatous figures may be coalesced, prior to her waking in the second, or headache, stage. On some occasions, the aura is followed by abdominal pain but no head-pain. Allied to the latter, but missing an aura, are pre-menstrual syndromes, in which a period of water-retention, constipation, and restlessness deliquesces into diuresis, diarrhoea, and menstrual flux: there may or may not be an associated vascular headache with these pre-menstrual syndromes. On some occasions she has had "grey-outs," or syncopes, usually though not invariably followed by migrainous headache. She is also subject to attacks of urticaria (hives) during periods of increased emotional stress. With successful treatment of her headache problems, the emphasis has shifted to increased abdominal attacks and urticaria.

DIFFERENTIAL DIAGNOSIS AND NOMENCLATURE

When the cardinal symptom of vascular headache is absent, the types of attack we have considered in this chapter may present formidable challenges in differential diagnosis; indeed, there is probably no field in medicine so strewn with the debris of misdiagnosis and mistreatment, and of well-intentioned but wholly mistaken medical and surgical interventions. Abdominal migraines, for example, no less than tabetic crises, must have afforded innumerable occasions for emergency laparotomies. It may not be justifiable to wait passively for the outcome of a mysterious but overwhelming attack of abdominal pain; it is doubtless better sense to perform a negative laparotomy in a case of abdominal migraine than be faced with a neglected appendicitis and peritonitis. The true diagnosis may only become apparent subsequently, with repetition of the attacks, and demonstration of their benign and transient nature. In many cases, therefore, the diagnosis of cryptic migraine equivalents requires prolonged observation, and may, in fact, be made only retrospectively.

We have limited our consideration, thus far, to relatively discrete, circumscribed, and strongly-marked paroxysmal attacks, and have selected, for the sake of emphasis, case-histories of an almost diagrammatic clarity. In practice, the symptoms experienced and the history obtainable may be altogether vaguer in terms of specific symptoms. Attacks characterised by little more than malaise are likely to be regarded as mild viral illnesses. Attacks characterised by alteration of affect and consciousness—mild drowsiness or depression—may be taken for purely emotional reactions. Both viral illnesses and emotional reaction *may*, indeed, share many clinical symptoms occurring in, though not pathognomonic of, migraines, and the differential diagnosis may never be clarified unless more specific symptoms, or determinants of the attacks, are elicited.

Beyond the sharp and artificial edges of "diagnosis" we enter a region of semantic ambiguity in which the definition of the term "migraine" is stretched to breaking-point. In the center, so to speak, we may place common migraine, clear and indisputable. Around this we may group the migraine equivalents, polymorphous in their manifestations, and representing various dissections, decompositions and agglomerates of different migraine components. Beyond this, we must recognise a penumbra of allied and analogous reactions, which may, as it were, do duty for a migraine.

Compact and clearly defined at its center, migraine diffuses outwards until it merges with an immense surrounding field of allied phenomena. The only boundaries which exist are those which we are forced to adopt for nosological clarity and clinical action. We construct such boundaries and limits, for there is none in the subject itself.

THREE

Migraine Aura and Classical Migraine

INTRODUCTION

We now come to the largest, strangest chapter in this book—for we must consider what lies at the very heart of migraine; here is the realm of its great wonders and secrets:

> We carry with us the wonders we seek without us: there is all Africa and her prodigies in us. . . .

Sir Thomas Browne's words perfectly fit this—the *aura* of migraine: here, inside us, is a veritable Africa of prodigies; here, by experience, exploration and reflection, one can chart a whole world—the cosmography of oneself.

The aura of migraine deserves a whole book to itself—or, at the very least, as in Liveing, it should form the centerpiece if a book is to be written on migraine. But, very puzzlingly, the reverse obtains; nobody has given the aura its due, since Liveing; and the more up-to-date the book, the less space it is given. The very words we use—*classical* migraine as opposed to *common* (the *classical* being a migraine with an aura)—imply that the aura is *uncommon*—and arcane.

This, as a start, is demonstrably untrue, and a consequence of inquiries which fly wide of the mark, and foolish assumptions which *make* them miss the mark. An acute and open-minded observer like Alvarez, putting together the experience of seventy years as a physician, considered the aura was far commoner than usually allowed; far commoner, indeed, than anything else in a migraine. And in this I find myself in complete agreement with him.

The following general points should first be made by way of introduction.

The aura itself is far from uncommon; adequate descriptions of it are extremely uncommon; good descriptions of the aura are vitally *needed*, because it is a phenomenon of the utmost importance, which can cast a great flood of light not only on migraine, but on the most elemental and fundamental mechanisms of the brain-mind; good descriptions are hard to obtain, because many aura phenomena are exceedingly strange—so strange as to transcend the powers of language; and good descriptions are made rarer still by the presence of something uncanny and fearful, the very thought of which causes the mind to shy.

This last, although neither analysed nor understood, was given a very striking emphasis by Liveing; it constituted a strange and incomprehensible barrier, over which neither he nor his patients could leap; so that, finally he could only say that "there are sufferers who cannot bear to think or talk of their attacks, and always refer to them with horror, though this is clearly not on account of the pain they occasion." Thus the subject of migraine aura is touched with the incomprehensible and the incommunicable: nay, this lies at its very center, its heart.

The term *aura* has been used for nearly two thousand years to denote the sensory hallucinations immediately preceding certain epileptic seizures.[10] The term has been employed, for somewhat over a century, to denote analogous symptoms which inaugurate certain attacks—the so-called classical migraine—or which may constitute, on occasion, the sole manifestation of a migraine attack.

We will have occasion to consider, as components of these auras, symptoms of an acuteness and a strangeness which sets them apart from anything we have thus far discussed. Indeed, if an aura were never followed by vascular headache, nausea, diffuse autonomic disturbance, etc., we might have great difficulty in recognising its migrainous nature. Such difficulties *do* arise, not uncommonly, when patients suffer from isolated auras lasting a few minutes, and not succeeded by headache or vegetative

---

[10] The derivation and original meaning of the term is described by Gowers as follows: "The word 'aura' was first used by Pelops, the master of Galen, who was struck by the phenomenon with which many attacks begin—a sensation, commencing in the hand or foot, apparently ascending to the head. The sensation having been described to him by patients as 'a cold vapour,' he suggested that it might really be such, passing up the vessels, then believed to contain air. Hence he named it πνευματικὴ αὔρα, 'spirituous vapour'."

disturbance. Such cases, as Gowers remarked, are very puzzling, of great importance and liable to be misunderstood.

Such uncertainties are reflected in a historical dichotomy, whereby accounts of (migraine) aura and accounts of (migraine) headache were separately published for centuries, without the making of any explicit connection between the two sets of phenomena.

The manifestations of migraine aura are exceedingly various, and include not only simple and complex sensory hallucinations, but intense affective states, deficits and disturbances of speech and ideation, dislocations of space- and time-perception, and a variety of dreamy, delirious, and trance-like states. The older medical and religious literature contains innumerable references to "visions," "trances," "transports," etc., but the nature of many of these must now remain enigmatic to us. Many different processes may have similar manifestations, and some of the more complex phenomena described may be hysteric, psychotic, oneiric, or hypnagogic in origin, no less than epileptic, apoplectic, toxic or migrainous in nature.

A single notable exception may be mentioned—the "visions" of Hildegard (1098–1179)—which were indisputably migrainous in nature. These are discussed in Appendix I.

Isolated accounts of such visual phenomena continued to appear throughout the Middle Ages, but we must move six hundred years before we find accounts of aura phenomena other than the visual, and the making of an *explicit* connection between such manifestations and migraine.

The following three accounts, all written in the early nineteenth century, and cited by Liveing, illustrate many cardinal characteristics of migraine aura, in its visual (scotomatous), tactile (paraesthetic) and aphasic forms. We may note, parenthetically, that many of the finest descriptions of the aura—from those of Hildegard in the twelfth century to those of Lashley and Alvarez in the present century—have been provided by introspective observers who themselves suffered from classical migraine, or, more commonly, isolated migraine auras.

> . . . I have frequently experienced a sudden failure of sight. The general sight did not appear affected; but when I looked at any particular object, it seemed as if something brown, and more or less opaque, was interposed between my eyes and it, so that I saw it indistinctly, or sometimes not at all . . .
>
> After it had continued a few moments, the upper or lower edge appeared bounded by an edging of light of a zigzag shape, and coruscating nearly at right angles to its length. The coruscation always appeared to be in one eye; but both it and the cloud existed equally whether I looked at an object with

one or both eyes open . . . The cloud and the coruscation . . . would remain
from twenty minutes, sometimes to half an hour . . . They were in me never
followed by headache . . . [but] generally went off with a movement in the
stomach producing eructation. (Parry)

Commencing in the tip of the tongue, at one part of the face, at the ends of
the fingers or toes, it [the paraesthesia] mounts little by little towards the
cerebrospinal axis, successively disappearing about those parts where it was
first developed . . . The thrilling sensation in the hands calls to mind the oscillatory movement of the visual image. (Piorry)

About a quarter of an hour after this [the blindness], she feels a numbness of
the little finger of the right hand, beginning at the point of it, and extending
very gradually over the whole hand and arm, producing a complete loss of
sensibility of the parts, but without any loss of the power of motion. The
feeling of numbness then extends to the right side of the head, and from this
it seems to spread downwards towards the stomach. When it reaches the side
of the head, she becomes oppressed and partially confused, answers questions
slowly and confusedly, and her speech is considerably affected; when it
reaches the stomach she sometimes vomits. (Abercrombie)

The elective sites of the paraesthesiae (tongue, hand, foot), and its
centripetal passage from the periphery, necessarily reminded the early
observers of the *aura epileptica*, and it remained for Liveing, writing
between 1863 and 1865, to make an absolutely clear distinction between
the two sets of phenomena.

We need proceed no further at this juncture with a historical account
of migraine aura, although we shall have to return to the older writings
when we come to consider (in Part III) the possible basis of its manifestations.

Our next task must be a systematic enumeration of the full range of
aural symptoms which may occur. Since they are exceedingly various,
we may consider them under certain general heads:

(a)   Specific visual, tactile, and other sensory hallucinations.

(b)   General alterations of sensory threshold and excitability.

(c)   Alterations in level of consciousness and muscular tone.

(d)   Alterations of mood and affect.

(e)   Disorders of higher integrative functions: perception, ideation,
      memory, and speech.

These categories are adopted purely for ease of discussion. They are in
no sense mutually exclusive. Migraine aura, like common migraine, is

composite in nature, and put together from a variety of possible components. Although a casual description may make reference to a single symptom only, such as a scintillating scotoma, a patient interrogation will nearly always reveal that the situation is more complex, and that several phenomena—some very subtle, and difficult of description—are happening simultaneously.

We shall first enumerate individual components of the aura *seriatim*, remembering that they are isolated only for purposes of exposition. This will be followed by a series of case-histories designed to illustrate the complex and composite nature of auras as they usually occur.

SPECIFIC SENSORY HALLUCINATIONS: VISUAL

A remarkable variety of visual hallucinations may be experienced during the course of a migraine aura.

The simplest hallucination takes the form of a dance of brilliant stars, sparks, flashes or simple geometric forms across the visual field. Phosphenes of this type are usually white, but may have brilliant spectral colours. They may number many hundreds, and swarm rapidly across the visual field (patients often compare them to the movement of radar "blips" across a screen). Sometimes a single phosphene may detach itself from the remainder, as in the following case (Gowers, 1892):

> One patient . . . with characteristic headaches preceded by hemianopia, complained of bright stars before the eyes whenever she had looked at a brilliant light; and sometimes one of the stars, brighter than the rest, would start from the right lower corner of the field of vision, and pass across the field, generally quickly, in a second, sometimes more slowly, and when it reached the left side would break up and leave a blue area in which luminous points were moving.[11]

At other times there may be only a single, rather elaborate phosphene in the visual field, which moves to and fro upon a set course, and then disappears suddenly, leaving a trail of dazzlement or blindness in its wake (Figure 2A). We may, once more, find the best descriptions of such phosphenes amongst Gowers's many writings on the subject (1904).

> . . . In another case a radial movement was presented by a stellate object which remained unchanged throughout. It appeared usually near the edge of the right half of the field just below the horizontal line, and consisted of about

---

[11] This case-history also draws attention to the specific capacity of light to provoke various forms of migraine aura, a subject more fully discussed in Chapter 8.

six pointed leaflike projections, alternately red and blue . . . [it] moved slowly towards the left and upwards, passing above the fixing-point, to a little beyond the middle line, then it returned to its starting place, retraced this path once or twice, and then passed to the right edge of the field . . . after two or three repetitions of the last course it suddenly disappeared . . . [on opening her eyes] the patient always found she could only see in the part of the field through which the spectrum had not passed.

Although such phosphenes may be confined to one half or one quadrant of the visual field, they not infrequently cross the midline (as in the case described above); rapidly-moving swarms of phosphenes are bilateral more often than not. Sometimes the phosphenes may be elaborated or interpreted by the patient as recognisable images; thus one patient (in Selby and Lance's series) described small white skunks with erect tails, moving in procession across one quadrant of the visual field.[12]

Other elementary hallucinations which are commonly experienced are rippling, shimmering and undulation in the visual field, which patients may compare to the appearance of wind-blown water, or looking through watered silk. (See Figure 5A and 5B, p. 77.)

During or after the passage of simple phosphenes, some patients may observe, on closing the eyes, a form of visual tumult or delirium, in which latticed, faceted and tessellated motifs predominate—images reminiscent of mosaics, honeycombs, Turkish carpets, etc., or moiré patterns. These figments and elementary images tend to be brilliantly luminous, coloured, highly unstable, and prone to sudden kaleidoscopic transformations.

These evanescent flitting phosphenes are usually no more than a preamble to the major portion of the visual aura. In most (though not all) cases the patient goes on to experience a longer-lasting and far more elaborate hallucination within the visual field—the migraine *scotoma*. Further descriptive terms are commonly used: the shape (and colours) of these scotomata lead us to speak of migraine *spectra*, and the structure of their margins (often reminiscent of the ramparts of a walled city) has given rise to the term *fortification spectra* (teichopsia). The term *scintillating scotoma* denotes the characteristic flickering of luminous migraine spectra, and the term *negative scotoma* denotes the area of partial or

[12] Hughlings Jackson makes the following comment on the tendency to elaborate images from elementary hallucinations when in physiologically abnormal states: "A healthy man has muscae from intra-ocular specks; they seem like moving dots and films in front of him. But suppose he undergoes dissolution (as in cases of delirium tremens), and that there is the first depth of dissolution, then he sees mice and rats. Speaking roughly, the muscae 'turn into' those animals for him."

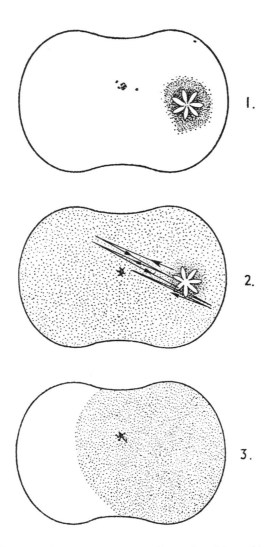

Fig. 2A.   Variants of migraine scotoma. Reproduced from Gowers (1904)
Mobile stellate spectrum

total blindness which may follow, or, on occasion, precede a scintillating scotoma.

The majority of migraine scotomata present as a sudden brilliant luminosity near the fixation-point in one visual half-field; from here the scotoma gradually expands and moves slowly towards the edge of the visual field, assuming the form of a giant crescent or horseshoe. Its sub-

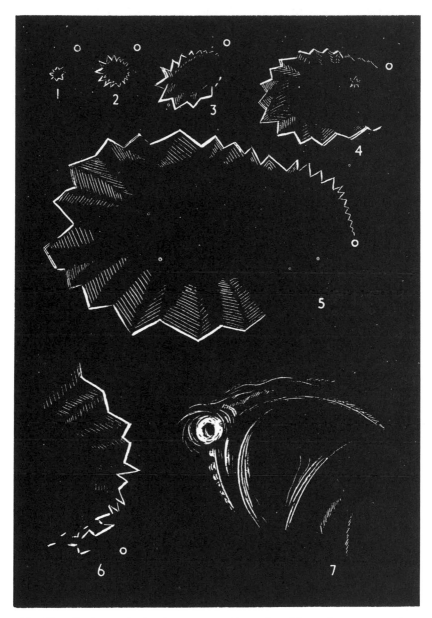

Fig. 2B.   Variants of migraine scotoma. Reproduced from Gowers (1904)
Expanding angular spectrum (Airy, 1868)

jective brightness is blinding—Lashley compares it to that of a white surface in noonday sunlight. Within this brilliance there may be a play of intense, pure spectral colours at the fringes of the scotoma, and objects seen through these fringes may be edged with a many-coloured iridescence. The advancing margin of the scotoma often displays the gross zigzag appearance which justifies the term fortification-spectrum (Figure 2B), and is invariably broken up, more finely, into minute luminous angles and intersecting lines—this *chevaux de frise* is particularly well shown in Lashley's sketches and is coarser in the lower portions of the scotoma (Figure 3). There is a characteristic boiling movement or scintillation throughout the luminous portions of the scotoma: the effect is vividly conveyed in a nineteenth-century description—

> it may be likened to the effect produced by the rapid gyration of small water-beetles as they are seen swarming in a cluster on the surface of the water in sunshine . . .

The rate of scintillation is below the flicker-fusion-frequency, yet too fast to count; its frequency has been estimated, by indirect methods, as lying between 8 and 12 scintillations per second. The margin of the scintillating scotoma advances at a rather constant rate, and usually takes between 10 and 20 minutes to pass from the neighbourhood of the fixation-point to the edge of the visual field (Figure 3B).

Perhaps the most detailed figures and descriptions ever given of migraine scotomata are those of Airy (1868); these are reproduced in detail both by Liveing and Gowers, and may without apology be cited once again. The stages of Airy's scotomata are shown in Figure 2B.

> A bright stellate object, a small angled sphere, suddenly appears in one side of the combined field . . . it rapidly enlarges, first as a circular zigzag, but on the inner side, towards the medial line, the regular outline becomes faint, and, as the increase in size goes on, the outline here becomes broken, the gap becoming larger as the whole increases, and the original circular outline becomes oval. The form assumed is roughly concentric with the edge of the field of vision . . . the lines which constitute the outline meet at right angles or larger angles . . . When this angled oval has extended through the greater part of the half-field the upper portion expands; it seems to overcome at last some resistance in the immediate neighbourhood of the fixing point . . . so that a bulge occurs in the part above, and the angular elements of the outline here enlarge . . . After this final stage occurs, the outer lower part of the outline disappears. This final expansion near the centre progresses with great rapidity, and ends in a whirling centre of light from which sprays of light seem flying off. Then all is over, and the headache comes on.

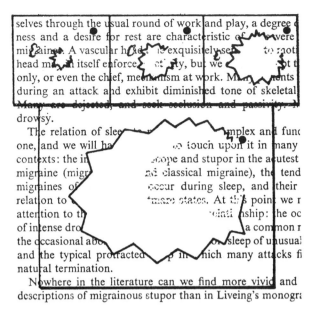

selves through the usual round of work and play, a degree
ness and a desire for rest are characteristic of ... were
migraine. A vascular head ... exquisitely se... to ...
head m... itself enforce ... ly, but we ... t
only, or even the chief, mechanism at work. M... ...nts
during an attack and exhibit diminished tone of skeletal
... ...
drowsy.

The relation of slee ... ...plex and fun...
one, and we will ha ... ...o touch upon it in many
contexts: the i... ...cope and stupor in the acutest
migraine (migr... ...d classical migraine), the tend
migraines of ... ...ccur during sleep, and their
relation to ... ...more states. At th... point we r
attention to t... ...nship: he oc
of intense dro... ...a common r
the occasional ab... ...r sleep of unusual
and the typical protracted ... ...p in which many attacks fi
natural termination.

Nowhere in the literature can we find more vivid and
descriptions of migrainous stupor than in Liveing's monogr...

Fig. 2C.   Variants of migraine scotoma. After Gowers (1904)
Expanding negative scotoma

Elsewhere Airy speaks of the rapid "boiling and trembling motion," and
the "bastioned" outline of the scotoma (he suggested the name "teichopsia"); he speaks of the "gorgeous chromatic edgings" to the figure, a
spectacle marred for him only by the anticipation of ensuing headache.

The margins of the luminous scotoma trail behind them a shadow-
crescent of total blindness, behind which is a penumbral region where
visual excitability is in process of restoration (Figures 2C and 3A). Airy
also makes reference (and the symptom is not an uncommon one) to the
occasional appearance of a second scintillating focus following within a
few minutes of the original scotoma, i.e., immediately upon the restitu-
tion of visual excitability near the fixation-point.

Such is the sequence in the commonest type of migraine scotoma (the
expanding angular spectrum of Gowers); there may occur, however,
many important variations on this theme, the existence of which must
be taken into account if any adequate theory of the scotoma is to be
derived. Not all scotomata commence near the fixation-point; a number
of patients consistently, and a few occasionally, experience scotomata
starting eccentrically or peripherally in the visual field (Gowers's radial

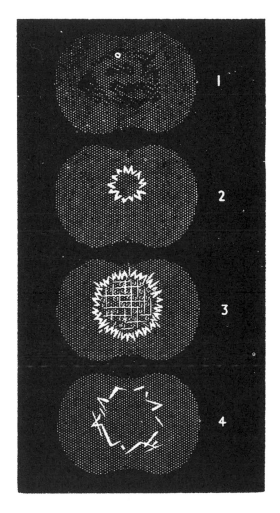

Fig. 2D.   Variants of migraine scotoma. Reproduced from Gowers (1904)
Pericentral spectrum

spectra). Expanding scotomata may appear alternately or simultaneously in both half-fields, and their continued alternation, in the former case, may give rise to an aura "status" lasting hours. Of great theoretical importance (and especial aesthetic appeal) are those bilateral scotomata whose evolution is exactly synchronised in both half-fields—the central and pericentral spectra of Gowers (Figure 2D). The existence of such scotomata poses very difficult problems to those who postulate a local,

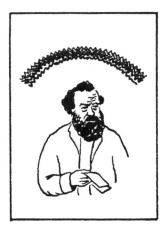

Fig. 2E. Variants of migraine scotoma. Reproduced from Gowers (1904)
Rainbow spectrum

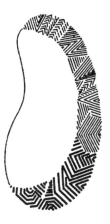

Fig. 3A. Course and structure of a scintillating scotoma. From Lashley
(1941). Fine structure of intersecting lines (*chevaux de frise*) at advancing
border of scintillating scotoma

unilateral process as the basis of migraine auras (see Chapters 10 and
11).[13] Luminous or negative scotomata may be not only central, but
quadrantic, altitudinal or irregular in their distribution. A particularly
pleasing pattern is that of a spectrum in the form of an arch, centrally
and bilaterally placed in the visual field (Figure 2E); Gowers considers

---

[13] Gowers, speaking of central negative scotomata, states: "Such a central loss, so perfectly symmetrical, seems inexplicable by an assumed disturbance of the function of one
hemisphere. It can only be explained . . . by a simultaneous functional inhibition (of both
hemispheres), perfectly symmetrical."

Course and
structure of a
scintillating
scotoma. From
Lashley (1941).
Enlargement and
evolution of
scotoma within
visual field
Fig. 3B.

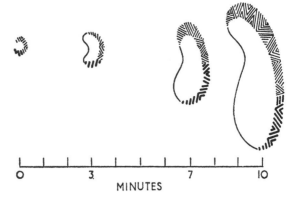

```
L_I_I_I_I_I_I_I_I_I_I_I_I
O        3        7       10
            MINUTES
```

Fig. 3B.   Course and structure of a scintillating scotoma. From Lashley
(1941). Enlargement and evolution of scotoma within visual field

these to be segments of a pericentral spectrum. Such a spectrum was
described by Aretaeus nearly two thousand years ago, and compared by
him to the appearance of a rainbow in the sky.

A *negative* scotoma generally follows a scintillating scotoma, but occasionally precedes it, and sometimes occurs in its stead. In the latter
event, as with all manifestations of cortical blindness, it may be discovered by accident, e.g. by suddenly observing the bisection of a face, or
the disappearance of certain words or figures on a page. It is important
to note, however, that observant patients consistently allude to a special
"dazzled" quality which appears to be an innate characteristic of negative scotomata. In the words of an old description cited by Liveing:

... "My sight suddenly becomes disordered, more on one side than the other,
like a person who has looked at the sun."

We cannot refrain from contrasting this "dazzled" quality with the
"blinding" brilliance of the scintillation if it occurs. The suspicion arises
that the extinction of vision and visual excitability may not, after all, be
a primary phenomenon, but a consequence of some preceding excitation
affecting the non-visual areas of the brain. This hypothesis will be explored later, and we may simply take note, at this stage, of descriptions
which *do* indicate some such antecedent excitation:

Case 67   A 32-year-old physician who has had classical migraines and isolated auras since childhood. The scotomata are always negative, but appear
to be preceded by a type of analeptic excitation. In the patient's words: "It
starts with a sort of excited feeling, as if I had taken an amphetamine. I know
that something is happening to me, and I start to look around. I wonder if

there is something the matter with the light. Then I notice that part of my visual field is missing."

Here we see that a negative scotoma can occur during and despite persistent analeptic excitement; other patients show the converse—scintillating scotomata associated with intense drowsiness. In such cases there is a *paradoxical concurrence of excitation and inhibition.*

TACTILE

Many of the observations which have been made with regard to the visual manifestations may be applied to the tactile hallucinations of migraine aura. There may be positive (paraesthetic) or negative (anaesthetic) hallucinations. The paraesthesiae have a characteristic thrilling or vibrato of the same frequency as the visual scintillations. Tactile hallucinations may coexist with scotomata, precede them, follow them, or occur in their absence, although they are appreciably less common than the visual manifestations. There is no constancy in this, even in repeated attacks in the same patient.

They most commonly announce their appearance in the most excitable and massively-represented portions of the tactile field—about the tongue and mouth, in the hand or hands, and less commonly in the feet—as the scotomata usually appear in relation to the macula or maculae of the visual field. Very occasionally they may start on the trunk, the thigh, or other portions of the tactile field.

Mild or fleeting paraesthesiae may remain at their point of origin; more commonly they spread centripetally, from the distal to the proximal portions of the limbs. It is entirely legitimate, therefore, to compare them to the Jacksonian march of an epileptic aura, if we remember two important differences. The centripetal passage of migraine paraesthesiae, like that of the scintillating scotomata, is far slower than the corresponding passage of epileptic paraesthesiae—a single "sweep" of the migraine aura occupies 20 to 30 minutes. Recurrent cycles of paraesthesiae may follow one another for hours on end, or alternate with cycles of scotomata, in a migraine "status." Secondly, in contradistinction to epileptic auras which start unilaterally in the vast majority of cases, the paraesthesiae of migraine aura start *bilaterally*, or become bilateral, in more than half of all cases. Bilaterality is particularly common with paraesthesiae of the lips and tongue. Indeed, one may go so far as saying that if a reliable witness insists that his or her aura symptoms have never departed from one or other side, the diagnosis of migraine must itself be regarded with some suspicion (*vide* Case 26, p. 107).

Migrainous paraesthesiae may spread in two ways, either by direct extension to contiguous portions of the body-surface (tactile field), or by the inauguration of new, separate foci elsewhere in the tactile field.

OTHER SENSORY HALLUCINATIONS

Hallucinations of the other special senses are uncommon in migraine aura, although I should judge them to be notably commoner than most accounts allow for. Auditory hallucinations generally take the form of hissing, growling, or rumbling noises, which may be succeeded or preceded by dullness or loss of hearing. Hallucinations of smell have been described to me by several patients: the smell is usually intense, unpleasing, strangely familiar yet unspecifiable, and often associated with forced reminiscence and feelings of *déjà vu*—symptoms reminiscent of those occurring in uncinate seizures. Hallucinations of taste are perhaps the least common of the special sense hallucinations.

A variety of visceral and epigastric symptoms may occur during migraine aura. The commonest, perhaps, is intense nausea of a quality which observant patients can distinguish from the subsequent nausea associated with headache, etc.

Other patients describe a variety of sensation in the epigastrium—one patient of mine had a sensation of "vibrating wires" in the pit of the stomach (see Case 19, p. 83)—sensations which may rise through the chest towards the throat, often accompanied by eructation or forced swallowing.

Hallucinations of motion may take two forms. Rarely, there may occur what Gowers has termed a "motor sensation," e.g. the feeling that a limb has moved, or the body has adopted a new posture, when in fact there has been no such movement. Far commoner, and perhaps the most intolerable of all aura symptoms, is intense sudden vertigo accompanied by staggering, overwhelming nausea, and frequently vomiting. The following description is taken from Liveing, and relates, yet again, to the unfortunate "Mr. A" who appeared subject to every conceivable symptom of migraine:

His megrim seizures usually commence with blindness, and giddiness is only exceptional and slight. On one or two occasions, however, he has suffered from short attacks of intense vertigo, which have appeared to him to replace the ordinary fit. On waking one morning, before moving or rising in bed, he was alarmed to see all objects in the room revolving with extraordinary velocity from right to left in vertical circles . . . an almost exclusively visual vertigo. Lying perfectly stiff with closed eyes, the attack passed off in about the same time as that occupied by the blind period of his ordinary seizures.

PSEUDO-OBJECTIVITY OF MIGRAINE HALLUCINATIONS

We have used the term "hallucination" to denote the sensory experiences which may occur during a migraine aura, and the use of this word—which carries pejorative implications to many ears—must be justified. The hallmarks of the hallucinatory experience are these: it is mistaken for reality, and it elicits a perceptual reaction, in Konorski's term a "targeting reflex" (Konorski, 1967, pp. 174 to 181). Thus dreams are true hallucinations because they are experienced as reality, and associated with targeting-reflexes of the eyes (the "rapid eye movements" of paradoxical sleep) as these scan the projected hallucinations. The abnormal sensations of a migraine aura, as opposed to those of dreams, are likely to be experienced in full waking consciousness (although they may also occur in twilight states, or in sleep), and most patients learn not to mistake them for reality. Nevertheless there exists, even in the most sophisticated patients, a *tendency* to objectivise the sensations of the aura. Patients with paraesthesiae may look down at the affected hand or rub it. Patient 67, a highly intelligent physician who had experienced many auras with negative scotomata, would invariably feel that the illumination in the room was at fault, before realising that she was experiencing a migraine aura. Many patients take off their spectacles and polish them carefully if they start to experience a migrainous shimmering. The sense of objectivity may be particularly striking where scintillating scotomata or olfactory hallucinations are experienced. Gowers (1904) remarks on the strength and stubbornness of this "involuntary sense of objectivity," and comments particularly on patients with pericentral scotomata who insist that they see a sort of angled crown or rainbow above the eyes (as drawn, by a patient, in Figure 2E, p. 62). Patient 75, a physician, who had had ample experience of the illusory nature of migraine auras, would always start searching for the cause of the smell when he experienced an olfactory aura. In the most severe auras, to be described below, the subjective sensations may completely overwhelm the patient and be experienced, like a dream, as total reality.

GENERAL ALTERATIONS OF SENSORY THRESHOLD

A *diffuse* enhancement or obfuscation of sensation may occur in addition to, or in place of, the specific sensory hallucinations we have described. Such changes have already been alluded to in the context of common migraine, but may reach an exalted intensity in migraine aura.

Some patients describe an overall brightening of vision. In the words of one of my patients, a man who had never experienced scintillating scotomata: "It was as if a thousand-watt bulb had been turned on in the room." Further evidence of such diffuse visual excitation is provided by the intense, protracted, sometimes almost dazzling, visual after-images which may occur at such times, and the furore of brilliant visual images which are seen if the eyes are closed. Analogous phenomena may occur with respect to hearing, the faintest sounds appearing overwhelmingly loud, and being followed by protracted echoing or reverberation for some seconds after they have ceased. The faintest touch, similarly, may be exaggerated and intolerable. This state is thus one of an excruciating overall sensitivity, patients being *assaulted* by sensory stimuli from their environment, or by internal images and hallucinations if they insulate themselves from their environment. Such states are often succeeded by a relative, and on occasion, absolute extinction of sensation, especially in severe auras where syncope occurs. Such a course is reminiscent of the much more acute sensory extinction which may occur in epilepsy, as in a case of Gowers: ". . . for a moment all was silent, then all was dark, then consciousness was lost" (*vide* Case 19, p. 83).

ALTERATIONS OF CONSCIOUSNESS AND POSTURAL TONE

It seems probable that all migraine auras commence with some degree of *arousal*, whether this is manifested as multiform positive hallucinations, or states of analeptic excitement (as in Case 67, p. 63 and Case 69, p. 85). Such states of arousal may be difficult to distinguish from hyperactive migrainous prodromes, and sometimes present themselves as the climax of such states.

As the positive are succeeded by the negative hallucinations, so a generalised arousal of consciousness and muscular tonus—the hyperalert, tense and vigilant phase—is succeeded by a waning of conscious level and tonus. In milder cases, this may be felt merely as a dullness and listlessness; in extreme cases there may be a total extinction of consciousness and/or an almost cataplectic loss of muscular tone.

Migrainous syncope is never of abrupt onset and offset, like a *petit mal* attack; the patient sinks into it over the course of a few minutes, and regains his faculties in the same gradual fashion. It is convenient to recognise three stages in this context: first a state of torpor and lethargy; secondly, a state of stupor in which the patient may suffer "forced" thought and imagery, generally with an unpleasing quality—Liveing speaks of "horrid trances" at this stage, in which vivid forced imagery is allied to akinesia (a state reminiscent of narcolepsy or "sleep paralysis"); thirdly, a state of coma, which is likely to be accompanied by incontinence, and, very occasionally, by seizure-activity.

It is difficult to assess the overall incidence of migraine syncope, for it may occur only once or twice in a lifetime in a given patient, and the fact of its occurrence may have been forgotten or suppressed. Thus Lees and Watkins report the following case under the label of "basilar migraine":

> A woman of 24 had had periodic attacks of bilateral visual disturbance, and numbness of the lips, tongue, and one arm, followed by frontal headache and faintness . . . *Once*, at the height of the attack, she became unconscious, and was incontinent of urine and faeces.

I myself have seen more than a hundred patients with migraine aura or classical migraine, and of these only four suffered syncopes with any regularity.

The incidence of *occasional* migraine syncopes may be very much higher. Thus, Selby and Lance found that "sixty patients (out of 396) had lost consciousness in association with attacks of headache," and that in 18 of these 60 the impairment of consciousness was profound, and accompanied by features suggestive of an epileptic seizure.

SPECIFIC MOTOR DISORDERS

". . . Features suggestive of an epileptic seizure": these features, in the minds of most patients, are unconsciousness and convulsions. We have discussed the incidence and quality of impaired or lost consciousness, as this occurs during migraine attacks, and we must now enquire whether true convulsions or spasms of epileptoid type may not also occur as a component of migraines. It is not denied that such motor symptoms, if their existence be accepted, are rare, far rarer than their epileptic counterparts; what we must question is the assertion, frequently and dogmatically made, that the higher disorders of migraine are exclusively sensory.

Accounts of muscular *spasms* may be found in many of the classical writings on the subject, particularly those of Tissot, Liveing, and Gowers:

> A young girl of 12 years became suddenly ill with a violent migraine that occupied her eye, the temple and ear of the left side of the head; at the same time she had a tingling sensation as if of swarms of ants that began with the little finger on the same side, soon reaching the other fingers, the forearm, the arm, the neck, causing a violent retraction of the head by spasmodic movements. The spasm involved her lower jaw, accompanied by a general weakness of her entire body, without, however, losing consciousness. This cruel access was terminated by vomiting bilious water. (Tissot, 1790)

> In one patient each attack of headache was preceded by sudden tingling in the calf, followed by painful cramp in the calf muscles, lasting a few minutes only. The same patient, however, had at other times attacks in which her face suddenly became crimson, sharp pains occurred in the head, and seemed to pass down the side to the leg, which was then "drawn up" in spasm for a few minutes. (Gowers, 1892)

If such spasms occur, Gowers remarks, "the case usually diverges very much from the type, and sometimes is of such a character as to render it doubtful whether it should be classed with migraine or not."

A transient motor weakness in a limb (as opposed to the protracted hemiplegias which are discussed in the following chapter) is not uncommon, and may follow the passage of paraesthesiae. In some such cases the apparent weakness resolves itself, on questioning or examining the patient, into an apractic rather than a paralytic deficit, but in other patients, of whom I have seen and examined a number during this stage of an aura, the limb may be toneless, areflexic and truly paralysed.

I have never witnessed a convulsion during a migraine aura, although I have been told by three patients (out of a total of 150 patients with classical migraine or isolated auras) that others had witnessed such convulsions during their attacks. The existence of such convulsions at the height of a migraine aura has been repeatedly attested by competent observers. Such accounts, indeed, may be traced into antiquity, the archetype of such attacks having been described by Aretaeus in the second century, a man in whom the appearance of a migraine spectrum was followed by loss of consciousness and convulsions.

How should we categorize such attacks? As atypical migraines with migrainous convulsions, as atypical epilepsies with migranoid features, or as attacks of epilepsy superimposed on migraines? Lennox neatly evades the dilemma by speaking of "hybrid seizures," and until we know more this is as good a term as any.

I have seen, on occasion, the onset of complex motor excitements in migraine aura, with the appearance of chorea, and sometimes tics as well, set against a background of extreme motor restlessness, irritability, and drive (akathisia).

Chorea—a twinkling movement or motor scintillation—does not have its origin in the cerebral cortex, but in the deeper parts of the brain, the basal ganglia and upper brainstem, which are the parts that mediate normal awakening. Thus these observations of chorea during migraine support the notion that migraine is a form of arousal disorder, something located in the strange borderlands of sleep—a disorder which has its origin deep in the brainstem, and not superficially, in the cortical mantle, as is often supposed (a matter further discussed in Part III of this book).

ALTERATIONS OF AFFECT AND MOOD

We have described the profound mood-disturbances which may precede and accompany successive stages of a common migraine or migraine equivalent. We must now consider symptoms altogether more acute, more dramatic, and different in quality from such mood-changes, notably the sudden eruptions of overwhelming "forced" affect which may occur in the course of severe migraine auras.

Like migrainous syncope, this is a relatively uncommon symptom, and rarely occurs with consistency in every attack the patient experiences; nevertheless most patients with severe frequent auras have occasionally experienced such sudden eruptions of affect. Thus one patient (Case 11), whose history is later detailed, who had had attacks of classical migraine or isolated aura since childhood which inconvenienced but rarely discomposed her, experienced on one occasion "a perfectly frightful sense of foreboding" during the course of an aura. She herself recognised that this was an exceptional feature of some of her attacks, and in no sense a mere anxious expectation of a banal sequence with which she was entirely familiar, and to which she was wholly inured.

Such states of sudden overwhelming affect have been richly documented in the earlier literature, especially by Liveing (with respect to migraine attacks) and by Gowers (in epilepsy). Thus Liveing observed that there were sufferers "who cannot bear to think or talk of their attacks, and always refer to them with horror, which is clearly not on account of the pain they occasion." Gowers observed in connection with epilepsy that the emotional aura usually took the form of *fear* ("vague alarm or intense terror"), although he provides case-histories of other types of affect being experienced. The most acute form of such fear may reach appalling intensity, and convey to the patient a sense of imminent destruction or death. This sense of mortal fear (which may also occur in association with attacks of angina, pulmonary embolism, etc.) was called by the older physicians "angor animi," a term which cannot be bettered. The affective reaction is not always in this direction. A few patients may experience a sense of mild *pleasure* or delight in the course of their auras (see Case 16, p. 84), and on rare occasions this may be exalted towards states of profound *awe* or *rapture* (see Appendix to this chapter). Again the affect, though intense, may lack the gravity of dread or rapture, and convey only a sense of fun or *hilarity* to the patient, or "silliness" to an observer (see Case 65, p. 84): Selby and Lance refer, rather curtly, to "apparently hysterical behaviour" in such cases.

Gowers records, in one epileptic patient, an access of pure moral feeling ("whatever was taking place before the patient would suddenly appear to be *wrong*—i.e. morally wrong") immediately prior to loss of consciousness and convulsion. A complex feeling which may also present itself with great force and suddenness, in these auras, is a feeling of *absurdity*. One of the commonest of these abrupt feeling-states (it cannot be called purely affective) is the sense of sudden *strangeness*, which may occur as an isolated feeling, or as an accompaniment of some of the affective states we have discussed: the sense of strangeness is frequently accompanied by a sense of profoundly-disturbed time-perception.

In summary, we may recognise the following features as characteristic of these affective states in migraine auras:

(a)   Their sudden onset.

(b)   Their apparent sourcelessness, and frequent incongruity with the foreground contents of consciousness.

(c)   Their overwhelming quality.

(d)   A sense of passivity, and of the affect being "forced" into the mind.

(e)   Their brief duration (they rarely last more than a few minutes).

(f)   The sense of stillness and timelessness they convey: such states
       may wax in depth or intensity, but this occurs despite the ab-
       sence of any experiential "happening."

(g)   Their difficulty or impossibility of adequate description.

Such states of overwhelming "forced" feeling may occur not only in
cerebral paroxysms as migraine and epilepsy, but in schizophrenic and
drug-induced psychoses, in feverish and toxic states, in hysterical, ecstatic and dream-states. We are inevitably reminded of William James's
listing of the qualities of "mystical" states: ineffability, noetic quality,
transiency, passivity.

ALTERATIONS OF HIGHEST INTEGRATIVE FUNCTION

It has been held by a number of eminent clinical observers that the cerebral disorders of migraine occur only at primitive levels, and that the
existence of subtler disorders, should they occur, is indicative of epilepsy
or of some organic pathology. This view is erroneous. An immense number of complex cerebral symptoms may occur in the context of indisputable migraines, symptoms fully as numerous and diverse as their epileptic
counterparts.

One might, indeed, suspect that alterations of higher cerebral function
occur in the majority of migraine auras, but may escape notice through
their subtlety or strangeness, or because the patient was not undertaking
any intricate intellectual or motor activity at the time of the aura. Thus,
Alvarez, a careful witness of his own migraines, has described how he
became aware, one day, that his auras were not merely "pure," isolated
visual phenomena:

> Often, when fuzzy-eyed and unable to read comfortably, I have employed my
> time writing a family letter, longhand. Later, on checking the letter, I had
> written words other than the ones I had thought I was writing.

It is easily understood how a subtle dyslexic or dysphasic deficit of
this type may fail to be noticed by a majority of patients. Leading questions will often be required to elicit the exact nature of such symptoms.
Many patients may confess that they feel "strange" or "confused" during
a migraine aura, that they are clumsy in their movements, or that they
would not drive at such a time. In short, they may be aware of *something*
the matter in addition to the scintillating scotoma, paraesthesiae, etc.,

something so unprecedented in their experience, so difficult to describe, that it is often avoided or omitted when speaking of their complaints. Great patience and minute exactitude are needed to define the subtler symptoms of migraine aura, and only if these are employed will the frequency and importance of such symptoms be realised.

It may be stated that the more complex disorders of cerebral function usually occur *after* the simpler phenomena (although this is not invariably so), and it may be possible to obtain descriptions of elaborate sequences: thus the simplest visual manifestations—dots, lines, stars, etc. —may be succeeded by a scintillating scotoma, and this in turn by bizarre alterations of perception (zoom vision, mosaic vision, etc.), finally culminating in elaborate illusory images or dream-like states. We may recognise the following important categories of disturbance:

(a)   Complex disorders of visual perception (conveniently described as Lilliputian, Brobdignagian, zoom, mosaic, cinematographic vision, etc.).

(b)   Complex difficulties in the perception and use of the body (apraxic and agnosic symptoms).

(c)   The entire gamut of speech and language disorders.

(d)   States of double or multiple consciousness, often associated with feelings of *déjà vu* or *jamais vu*, and other disorders and dislocations of time-perception.

(e)   Elaborate dreamy, nightmarish, trance-like or delirious states.

These categories are isolated for convenience only, and, far from being mutually exclusive, they overlap at many levels; many or all of these disorders may occur simultaneously in the course of a severe migraine aura. We may first describe some of these symptoms in greater detail, and then proceed to the presentation of illustrative case-histories.

Lilliputian vision (micropsia) denotes an apparent diminution, and *Brobdignagian vision* (macropsia) an apparent enlargement, in the size of objects, although the terms may also be used to denote the apparent approach or recession of the visual world—these representing alternative descriptions or hallucinations or disordered size : distance constancy. If such changes occur gradually rather than abruptly, the patient will experience *zoom vision*—an opening-out, or closing-down, in the size of objects as if observing them through the changing focal lengths of a

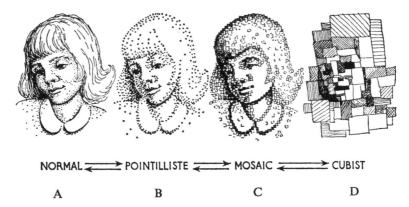

Fig. 4.   The stages of "mosaic" vision, as experienced during migraine
aura (see text)

"zoom" lens. The most famous descriptions of such perceptual changes
have, of course, been provided by Lewis Carroll, who was himself subject
to dramatic classical migraines of this type. A scintillating scotoma itself
has no external location, and may therefore be projected as an "artefact"
of any size, at any distance (see Case 69, p. 85, and Figure 2E, p. 62).

MOSAIC AND CINEMATIC VISION

The term *mosaic vision* denotes the fracture of the visual image into
irregular, crystalline, polygonal facets, dovetailed together as in a mosaic. The size of the facets may vary greatly. If they are extremely fine,
the visual world presents an appearance of crystalline iridescence or
"graininess," reminiscent of a pointillist painting (shown schematically
in Figure 4B). If the facets become larger, the visual image takes on the
appearance of a classical mosaic (Figure 4C), or even a "cubist" appearance (see Plate 6). If they compete in size with the total visual image, the
latter becomes impossible of recognition (Figure 4D), and a peculiar
form of visual agnosia is experienced.

The term *cinematographic vision* denotes the nature of visual experience when the illusion of motion has been lost. At such times, the patient
sees only a rapidly-flickering series of "stills," as in a film run too slowly.
The rate of flickering is of the same order as the scintillation-rate of
migrainous scotomata or paraesthesiae (6 to 12 per second), but may
accelerate during the course of the aura to restore the appearance of

normal motion, or (in a particularly severe, delirious aura) the appearance of a continuously-modulated visual hallucination.[14]

Both of these rare symptoms have been recorded as occurring in the course of epileptic seizures, and, more commonly, during acute psychoses, whether drug-induced or schizophrenic. The famous cat-painter Louis Wain experienced a variety of visual misperceptions during phases of acute schizophrenic psychosis, including mosaic vision, and was able to provide remarkable records of the experiences (Figure 5).

The phenomena of "mosaic" and "cinematic" vision are of extreme importance. They show us how the brain-mind constructs "space" and "time," by demonstrating to us what happens when space and time are broken, or *unmade*.

In a scotoma, as we have observed, the idea of space itself is extinguished along with the extinction of the visual field, and we are left with "no trace, space, or place." In mosaic and cinematic vision we seem to be presented with an intermediary state which has an inorganic, crystalline character, but no organic personal character, no "life."

This too, like scotomata may inspire a strange horror.[15]

OTHER DISTURBANCES

Many other forms of visual misperception have been described in migraine auras. Objects may appear to have unnaturally sharp contours, to be diagrammatic, to be flattened and without a third dimension, to be set in an exaggerated perspective, etc.[16] Occasionally a patient may

[14] An extremely detailed personal account of mosaic and cinematic vision, as experienced in a severe attack of migraine, is given in my book *A Leg to Stand On*, pp. 95–101.

[15] A recent exhibit entitled "Mosaic Vision"—paintings by migraine sufferers of their own visual experiences in attacks—indicates that mosaic vision, to some degree at least, is not uncommon during severe migraine auras. At first, these paintings would seem to indicate, there may be an appearance like a polygonal latticework over part or all of the visual field, and then the image itself becomes "polygonized." The breakage of time and space in these very gross disturbances of perception seems to go with the emergence of fractional dimensions, or fractality, in the perceptual/cortical field. (See Chapter 17, Migraine Aura and Hallucinatory Constants.)

[16] A particularly detailed description of complex visual hallucinations in migraine has been provided by Klee (1968); unfortunately this was not available to me until after the completion of my own work. Klee describes many forms of *metamorphopsia* occurring during migraine auras: distortion of contours, monocular diplopias, reduced discrimination of contrast (leading, on occasion, to effective blindness), waviness of linear components in visual images and formation of concentric haloes (compare Figure 5B), etc. He also records examples of colour changes in visual images, and eccentric misplacements within the visual field other than micropsia and macropsia. Classical scotomata, positive and negative, are relatively infrequent in Klee's series. Both simple and complex visual hallucinations, Klee observes, are much more commonly diffuse than unilateral in their

suffer from *simultagnosia*—an inability to recognise more than one object at a time, and thus to construct a complex visual picture.[17]

Analogous phenomena may occur with reference to body-image and body-movements. Sometimes (especially after the passage of intense paraesthesiae in a limb) a portion of the body may feel magnified, diminished, distorted, or absent. It may be impossible to examine or perceive adequately the nature of an object held in the hand (one cannot clearly distinguish the sensory from the motor components in such cases, for sensation is always active and exploratory: one should perhaps speak of *apractagnosia* in this context). Higher sensory and motor deficits of this type are often mistaken for elementary anaesthesias and paralyses. One must consider separately difficulties in planning complex sensory-motor tasks; Pribram has called these *scotomata of action*. These are of great practical importance, and may underlie, for example, the patient's discovery that he cannot drive a car or organise a long sentence or a complex sequence of actions, during the course of a migraine aura.

Speech difficulties of this type have been termed (by Luria) dynamic aphasias. Other types of aphasia may also occur in the course of a migraine aura. The commonest of these is the occurrence of an expressive aphasia, which may be associated with bilateral paraesthesiae of the lips and tongue, and apractic difficulties using the oral and vocal muscles. Occurring sometimes in the wake of auditory misperception or halluci-

---

distribution; this finding is in accordance with my own experience, though at odds with most other published accounts.

[17] I have recently seen a patient who gives an extremely clear description of such a visual agnosia following a scintillating scotoma. In this state he finds it very difficult, for example, to tell the time from looking at his watch. He must first gaze at one hand, then at the other, then at all the figures in turn, and in this way, very slowly and laboriously, he will "puzzle out" the time. If he just glances at the watch-face, as he would normally do, it appears absolutely unintelligible to him. In effect the watch has lost its physiognomy, its "face." It can no longer be perceived as an organic whole, synthetically, but has to be broken down, analyzed, feature by feature, part by part. Such a loss of qualititative or "synthetic" perception may occur rather commonly, and disconcertingly, in migraine.

A particularly striking and disconcerting form of this disorder is the sudden inability to recognize a *face*, to see it as familiar, as a whole, indeed *as* a face. This singular (and frightening and sometimes comic) disorder is termed *prosopagnosia*. (I describe this in detail in the title story of *The Man Who Mistook His Wife for a Hat*.) Similar breakdowns in synthetic perception may also occur in the sphere of audition. Voices may seem to lose their characteristic quality, become inexpressive and toneless, completely unvoicelike. Music similarly may apparently lose its tonality and musical character, becoming an unintelligible mere noise, during a migrainous *amusia*. At such time, the very *idea* of music is lost, as in prosopagnosia the very idea of faces is lost; and in our patient bewildered before his watch, the very idea of a time-telling watchface.

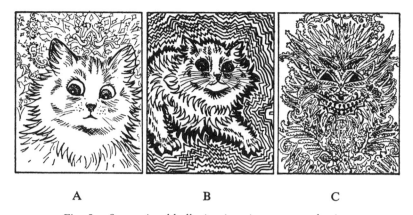

A   B   C

Fig. 5. Some visual hallucinations in acute psychosis
These drawings of cats, depicted by a schizophrenic artist (Louis Wain) during a very acute psychosis, formalise certain perceptual alterations which may also occur during migraine aura. In Figure 5A, the face is set upon a background of swarming brilliant star-like figures: in Figure 5B, concentric shimmering waves expand from the point of fixation: in Figure 5C, the entire image has been transformed to a mosaic pattern.

nation, there may occur a sensory aphasia, in which speech sounds like "noisc," and the perception of its phonemic structure is lost.[18]

Among the strangest and most intense symptoms of migraine aura, and the most difficult of description or analysis, are the occurrence of feelings of sudden familiarity and certitude (*déjà vu*), or its opposite, feelings of sudden strangeness and unfamiliarity (*jamais vu*). Such states are experienced, momentarily and occasionally, by everyone; their occurrence in migraine auras (as in epileptic auras, psychoses, etc.) is marked by their overwhelming intensity and relatively long duration. These states are sometimes associated with a multitude of other feelings: the thought that time has stopped, or is mysteriously recapitulating itself;

[18] We are describing certain sensory, motor, and conceptual symptoms of migraine aura in their severest forms, in order to clarify the type of cerebral disturbance which is involved. Frequently, however, such symptoms may present themselves as no more than a very mild disturbance, in particular as a tendency towards *mistakes* of various kinds: mishearing, mislaying, misreading words, slips of the tongue, slight lapses of memory, etc. Freud, himself a sufferer from classical migraines, comments on such errors: "Slips of the tongue do indeed occur most frequently when one is tired, or has a headache, or feels an attack of migraine coming on. Forgetting proper names very often occurs in these circumstances; many people are habitually warned of the onset of an attack of migraine by the inability to recall proper names" (Freud, 1920). Freud, indeed, was not only a sufferer from migraine, but was fascinated by its exemplary status as a psychophysical and biological reaction. In March of 1895 he summarized many of his ideas on its nature and causation, and sent a copy of these to Fliess; one can only regret that he never went on to publish on the subject.

the feeling that one is dreaming, or momentarily transported to another world; feelings of intense nostalgia, in *déjà vu*, sometimes associated with an uprush of long-forgotten memories; feelings of clairvoyance, in *déjà vu*; or of the world or oneself being newly-minted, in *jamais vu*; and in all cases, the feeling that consciousness has been doubled.

> There is (1) the quasi-parasitical state of consciousness (dreamy state), and (2) there are remains of normal consciousness and thus, there is double consciousness . . . a mental diplopia.

Thus Hughlings Jackson describes the doubling of consciousness.[19] No description is ever adequate for the elaborate yet unmistakable sensations of *déjà vu* and all that goes with it, and the most vivid descriptions are found outside medical literature:

> We have all some experience of a feeling which comes over us occasionally, of what we are saying and doing, having been said or done before, in a remote time—of our having been surrounded, dim ages ago, by the same faces, objects, and circumstances—of our knowing perfectly what will be said next, as if we suddenly remembered it. (Dickens: *David Copperfield*)

> Moreover, something is or seems
> That touches me with mystic gleams,
> Like glimpses of forgotten dreams—
>
> Of something felt, like something here;
> Of something done, I know not where;
> Such as no language may declare.
>   Tennyson: *The Two Voices*

> One of the wonders of opium is to transform instantaneously an unknown room into a room so familiar, so full of memories, that one thinks one has always occupied it. (Cocteau: *Opium*[20])

---

[19] A variety of psychological and physiological theories have been advanced to explain *déjà vu* and the symptoms with which it is commonly linked. Thus Freud ascribes the uncanniness of the experience to a sudden return of repressed material, while Efron sees *déjà vu*, aphasia, and subjective time-distortions—when linked together—as representing an alteration of "time-labelling" in the nervous system. These two theories are in different dimensions of explanation, and are perfectly compatible with one another.

[20] A number of people, learning that forced reminiscence and *déjà vu* experiences are particularly common in epilepsy, migraine, psychosis, etc., become alarmed for their own health or sanity. They may be reassured in the words of Hughlings Jackson: "I should never . . . [he writes] diagnose epilepsy from the paroxysmal occurrence of 'reminiscence' without other symptoms, although I should suspect epilepsy, if that super-positive mental state began to occur very frequently . . . I have never been consulted for 'reminiscence' only; there have always been in the cases I have seen, at the time I have seen them, with this and

The terms "dreamy state" and "delirium" require some clarification in the context of migraine auras. One type of dreamy state is that associated with *déjà vu* and doubling of consciousness; in such cases there may be "forced reminiscence," or the unfolding of a stereotyped, unchanging, reiterative dream-sequence or memory-sequence in every attack. Such sequences are perhaps commoner in (psychomotor) epilepsy than in migraine, but they undoubtedly occur in the latter. Penfield and Perot (1963), who have investigated these phenomena in remarkable detail, and have succeeded in eliciting such reiterative sequences by the stimulation of certain cortical points, regard them as "fossilised" dream-sequences preserved as such in the cortex, precise replicas of past experience; they appear to be mnemic images which unfold, given the initial activation (epileptic, migrainous, experimental, etc.) at the same rate as the initial perceptual experience.

Different from these stereotyped, reiterative sequences, but with something of the same coercive quality, are free-wheeling states of hallucinosis, illusion or "dreaming" which may be experienced during intense migraine auras, and be manifest as confused or confabulatory states of which the patient retains imperfect recollection. These states are composed of coherent, dramatically-organised series of images, and arc usually compared by patients to intense, involuntary daydreams or daymares (see Cases 72 and 19, p. 83).

It is impossible to make a clear dividing line between these "dreamy states" and migrainous deliria or psychoses. The degree of disorganisation in a delirium is greater, and the patient may experience only an effervescence of elementary sensations (dots, stars, lattices, tessellated forms,[21]

---

other forms of 'dreamy state,' ordinary, although often very slight, symptoms of epilepsy." Such states of dreamy reminiscence are quite frequent in classical migraines. The most detailed accounts of them have been given to me, however, in the context of epilepsy (see "Reminiscence," in *The Man Who Mistook His Wife for a Hat*).

[21] A vivid account of tessellated hallucinations is provided in Klee's monograph, one of his patients experiencing, on one occasion, a vision of red and green triangles moving towards her, on other occasions hexagonal black figures surrounding a shining circle, and on many occasions a shimmering of red and yellow, which looked like a waving, checked blanket.

In a fascinating article based partly on his own experiences ("The Fortification Illusions of Migraine," 1971), Dr. W. Richards describes repeating hexagonal motifs as a highly characteristic feature of migraine hallucinations and speculates that this reflects the functional organisation of the visual cortex in hexagonal units. Repeating geometrical and especially hexagonal patterns have been reported in almost all forms of primitive visual hallucinations, and are regarded by Kluver as "hallucinatory constants." (See Chapter 17, Migraine Aura and Hallucinatory Constants.)

tinnitus, buzzing, formication, etc.), which have not been elaborated to
the level of concrete images. In profound migraine deliria, the patient
presents a muttering, restless (twitching or tossing) picture strongly reminiscent of a febrile delirium or delirium tremens. Gowers (1907) observes
that migraine is ". . . often attended by quiet delirium of which nothing can
be subsequently recalled," and describes one such patient who at the height
of her attack ". . . passed into a delirious state, making strange statements,
of which she afterwards remembered nothing. Her condition was described by a doctor who saw her as resembling epileptic mania."[22]

The swarming figments of delirium are occasionally organised into a
multitude of minute (Lilliputian) hallucinations, as in the following case-
history provided by Klee (1968):

> The patient . . . was a 38-year-old man who suffered from attacks of severe
> migraine associated with sub-acute delirious state and delirium. As a rule he
> had amnesia for the greater part of the time during which the attacks lasted.
> During his admission he was, however, able to report that during his attacks
> he had on one occasion seen 20 cm. high, greyish-coloured Red Indians
> crowding round in the room in which he lay. He was not afraid of them, as
> they did not seem to have anything to do with him. On another occasion he
> lay and picked up hallucinatory musical instruments from the floor.[23]

Very rarely, the profound delirium of a migraine aura may last
throughout the ensuing (classical) migraine, and in such cases—as with

[22] Some clarification of this complex twilight zone in which "delirium," "mania,"
"dreamy states," and "confusion" have been reported is perhaps afforded by the very
recent recognition that so-called transient global amnesia (TGA) may occur with significant frequency in classical migraine attacks. Indeed it has been suggested that this spectacular syndrome—in which the patient may not only lose all short-term memory but may
develop a profound retrograde amnesia—may be chiefly or exclusively migrainous in nature. In such an amnesia the patient may not only lose the ability to recognise family,
friends, people, and place from the present, but may after recovery have no recollection of
headache, nausea, scotomata, etc., of which they complained when in the throes of the
attack (Crowell 1984). I have written at length about the almost incredible effects of
profound retrograde amnesia in "The Lost Mariner," in *The Man Who Mistook His Wife
for a Hat*, and in "The Last Hippie," an essay in the *New York Review of Books*.
[23] Lilliputian hallucinations are notoriously associated with alcoholic deliria, and, less
commonly, with intoxication by ether, cocaine, hashish, or opium—Theophile Gautier
has provided delightful descriptions of such hallucinatory, drug-induced elves. Myriads of
minute hallucinations may occur in the excitements of general paresis (Baudelaire). Sufferers from feverish deliria may experience Lilliputian hallucinations, as described by de
Musset. Fasting, inanition, and infected flagellations may have played a part in causing the
minute hallucinations of certain mystics (e.g. Joan of Arc). Leroy (1922), reviewing the
subject, observes that whereas "ordinary toxic visions may produce a feeling of fear and
terror, Lilliputian visions are accompanied, on the contrary, by a feeling of curiosity and
amusement." Cardan used to have almost daily attacks, or conjurings up, of Lilliputian
hallucinations. (See Appendix II: Cardan's Visions.)

all extended deliria—may be structured into the form of an acute hallucinatory psychosis. Mingazzini (1926) provided classical descriptions of such states ("hemikranischen Psykosen"), and a particularly vivid case-history has recently been provided by Klee (1968):

> . . . During a particularly severe attack which lasted for a week, the patient became psychotic and it was necessary to admit her to a mental hospital. The patient has amnesia for the episode . . . It appears that during the day preceding her admission she had been increasingly restless with clouding of consciousness, she had heard her neighbours making unpleasant comments about her, and also she believed that she had been stuck with knives. During the first days of her admission she was disoriented, restless, and presumably hallucinated in both hearing and sight: she heard children's voices and the voice of her general practitioner, she believed that her legs had been amputated, and that people were shooting at her through the window. This psychotic episode disappeared within a few days . . .

It must be emphasised that a migrainous psychosis of this magnitude is exceedingly rarely seen: Klee, in his unique series of 150 patients with migraine severe enough to warrant hospital admission, observed recurrent migraine psychoses in only two of these. I have seen only a single such case myself, in a patient who was schizophrenic: his acute psychoses, however, occurred only in the context of intense classical migraines.

Transient states of *depersonalisation* are appreciably commoner during migraine auras. Freud reminds us that ". . . the ego is first and foremost a body-ego . . . the mental projection of the surface of the body." The sense of "self" appears to be based, fundamentally, on a continuous inference from the stability of body-image, the stability of outward perceptions, and the stability of time-perception. Feelings of ego-dissolution readily and promptly occur if there is serious disorder or instability of body-image, external perception, or time-perception, and all of these, as we have seen, may occur during the course of a migraine aura.

CASE HISTORIES

The following three case-histories are taken from Liveing's monograph, and are presented *in extenso* in view of their clarity and graphic power.

> *Forced reminiscence, time-distortion, and doubled consciousness*
> . . . As the visual phenomena passed off, he experienced a singular disorder of ideation; circumstances and events which had occurred long before were

brought back to him as if actually present; his consciousness appeared to be doubled, and the past and the present confounded.

Forced thinking, confusion, and multiple dysphasic symptoms
. . . For about half an hour, one series of ideas forced themselves involuntarily on my mind. I could not free myself from the strange ideas which existed in my head. I endeavoured to speak . . . but found that I spoke uniformly other words than those intended . . . It became necessary that I should write a receipt for some money that I had received on account of the poor. I seated myself and wrote the first two words, but in a moment found that I was incapable of proceeding, for I could not recollect the words which belonged to the ideas which were present in my mind . . . I tried to write one letter slowly after the others . . . but remarked that the characters I was writing were not those which I wished to write . . . For about half an hour there reigned a kind of tumultuary disorder in my senses . . . I endeavoured, as much as lay in my power, considering the great crowd of confused images which presented themselves to my mind, to recall my principles of religion, of conscience, of future expectation . . . Thank God, this state did not continue very long, for in about half an hour my head began to grow clearer, the strange and tiresome ideas became less vivid and turbulent . . . At last, I found myself as clear and serene as in the beginning of the day. *All that remained now was a slight headache.*

When migraine auras reach their ultimate intensity, the "great crowd of confused images," of which the above patient speaks, assume hallucinatory form, and blot out the world around him. Jones has reminded us that "attacks in every way indistinguishable from the classical nightmare may not only occur but may run their whole course during the waking state," and such "daymares"—as they have been called—in their quality (feelings of dread, horror, paralysis) and duration (a few minutes) bear a remarkable similarity to delirious migraine auras. This clinical affinity does not, of course, imply that similar physiological mechanisms are necessarily involved.

Delirious migraine aura
He had been somewhat overworked at school, and on returning home early one day, was suddenly seized with what he called a "day nightmare." He lost all conscious perception of the room and objects about him, and he felt himself hanging on the brink of a precipice, and other horrors which he could not remember or describe. His relatives were alarmed by hearing him cry out, and found him on the stairs in a kind of somnambulistic state, vociferating loudly. He recovered himself in about 10 minutes, but remained a good deal shaken and distressed . . . The second attack was of much the same kind, but occurred shortly after going to bed at night . . . It was shortly after these attacks . . . that his megrim became fully established.

I shall pass now to a number of illustrative case-histories taken from my own records.

Case 72   *Dreamy state*

This 44-year-old man had suffered from very occasional classical migraines since adolescence. His attacks would be ushered in by scintillating scotomata. In one attack, a profound dream-like state followed the visual phenomena. He has described this as follows:

A very strange thing happened, shortly after my vision came back. First I couldn't think where I was, and then I suddenly realised that I was back in California . . . It was a hot summer day. I saw my wife moving about on the verandah, and I called her to bring me a Coke. She turned to me with an odd look on her face, and said: "Are you sick or something?" I suddenly seemed to wake up, and realised that it was a winter's day in New York, that there was no verandah, and that it wasn't my wife but my secretary who was standing in the office looking strangely at me.

Case 19   *Scotomata, paraesthesiae, visceral aura and forced affect: Occasional delirious auras: Occasional aura "status"*

This patient was a young man of 16 who had been prone to classical migraines and isolated auras since childhood. He has attacks with many different formats.

Most commonly they start with paraesthesiae in the left foot, rising towards the thigh. When these have reached the knee, a second focus of paraesthesiae starts in the right hand. As the paraesthesiae die away, there occurs a curious distortion of hearing, in which there appears to be a roaring sound in the ears, as if they were cupped by shells. Following this, he tends to get bilateral scintillating scotomata confined to the lower halves of both visual fields . . .

On a few occasions, this patient has suffered from an aura "status" lasting as much as five hours, constituted of alternating paraesthesiae in the feet, hands, and face.

On other occasions, the aura has started with a sensation of "tingling—like vibrating wires" in the epigastrium, associated with an intense sense of foreboding.

Yet other attacks, usually nocturnal, have a nightmarish quality. The initial symptoms are of compulsion and restlessness—"I feel edgy—like I got to get up and do something." Subsequently there develops a profound hallucinatory state: vertiginous hallucinations, hallucinations of being trapped in a speeding car, or of seeing heavy figures made of metal advancing upon him. As he emerges from this delirious state, he becomes conscious of paraesthesiae and sometimes scotomata. These delirious auras are usually succeeded by intense headache.

This patient has also suffered a number of syncopal attacks in severe auras, in which the positive hallucinations have been followed by a simultaneous

"fading" away of sight and hearing, a sense of faintness, and then unconsciousness.

Case 11   Classical migraine: Loss of headache component in pregnancy: Scintillating scotomata and Negative scotomata; Photogenic attacks: Occasional "angor animi"

This patient was an extremely self-possessed and intelligent woman who had
suffered from attacks of classical migraine, 6 to 10 attacks yearly, except
during pregnancy—when she had only isolated auras, and occasional periods
of up to two years, when she had abdominal instead of cephalgic migraines.

The attacks were almost always ushered in by scintillating scotomata in
either or both half-fields. The period of scintillation was found to be associated, if the patient closed her eyes, by exaggerated visual after-images and
tumultuous visual imagery. Flickering light of certain frequencies would invariably elicit a scintillating scotoma. The visual aura would be followed by
a "thrilling" sensation in the nose and tongue, and occasionally the hands.
On a few occasions this patient experienced a "perfectly frightful sense of
foreboding" during the aura. Negative scotomata were rare, always invested
with intensely unpleasant affect, and invariably followed by a particularly
severe headache.

Case 16   Visual aura: Forced thinking and reminiscence: Pleasurable affect: Protracted sensory prodrome

A 55-year-old man with onset of classical migraine and isolated auras in
childhood. He describes his auras with a certain fervour. "There is greater
depth and speed and acuity of thought," he maintains. "I keep recalling things
long forgotten, visions of earlier years will spring to my mind." He enjoys his
auras, provided they are not succeeded by a migraine headache. His wife,
however, is less impressed with them; she remarks that during his auras her
husband "walks back and forth, talks in a repetitive manner in a sort of
monotone; he seems to be in a trance, and is quite unlike his usual self."

This patient has consistently observed "luminous spots" fleeting across his
visual fields for two to three days before each attack, and this visual excitation
may be accompanied by prodromal excitement and euphoria.

Case 65   Aphasic and paraesthetic aura accompanied by "silly" affect and forced laughter

This patient was a normally self-possessed girl of 15 subject to infrequent
classical migraines of great severity. For a period of 45 minutes, in my consulting-room, she experienced an aura during which she giggled without in-
termission. During this time she was severely aphasic, and had paraesthesiae
flitting from one limb to another. When she recovered from this state, she
apologised in these terms: "I don't know what I was laughing at—I just
couldn't help it—everything seemed so funny, like laughing gas."

Case 69   Complex visual aura, preceded by intense arousal

A 23-year-old man with attacks of classical migraine and isolated aura since early adolescence. The onset of the attacks is heralded by hyperactivity and elation of almost maniacal intensity. Thus, on one morning, the patient—normally a sober motorcyclist—found himself driven to speed wildly, and to shout and sing while he did this. This was followed by a scintillating scotoma, accompanied by perceptual changes of higher order. He describes the concentric lines of the scotoma as like "the furrows in a ploughed field . . . I could see them between the lines of the book I was reading, but the book looked huge, and the furrows seemed like great chasms, hundreds of feet behind the lines of print." As the scintillations died away, he experienced a "let-down, empty feeling, like after taking benzedrine."

On this occasion, the patient experienced a typical vascular headache and intense abdominal pain for the ensuing 10 hours. These symptoms finally passed away, rather suddenly, and were succeeded by "a marvellous calm feeling."

Case 70   Mosaic and cinematographic vision

A 45-year-old man who had experienced frequent migraine auras and occasional classical migraines since childhood. The aura generally took the form of scintillating scotomata and paraesthesiae, but on a number of occasions he had experienced mosaic vision as a chief symptom. During these episodes he has observed that portions of the visual image, in particular faces, may appear "cut-up," distorted and disjointed, being composed of sharp-edged fragments. He compares this appearance to that of an early Picasso. More frequently he has experienced cinematographic vision, this type of aura being particularly prone to be evoked by flickering light of certain frequencies, e.g. if his television-set is improperly adjusted. The cinematographic vision may also be elicited, experimentally, by the flickering illumination of a "strobe" lamp. In either case, it will continue for several minutes following cessation of the provocative stimulus, and is generally followed by a severe classical migraine.

Case 14   Multiple aura equivalents

A 48-year-old woman who suffered from classical migraines until the age of 20, but has had only isolated auras and migraine equivalents since this time. She has frequent attacks of scintillating scotomata unaccompanied by paraesthesiae, and occasional attacks of paraesthesiae, in the lips and hands, unaccompanied by scotomata. Severe scotomatous auras are accompanied by intense "angor animi," and are followed by syncope. She has, however, also suffered from syncopes of slow onset and offset, and also from attacks of intense angst, unaccompanied by sensory hallucinations, and lasting 10 to 20 minutes. All these appear to be variants of migraine aura.

Further varieties of migraine aura, as experienced at different times by the same individual, are quoted below through the courtesy of a colleague, who has suffered from frequent migraine auras, and occasional classical migraines, since childhood. He has provided short notes on a number of his attacks, and an elaborate description of two unusual attacks.

Case 75   (a) Nightmare, followed by sudden appearance of two white lights, blinking, drawing nearer with a jerking motion. Affect of intense terror, with feeling of incongruity with nightmare contents. Subsequent evolution of classical migraine.
(b) Nightmare, suddenly changing to cinematographic vision of flickering stills persisting for 10 minutes in waking state.
(c) "Daymare" intruding on waking consciousness, with great anxiety, forced reminiscence, and dysphasia on attempting to speak. Duration about 30 minutes: no sequel.

The following description is quoted *in extenso*:

It was a late summer afternoon, and I was winding along a country road on my motorbike. An extraordinary sense of stillness came upon me, a feeling that I had lived this moment before, in the same place—although I had never travelled on this road before. I felt that this summer afternoon had always existed, and that I was arrested in an endless moment. When I got off the bike, a few minutes later, I had an extraordinarily powerful tingling in my hands, nose, lips and tongue. It seemed to be a continuation of the vibration of the motorbike, and at first I took this to be some simple after-effect. But no such explanation was tenable, for the vibrating sensation was growing stronger every moment, and appeared to be spreading, very slowly, from my finger-tips to the palms of my hands, and then upwards. My sense of vision was then affected; a feeling of motion was communicated to everything I saw, so that the trees, the grass, the clouds, etc., seemed to exhibit a silent boiling, to be quivering and streaming upwards in a sort of ecstasy. The hum of crickets was all around me, and when I closed my eyes, this was immediately translated into a hum of colour, which seemed to be the exact visual translation of the sound I heard. After about 20 minutes, the paraesthesiae, which had ascended to my elbows, retraced their course and disappeared, the visual world resumed its normal appearance, and the sense of ecstasy faded. I had a "come-down" feeling, and the beginnings of a headache.

There are many points of interest in this detailed description; the elicitation of Jacksonian paraesthesiae apparently in resonance with the oscillation of the motorbike, a phenomenon which appears analogous to the elicitation of a scintillating scotoma by flickering light of the same frequency, the "boiling" motion of visual images, the sense of timelessness and *déjà vu*, and not least the experience of a synaesthetic equivalence between auditory stimuli and visual images.

The following account is also quoted at length, because it conveys the typical quality of a migrainous delirium:

> It started with the wallpaper, which I suddenly observed to be shimmering like the surface of water when agitated. A few minutes later, this was accompanied by a vibration in the right hand, as if it were resting on the sounding-board of a piano. Then dots, flashes, moving slowly across the field of vision. Patterns, as of Turkish carpets, suddenly changing. Images of flowers continuously raying and opening out. Everything faceted and multiplied: bubbles rising towards me, apertures opening and closing, honeycombs. These images are dazzling when I close my eyes, but still visible, more faintly, when the eyes are opened. They lasted 20 or 30 minutes, and were succeeded by a splitting headache.

STRUCTURE OF THE AURA

Migraines are often described, and misunderstood, because they are described in terms of a single symptom. Thus, a common migraine may be equated with a headache, and a migraine aura with a scotoma: such descriptions are ludicrously inadequate in a clinical sense, and permit the formulation of equally absurd physiological theories (these are discussed in Chapter 10). The discussion and case-histories presented in this chapter indicate the richness and complexity of aura symptoms. It is as rare to encounter a single symptom in the course of a migraine aura, as in a common migraine. Careful interrogation and observation will usually reveal that two, five, or a dozen manifestations are proceeding in unison. Nor are all of these manifestations likely to be on the same functional level (in the sense that scotomata and paraesthesiae may be presumed to be): simple circumscribed hallucinations projected on to the visual or tactile field are likely to be accompanied by sensory alterations of greater complexity (e.g. mosaic vision), disorders of arousal mechanisms (conscious level, etc.), of affect, and of highest integrative function.

Further, the symptoms of migraine aura are variable, even in successive attacks in the same patient: sometimes the emphasis may be on the scotomatous manifestations, sometimes on the aphasic, sometimes on the affective, etc., allowing as great a variety of "equivalents" as we have encountered in the decompositions and recompositions of the common migraine. Thus, migraine aura, like common migraine, has a *composite* structure; it is put together from a variety of components or *modules* arranged in innumerable different patterns.

It must also be emphasised that migraine aura has a *sequence* like common migraine, and cannot be adequately portrayed in terms of the symptoms present at any one time. We may readily recognise both excitatory and inhibitory phases, the former manifest as scintillations and paraesthesiae, diffuse sensory enhancement, arousal of consciousness and muscular tonus, etc., and the latter as negative hallucinations, loss of muscular tone, syncope, etc. The time-scale of the aura is much contracted, the sequence of excitation-inhibition-re-excitation, etc., taking only 20 to 30 minutes, as opposed to a cycle of hours or days in a common migraine. Finally, we observe that the symptoms of the aura are central and cerebral, whereas many (but not all) of the symptoms of a common migraine are peripheral and vegetative.

INCIDENCE OF MIGRAINE AURA

The incidence of migraine aura is almost impossible to assess. It has been estimated that the incidence of classical migraine is less than one per cent in the general population, but this gives us no information concerning the incidence of isolated auras, which may not form the grounds of complaint, or be recognised for what they are by either patient or physician.[24] Thus Alvarez, in a study of over 600 migraine scotomata, estimated that more than 12 per cent of his male patients experienced solitary scotomata. In a more sophisticated group (comprised of 44 physicians) he found that no less than 87 per cent of them had experienced "many solitary scotomata with never a headache." If we also take into consideration the occurrence of negative scotomata (which may pass unnoticed by the patient), of isolated paraesthesiae, attacks of faintness and drowsiness, of altered affect, and of disordered highest functions, etc.—all of which may occur as manifestations of aura, but by their subtlety or ambiguity elude diagnosis—we may reasonably suspect the incidence of migraine aura to be far in excess of the quoted incidence of classical migraine.

[24] I happened to be discussing the subject with a colleague, a zoologist, who immediately recognised my diagram of a scintillating scotoma, and said: "I often had it as a young man, usually when I was in bed at night. I was delighted by the colours and their expansion—it reminded me of the opening of a flower. It was never succeeded by a headache or other symptoms. I presumed everybody saw such things—it never occurred to me that it was a 'symptom' of anything."

THE DIFFERENTIAL DIAGNOSIS OF MIGRAINE AURA:
MIGRAINE VERSUS EPILEPSY

The differentiation of migraine aura from other paroxysmal states, in particular epilepsy, is a vital diagnostic exercise. It is frequently asserted, either on clinical or statistical grounds, that the two maladies are closely related to one another; opposed to this school of opinion are those who vehemently deny the existence, or even the possibility, of such a relation. It is evident that there is much doubt (assertion and denial imply doubt), and that the matter carries too great an emotional charge for cool discussion. Doubt springs from the inadequacy of our definitions, and emotional charge from the sinister and pejorative reputation so often attached to epilepsy. We have already referred to certain clinical associations (Gowers's "borderlands of epilepsy," and Lennox's "hybrid seizures"), and the time has come to clarify the meaning of such terms.

The crux of the matter, as Hughlings Jackson repeatedly stated, lies in the distinction between two frames of reference: roughly speaking, theory and practice. Thus Jackson writes:

> While scientifically migraine is, I think, to be classified with epilepsies . . . it would be as absurd to classify it along with ordinary cases of epilepsy as to class whales with other mammals for purposes of practical life. A whale is in law a fish; in zoology it is a mammal.

In practice, it is easy to differentiate migraines from epilepsies in the vast majority of cases. Doubt is only likely to arise in the case of complex auras, especially if they occur as isolated events. Doubt may be exacerbated if there is any personal or family history of epilepsy, if the patient loses consciousness during the aura, and, above all, if he is alleged to have had a convulsion while unconscious. It may be instructive, therefore, to compare certain specific phenomena as they occur in epilepsy and in migraine, and in so doing we may reinforce personal experience with the most reliable figures in the older literature—those of Liveing (1873) in relation to migraine, and of Gowers (1881) in relation to epilepsy.

Visual symptoms are far commoner in migraine, and often assume a very specific form—scintillating and negative scotomata—not seen in epileptic auras; visual symptoms were recorded in 62 per cent of Liveing's cases (this included both common and classical varieties, but predominantly the latter), but only 17 per cent of Gowers's cases. *Paraesthesiae* of Jacksonian distribution occur with somewhat greater frequency in migraine (35 per cent of Liveing's cases, 17 per cent of Gowers's), but are very rarely bilateral in epilepsy, whereas they are frequently so in migraine, especially in the lip and tongue areas; a crucial differentiation is given by the rate of passage of such paraesthesiae, those of migraine being, very roughly, a hundred times slower than their epileptic counterparts. *Convulsions* are common in epilepsy, but are so rare in migraine as to cast doubt on its diagnosis: post-ictal weakness is the rule in motor epilepsies, but does not occur in migraines save in the very special case of hemiplegic attacks (see following chapter). *Loss of consciousness* is common in epilepsy (it occurred in 50 per cent of Gowers's 505 cases), but it is a distinct rarity in migraine; further it is generally abrupt in onset in epilepsy (save in psychomotor seizures), but gradual in onset in migraine. Complex *alterations of higher integrative functions and affect* are recorded by both authors as occurring in more than 10 per cent of their patients; it is, however, rare for the dreamy or dissociated states of migraine aura to reach the intensity of those occurring in certain temporal lobe seizures (e.g. automatism followed by amnesia), and, conversely, rare for epileptics to experience the protracted delirium or quasi-delirium which may accompany and greatly outlast migraine auras.

By these and similar criteria we may achieve diagnostic certainty, or at least diagnostic probability, in a majority of cases. There remain for consideration those patients who appear to experience both epileptic and migrainous attacks, or the evolution of one into the other; those patients with true "hybrid" attacks; and, finally, those patients in whom attacks are of such ambiguous nature as to defeat clinical diagnostic methods. The reader must be referred to the exceedingly detailed writings of Gowers (1907) and of Lennox and Lennox (1960) for a full discussion of this twilight region, and for a tally of case-histories which plays havoc with our rigid nosologies.

Gowers provides several case-histories of migraines and epilepsies alternating in the same patient, one set of symptoms usually ousting the other at different periods in the life-history. More dramatic are his cases "in which there is an actual passage of the symptoms of one into the other": thus in one such patient, a girl who had been subject to classical migraines since the age of five, the headache component by degrees disappeared and was replaced by convulsions. (We will recollect that Aretaeus first described such a hybrid attack of migraine spectrum followed by convulsion.) Gowers ascribes the onset of epilepsy in such cases to the effects of migrainous pain and cerebral disturbance: Liveing, more plausibly, if more enigmatically, speaks of the perpetual possibility of "transformations" from one paroxysm to another.

Lennox and Lennox provide more case-histories of this type, in which the epileptic component, where present, could be further substantiated by electroencephalographic findings. In one such case a patient with elaborate visual disturbances (yellow whirling stars and Lilliputian vision) might suffer either a *grand mal* convulsion or a classical migraine headache in their wake. Another patient with protracted visual and paraesthetic symptoms, would then suffer severe headache, and, finally, a generalised convulsion, the headache still being present after the convulsion had terminated. Lennox terms this attack a "migralepsy."

It is clear that in a majority of instances questioning and observation will resolve the problem as to whether an acute paroxysmal attack is migrainous, epileptic, or of any other type. There are occasions, however, when the greatest clinical acumen may fail to clarify the issue: we have described, for example, migraine auras characterised by hallucinations of smell, feelings of *déjà vu*, and sometimes forced reminiscence and forced affect, which may be indistinguishable from epileptic "uncinate attacks" unless further differential features are present.

Case 98   A 42-year-old woman with complex attacks since the age of nineteen, gradually becoming more severe, frequent, and elaborate. The attacks start with "a vague but all-pervasive perceptual shift in the sense of time and space . . . a certain strangeness . . . a feeling of 'static' or energy." This is followed by "visual streaking," and sometimes a sharp visual field cut affecting the upper temporal quadrant of the hemifield on the left. This state of heightened sensory stimulation, with perhaps specific visual field cuts, is often followed by a complex dreamlike or hallucinatory state: "There are moiré patterns . . . entity hallucinations . . . a face, a voice, here, there, they appear and disappear very quickly." Attacks sometimes terminate at this point. At other times the patient experiences "a metallic taste on the tongue . . . the same taste each time," and this is followed by falling and loss of consciousness, or a fugue-like automatism of which she retains no memory.

There is a very strong family history of classical (and sometimes complicated) migraine on the father's side. The patient's father gets "kidney-shaped dazzles, zigzags and blindness"; his sister sometimes becomes aphasic in migraines; his mother has severe, light-induced seizures and migraines. The patient herself shows strong reactions to photic stimulation, with photomyoclonus, photoconvulsive reactions *and* photic migraines (induction of scotomata by flickering light). Brain imaging has shown a vascular malformation (a venous angioma) in the right temporal lobe.

These complex attacks were called "migralepsies" by a colleague, because they had features of both migraines and temporal lobe epilepsies. They were helped, somewhat, by taking ergotamines, but only diminished in frequency when anti-convulsants were prescribed.

The most ambiguous region is that occupied by paroxysmal dream-like or trance-like states accompanied by intense affect (terror, rapture, etc.) and elaborate alterations of highest mental functions. The differential diagnosis in such cases must include the following states:

Migraine Aura

Epileptic Aura or Psychomotor Seizure

Hysterical Trances or Psychotic States

Toxic, Metabolic, or Febrile delirious or hysteroid states

Sleep and arousal disorders: e.g. Nightmares, Daymares, atypical narcolepsies or sleep-paralyses, etc.

We may thus encounter what has already been described in relation to the differential diagnosis of certain migraine equivalents: a region where a number of clinical syndromes appear to coalesce and to become indistinguishable from one another with the means at our disposal. Finally the problem may cease to be one of clinical or physiological differentiation, and become one of semantic decision: we cannot name what we cannot individuate.

> Either a thing has properties which no other thing has, and then one has to distinguish it straight away from the others by a description and refer to it; or, on the other hand, *there are several things which have the totality of their properties in common, and then it is not possible to point to any one of them.*
>
> For if a thing is not distinguished by anything, I cannot distinguish it—for otherwise it would be distinguished. (Wittgenstein)

CLASSICAL MIGRAINE

A lengthy consideration of migraine aura has left us with relatively little to say about classical migraine. A certain proportion of patients may proceed from the aura to a protracted vascular headache, with nausea, abdominal pain, autonomic symptoms, etc., of many hours' duration. The repertoire of such symptoms in a classical migraine is no different from that of a common migraine, and requires, therefore, no specific description.

There tend, however, to be some general differences of format. Classical migraines tend to be more compact and intense than common migraines, and rarely have a duration in excess of twelve hours; frequently the attack may last only two or three hours. The termination of the attack may be similarly incisive, and followed by an abrupt return to normal function, or post-migrainous rebound. As Liveing writes in this context:

> The abrupt transition from intense suffering to perfect health is very remarkable. A man . . . finds himself, with little or no warning, completely disabled, the victim of intense bodily pain, mental prostration, and perhaps hallucinations of sense or idea . . . and in this state he remains the greater part of the day; and yet towards its close . . . he awakes a different being, in possession of all his faculties, and able to join an evening's entertainment, to get up a brief, or take part in a debate.

The protracted course of some common migraines, in which the patient may spend day after day in a state of wretched malaise, is rarely seen in a classical attack.

We will consider the frequency and antecedents of migraines in Part II, but we may notice, at this point, that classical migraines tend to be less frequent than common migraines, and often have a "paroxysmal" rather than a "reactive" quality. This does not represent an absolute "rule," but is nevertheless a frequent distinguishing characteristic of the two types of attack.

There is a strong tendency for patients to adhere to a given clinical pattern; patients with classical migraine rarely have common migraines, and vice versa. Again, there are no absolutes—I have seen at least 30 patients who suffer from both types of attack, the two types existing either concurrently or in alternation.

We have already noted that some patients who were prone to classical migraines at one time may "lose" the headache component, and thereafter suffer from isolated auras (*vide* Case 14, p. 85).[25] Conversely, there are also a considerable number of patients who lose their auras, and thereafter suffer from attacks similar to common migraine.

The headache of a classical migraine characteristically comes on as the aura draws to its close, and rapidly attains climactic intensity It may affect either or both sides of the head, and its location bears no consistent relationship to the lateralisation of the aura. Indeed, further attacks of aura may occur after the headache has been established. We have seen that the aura and the headache stages may become spontaneously dissociated in a variety of circumstances (*vide* Case 11, p. 84), and they are

---

[25] A number of patients who have suffered from classical migraines for many years have proceeded to "lose" their headaches while under my care, despite the fact that no specific medication has been given. I suspect that this modification of migraine-format is due to suggestion, a consequence of my showing extreme interest in their aura symptoms, and rather less interest in their headaches.

also readily separated by ergot derivatives and other drugs which "abort" attacks of classical migraine.

We thus have a number of reasons for thinking of classical migraine as a sort of hybrid in which the aura and the headache stages have a contingent link, or tendency to be associated, but no necessary or essential connection. Thus the classical migraine is an aggregate structure itself composed of aggregate structures.[26]

POSTSCRIPT (1992)—THE ANGST OF SCOTOMA

A peculiar *horror*—perhaps this is part of the horror of which Liveing speaks—may be associated with negative scotomata, which may be felt, not just as a failure of sight but a failure of reality itself.

This feeling, full of fear and deeply uncanny, is indicated in the following case histories:

Case 90   A highly gifted physician, a psychoanalyst, who has had occasional negative scotomata, or hemianopia, coming two or three times a year since early childhood. These are frequently, but not invariably, followed by migraine headaches.

Although this man is taken daily into the depths of the soul and its primeval terrors by his calling and profession, and although he boldly faces all the monsters of the unconscious, he has never become inured to his own scotomata, which introduce a realm or category of the unbearable and uncanny, beyond anything he has encountered in the realms of psychiatry. In his own words:

"I may be seeing as a patient someone I know well, sitting across the desk, with my gaze fixed upon them. Suddenly I become aware that something is wrong—although at this point I cannot say what it is. It is a sense of something *fundamentally* wrong—something impossible and contrary to the order of nature.

"Then I suddenly 'realize'—*part of the patient's face is missing*: part of their nose, or their cheek, or perhaps the left ear. Although I continue to listen and speak, my gaze seems transfixed—I cannot move my head—and a sense of horror, of the impossible, steals over me. The disappearance continues—usually until half the face has disappeared and, with this, that same half of

---

[26] There has been a recent change in terminology, the terms "classical" and "common" migraine having been replaced by migraine *with* and *without* aura. Some investigators (e.g. Olesen *et al.* in Denmark) feel there may be important hemodynamic differences between common and classical migraine, but the opinion now, increasingly, is that there is no essential difference—epidemiologically, clinically, physiologically—between the two (see Ranson *et al.*, 1991). Many patients have sometimes one, sometimes the other, and sometimes attacks with great visual excitability throughout, but no aura, which seem to be intermediate between the two.

the room. I feel paralyzed and petrified in some sort of way. It never occurs to me that something is happening to my vision—I feel something incredible is happening to the *world*. It doesn't occur to me to move my head or eyes to 'check' on the existence of what seems to be missing. It never occurs to met that I am having a migraine, even though I have had the experience dozens of times before. . . .

"I don't exactly feel that anything is 'missing,' but I fall into a ridiculous obsessive doubt. I seem to lose the *idea* of a face; I 'forget' how faces look—something happens to my imagination, my memory, my thinking. . . . It is not that half the world mysteriously 'disappears,' but that I find myself in doubt as to whether it was ever there. There seems to be a sort of hole in my memory and mind and, so to speak, a hole in the world; and yet I cannot imagine what might go in the hole. There is a hole and there isn't a hole—my mind is utterly confounded. I have the feeling that my body—that *bodies* are unstable, that they may come apart and lose parts of themselves—an eye, a limb, amputation—that something vital has disappeared, but disappeared *without trace*, that it has disappeared *along with the 'place' it once occupied*. The horrible feeling is of nothingness nowhere.[27]

"After a while—perhaps it is only a minute or two, but it seems to last forever—I realize that there is something wrong with my vision, that it is a natural, physiological disturbance in my vision, and not some grotesque, unnatural disturbance in the world. I realize that I am having a migraine aura—and an immense sense of relief floods over me. . . .

"But even knowing this does not *correct* the perception. . . . There is still a certain residue of dread, and a fear that the scotoma may go on forever. . . . It is only when there is full restoration of the visual fields that the sense of panic, and of something wrong, finally goes away. . . .

"I have never experienced this sort of fear except in regard to a migraine scotoma."

Case 91   This woman of 75 has frequent attacks—variously called "migraine auras" or "epilepsies" or sometimes "migralepsies"—which have a clear physiological basis in a discharging lesion, a scar, in her right parietoccipital area due to an injury sustained in infancy.

In these attacks the left side of her body seems to disappear and everything normally seen on the left disappears. She says. "There is nothing there any more, just a blank, just a hole"—a blank in her visual field, in her body, in the universe itself, and in that state she cannot trust herself to stand, and must sit down before it gets worse. She also experiences a feeling of mortal terror when she has these attacks. She feels the "hole" is like death, and that one day it will get so large that it will "swallow" her completely. She had these attacks as a child but was called a "liar" when she described them.

In severe attacks, it is not only the left side of her body which seems to

---

[27] Compare Hobbes: "That which is not Body is no part of the Universe . . . and since the Universe is All . . . that which is not Body is Nothing . . . and Nowhere." Hobbes, *The Kingdome of Darknesse*.

disappear, but she is deeply confused about her *whole* body, and cannot be sure where anything is—or *that* it is.

She feels quite unreal (this is one of the reasons for her fears of engulfment). Also in such severe attacks she cannot make sense of what she *can* see (visual agnosia) and, specifically, she may be unable to recognize the faces of familiar people—either their faces seem "different" or, more commonly, they seem "faceless," for example, they have features which bear no expression (prosopagnosia). In the worst attacks this extends to voices too—they are heard, but lose all tonality and "character"; a sort of auditory agnosia.

Such privations of sense go on to complete darkness and silence—as in cases recorded by Gowers—and she might be said to lose consciousness, although essentially it is a dissolution of her sensorium in which she gradually sinks to deeper and deeper "senselessness" until finally she is completely insensible. It is not surprising that attacks so dreadful and so real are experienced as deathlike.

The word *scotoma* means darkness or shadow, and we can understand from the above history something of the quality of this shadow. In the case of *bilateral* scotoma, there may be even more horrifying experiences; thus a bilateral, central scotoma causes the middle of the visual field, the world, to disappear—and faces, at such times, have the center punched out, and become a ring of flesh surrounding a void (a condition termed *doughnut* or *bagel* vision).

If there is a complete bilateral scotoma, with total loss of the visual fields, and (as may happen, from the proximity of the visual and tactile areas in the brain) total loss of the body-fields, or sense of the body, a most terrifying sense of extermination may occur.

The sense of violation, of the uncanny, of horror, only occurs if the situation is acute, and there is some remainder of the person to see what has happened (or, rather, what is no longer happening). A scotoma may be missed, even when acute, and with an acute observer—as, at first, in case 90. And it is almost invariably "missed" (the person fails to miss what is "missing") when it is long-standing, persistent, or chronic: a situation one not uncommonly sees with some strokes. The following case-history illustrates this:

Case 92   An intelligent woman in her sixties who had suffered a massive stroke, affecting the deeper and back portions of her right cerebral hemisphere. She has perfectly preserved intelligence—and humor.

She sometimes complains to the nurses that they have not put dessert or coffee on her tray. . . . When they said: "But, Mrs. X, it is right there, on the left," she seems not to understand what they say, and does not look to the left. If her head is gently turned, so that the dessert comes into sight, in the preserved right half of her visual field, she says: "Oh there it is—it wasn't there before." She has totally lost the *idea* of "left," both with regard to the world, and also her own body. Sometimes she complains that her portions are too small—but this is because she only eats from the right half of the plate—it does not occur to her that it has a left half as well. Sometimes, she will put on lipstick, and make up the right half of her face, leaving the left half completely neglected: it is almost impossible to treat these things, because her attention cannot be drawn to them ("hemi-inattention"), and she has no conception that they are "wrong." She knows it intellectually, and can understand, and laugh; but it is impossible for her to know it *directly*.

Macdonald Critchley, in his fascinating history of migraine (Critchley, 1966), reminds us that

Blaise Pascal . . . was prey to periodic illusions of a terrifying character. From time to time he would imagine that a cavity or precipice was yawning on his left-hand side. To reassure himself he would often manoeuvre a piece of furniture to that side. . . . This periodic illusion was spoken of by his contemporaries as l'Abime de Pascal. . . . [There is] interesting evidence to suggest that this recurring precipice was actually a transitory left hemianopia.

Critchley thinks it probable that Pascal's hemianopia was migrainous in character. It is clear from the description—and the use of such words as "abyss" or "cavity"—that there was a profound, almost metaphysical, angst, a sense that part of space itself had vanished. This bewilderment is exactly like the cosmic "hole"—the hole in consciousness—described by the patient in Case 91, and the personal experience I myself describe in *A Leg to Stand On*.

Patients such as this, then, may suddenly find they have lost half the universe, in an unaccountable and terrible way. There is retained some higher order function—an observer who can (at least intermittently) report on what is happening. But if the disorder is more chronic or extensive, there is lost all sense that anything has happened, and all memory that anything was ever different. Such patients now *live* in a half-space, a half-universe, but their consciousness has been reorganised, and they do not know it.

Such conditions, which are almost too strange to be imagined (except by those who have actually experienced them), have often been regarded as "illusory" or "crazy," an opinion which can add greatly to the distress of the sufferer. But it is only very recently, with the new biological or neuropsychological concepts of consciousness provided by Gerald Edelman, that such syndromes have started to become intelligible, to make sense.

Edelman sees consciousness as arising in the first place from a perceptual integration, coupled with the sense of historical continuity, a continuous relating of past and present. "Primary" consciousness, as he terms it, is thus constituted by the perception of a coherent body and world, extended in space (as a "personal" space) and in time (as a "personal" time, or history). In a deep scotoma all three of these disappear: one can no longer claim for oneself (the left half of) one's body or visual world; it disappears, taking its "place" with it, and it disappears taking its *past* with it.

Such a scotoma, then, is a scotoma *in* primary consciousness, as well as in one's body-ego or primary self. Such a scotoma will indeed fill one with horror, for one's higher consciousness, higher self, can observe what is happening, but is impotent to do anything about it. Fortunately, such profound alterations of "self" and consciousness only last for a few minutes in migraine. But in these few minutes one gets an overwhelming impression of the absolute identity of Body and Mind, and the fact that our highest functions—consciousness and self—are not entities, self-sufficient, "above" the body, but neuropsychological constructs—processes —dependent on the continuity of bodily experience and its integration.

FOUR

Migrainous Neuralgia ("Cluster Headache")— Hemiplegic Migraine— Ophthalmoplegic Migraine— Pseudo-Migraine

These variants of migraine are considered in the course of a single chapter because they have one characteristic in common: the occurrence of neurological deficits which may be of considerable duration. Other than this accidental characteristic, they bear no special affinity to one another.

MIGRAINOUS NEURALGIA

Migrainous neuralgia has been redescribed and renamed a dozen times since Möllendorff's original account in 1867. Among its synonyms are "ciliary neuralgia," "sphenopalatine neuralgia," "Horton's cephalalgia," "histamine headache," and "cluster headache".

The syndrome is a very distinctive one, and its affinities to other forms of migraine have appeared questionable to some observers. There is usually an extremely acute onset of pain referred to the temple and the eye on one side; less frequently, pain may be felt in or behind the ear, or in the cheek and nose. The intensity of the pain may be overwhelming (one patient described it to me as an "orgasm of pain"), and may drive patients into a frenzy. Whereas the majority of migraine patients sit or lie down, or wish to do so, the sufferer from migrainous neuralgia tends to pace up and down in a fury, clutching the affected eye and groaning. I have even seen patients beat their heads against the wall during an attack.

The pain tends to be accompanied (and, on occasion, preceded) by a number of striking local symptoms and signs. The affected eye becomes bloodshot and waters, and there is blockage or catarrh of the nostril on the same side. Sometimes the attack is accompanied or heralded by a flow of thick saliva, rarely by recurrent coughing. There may be a partial or complete *Horner's syndrome* on the affected side, and this may occasionally persist as a permanent neurological residue. The duration of the attacks may be as little as two minutes, and is rarely more than two hours.

A majority of attacks are nocturnal and wake the patient from deep sleep; some come on within a few minutes of waking in the morning, before the fogs of sleep have lifted; diurnal attacks, when they occur, tend to come during periods of rest, exhaustion, or "let-down." They are uncommon when patients are fully aroused and going "full blast." It is rarely possible to identify any *trigger* of the attacks, other than alcohol: during susceptible periods (see Case 1, p. 101) the sensitivity to alcohol is so consistent that it can afford a diagnostic test when the history is equivocal.

I have seen 74 cases of migrainous neuralgia in a total of nearly 1,200 migraine patients. This figure probably conveys a disproportionately high incidence, and reflects the fact that the unfortunate sufferers from this symptom are usually forced to seek medical help, and may wander from one physician to another, finally coming to a headache specialist, in order to secure relief from a stubborn and terrible symptom.

Two other peculiarities of incidence may be noted. Migrainous neuralgia is almost ten times commoner in men than in women (the sex-incidence of other forms of migraine is probably equal), and it is rarely familial; only 3 of the 74 cases I have seen had a family background of similar attacks, whereas other forms of migraine are commonly familial.

Finally, we must notice the singular format of attacks in many patients, a format which justifies the name of "cluster headache" for this variant of the syndrome. One sees, in such patients, a close-packed grouping of attacks lasting for several weeks (there may be as many as 10 attacks daily) and this is followed by a remission lasting months, or even years. Some patients tend to have annual clusters with some regularity (Easter is the usual cluster season) while others may go 10 years or more between clusters. During these remissions, patients appear to be entirely immune from attack, and may, in addition, take indefinite quantities of alcohol with impunity. Sometimes the cluster is of abrupt onset, but more commonly it builds up by degrees to a climactic intensity over the course of a few days. Sometimes there is a distinct prodromal period, in which the patient may note a vague burning or discomfort on one side, not amounting to frank pain. Sometimes the imminence of a cluster is announced by the development of alcohol-sensitivity. Some clusters taper off by degrees, although the usual pattern is of sudden, dramatic cessation of the attacks.

There are other sufferers from migrainous neuralgia who never enjoy the blessing of intermittent remission, but have continued attacks, often several a week, for years on end. Attacks are almost invariably confined to one side; I have seen only two patients who have had attacks on alternating sides. A few patients demonstrate tenderness and induration of a superficial temporal artery during a "cluster," or permanently.

The best evidence for the relation of such attacks to common migraine lies in the occurrence of "transitional" attacks which combine features of both (*vide* Case 1, below). Their identification with migraine is further fortified by consideration of their physiological substrates (Part III), and their response to medication (Part IV).

ILLUSTRATIVE CASE-HISTORIES

Case 1   Atypical cluster attacks. The initial attacks are of lancinating severity, very brief duration, and entirely local in their manifestations. As the cluster proceeds, the individual attacks become longer, less intense in severity, and accompanied by abdominal pain, diarrhoea, and varied autonomic symptoms, i.e. indistinguishable from common migraines. There is intense alcohol-sensitivity during, and only during, the clusters. Clusters come annually, with considerable regularity, and have only failed to come at the expected time when this patient was pregnant.

Case 2   A 28-year-old man who had suffered incessant attacks of migrainous neuralgia from the age of 18 to 25, but subsequently differentiated a cluster-pattern. His younger brother is similarly affected. This patient provides an instructive account of the times and circumstances at which he is liable to an attack, viz. in the middle of the night, when "napping" before the television set, when resting after work or a heavy meal, or following an orgasm.

Case 3   A 40-year-old man with migrainous neuralgia who presents a number of unusual features. Lacrimation constitutes an invariable "warning" of an impending attack, and may precede the onset of pain by one or two hours. The majority of attacks are right-sided, but about one in twenty occurs on the left side. The implacable frequency of his attacks has been successfully broken up by the use of monthly injections of histamine. The histamine-reaction is immediately followed by a true attack of migrainous neuralgia, and this, apparently, "defuses" the patient, exempting him from further attacks until his next injection.

Case 5   A 36-year-old woman who suffers from both classical migraines *and* cluster headache. Her attacks of migrainous neuralgia are invariably nocturnal, and are remarkable for the profuse and viscid salivation which accompanies them.

Case 6   A 47-year-old man, paranoid, masochistic and depressed. He too suffers from two forms of migraine—attacks of migrainous neuralgia nightly, and attacks of common migraine at weekends. He demonstrates a permanently tender and indurated superficial temporal artery on the affected, right side.

Case 7   A 37-year-old man with a 12-year history of cluster headache. Each cluster is preceded by a prodromal period of about a week, during which there is a diffuse burning feeling in the right temple and tender induration of the superficial temporal artery on this side. He displays a permanent partial Horner's syndrome. Individual attacks are accompanied by intense restlessness, frequency of urination and polyuria.

Case 8   A 55-year-old man who has suffered from annual clusters of migrainous neuralgia since the age of 12, his sole remission being for a period of five years when he was undergoing psycho-analysis.

Case 9   A 30-year-old man who when first seen was in the middle of an attack of migrainous neuralgia, with a half-closed eye and a Horner's syndrome on the right side, running of the nose, and an enlarged, throbbing temporal artery on this side. He was in great pain, very pale, with a small, slow pulse, and a look of having been "beaten," of defeat. He told me that he had been humiliated, not an hour before, by his boss, who had found fault with him, and been sarcastic with him in front of his fellow workers. As he related this, he became angry, even furious; he lost his "beaten," defeated look, and now looked bellicose and aggressive; he lost his pallor, and flushed beet-red; and with this his right pupil dilated, his eyelid lifted, he lost his Horner's syndrome—*and he lost his pain*. Then, as his anger passed, and the moral-physiological surge which went with it, he became fearful and dejected, became pale again, developed his Horner's syndrome once again, and fell right back into the depths of his migrainous neuralgia. This is as striking a case as I have ever seen of a strong emotion, a fighting feeling, a sympathomimetic surge, overcoming and temporarily "curing" an attack of migrainous neuralgia.

HEMIPLEGIC MIGRAINE

The term "hemiplegic migraine" is often loosely used to denote ordinary attacks of classical migraine with transient neurological symptoms, as well as attacks in which a true motor hemiplegia of hours' or days' duration is seen. We shall here be using the term *in sensu stricto*.

The earliest clear description of hemiplegic migraine of which I am aware is to be found in Liveing's monograph:

> A young gentleman, 24 years of age . . . was attacked with what, according to the custom of the day, was called an "apoplectic seizure," commencing with imperfect articulation and mental confusion of a very transient character, but followed by right hemiplegia which was more lasting . . . [on a second occasion] he was again attacked, but this time with a great drowsiness and some degree of right hemiplegia, while his pulse fell to 40. The drowsiness had disappeared by the next morning, and the pulse had risen, but the hemiplegic symptoms increased, and the power of utterance was almost extinguished . . . and only gradually restored.

In summary, this patient experienced a classical migraine which was followed, unexpectedly, by a hemiplegia of one day's duration, and an aphasia of one week's duration.

Infrequent accounts of such attacks were published, but not until 1951, when Symonds provided an extremely detailed account of two cases, did the nature of the attack begin to be clarified. One of Symonds's patients exhibited a left hemiplegia and coma for five days, following a classical migraine.

Both his father and grandfather had had similar attacks. The spinal fluid showed a pleocytosis of 185 polymorphs/mm^3, which disappeared after two days. Electroencephalography showed slow-wave activity of the entire right hemisphere, which was similarly transient. Angiography at the height of the hemiplegia failed to reveal any detectable abnormality.

Similar cases have been described by Whitty *et al.* (1953), who stress the strong family history generally obtainable in such cases. Three of Whitty's cases also exhibited a transient cellular response in the spinal fluid. Harold Wolff also described a number of cases, and was able to demonstrate a transient pineal shift in one such case.

The clinical and electrical pictures in such cases indicate profound though transient cerebral dysfunction, usually confined to one hemisphere. The occasional precipitation of such attacks by angiography, or by ergot overdosage, suggests the likelihood of vascular spasm or reversible damage. The failure to demonstrate such changes on angiography suggests that only vessels of arteriolar calibre may be involved. The occurrence of pineal shift is compatible with oedema of a hemisphere, and the cellular response in the spinal fluid indicates the likelihood of a sterile inflammatory response, probably in the involved vessels.

Whatever the findings in a few cases, there is not enough evidence to support the notion of an ischaemic or inflammatory response as the basis of cerebral dysfunction in all cases. There is also the possibility that a violent migraine, or crescendo of violent attacks, may lead to a prolonged functional depression of cerebral activity, something analogous to, though far more protracted than, a post-epileptic (Todd's) paralysis.

Hemiplegic migraine (and a minor variant sometimes termed "facio-plegic migraine") is exceedingly rare. I have seen only the following two cases:

Case 23   A 43-year-old woman who has had classical migraine since the age of 12 (6 to 10 attacks yearly), and occasional hemiplegic attacks—5 in all. Similar hemiplegic attacks had also occurred in her mother and in a maternal aunt. I was enabled to examine her in one attack, at which time she demonstrated a left-sided hemiparesis with impaired cortical sensation and an extensor plantar response. This hemiparesis cleared in three days. She was subsequently admitted for detailed neurological investigation: angiography and contrast-studies failed to visualise any anatomical lesion.

Case 25   A 14-year-old boy who had suffered repeated "bilious attacks" between the ages of 5 and 11, and infrequent classical migraines of great severity since their termination. The majority of his attacks were precipitated by a combination of extravagant exercise and exertion, and tended to come immediately after cross-country races at school.

A number of his attacks were accompanied by a lower facial weakness of many hours' duration, and on one occasion of three days' duration. The father experienced severe attacks of classical migraine without a facio-plegic component.

OPHTHALMOPLEGIC MIGRAINE

Ophthalmoplegic migraine is also exceedingly rare (Friedman, Harter and Merritt (1961) were able to find only 8 cases in a population of 5,000 migraine patients). The majority of patients have usually experienced many common or classical migraines, of which a few attacks have been followed by ophthalmoplegic symptoms. It need hardly be emphasised that this diagnosis should only be made after careful neurological investigation, and the exclusion of possible anatomical abnormalities (aneurysms, angiomas, etc.).

The third cranial nerve is most frequently involved, but the fourth and sixth nerves may also be affected on occasion, leading to total ophthalmoplegia. These neurological deficits usually take several weeks to clear. Involvement in repeated attacks is always unilateral. It has been suggested that the involvement of cranial nerves is due to oedema in the intracavernous portion of the internal carotid artery, but there is no supporting evidence for this supposition.

I have seen three cases of ophthalmoplegic migraine in a total of 1,200 migraine patients:

Case 24   This 34-year-old woman has had infrequent common migraines since childhood, and a total of three ophthalmoplegic attacks at widely separated intervals (1943, 1953, and 1966). All of these were preceded by a series of common migraines of increasing severity, and in rapid succession to one another. The culminating attack would be followed, the next day, by the development of an ophthalmoplegia. In her 1966 attack, a series of intense left-sided headaches was followed by the development of third- and fourth-nerve paralyses. The patient experienced complete ptosis for three weeks, and diplopia for a further month. When I examined her, 10 weeks after the start of her ophthalmoplegia, she exhibited a dilated pupil on the affected side, but no ptosis or external palsy. Bilateral carotid angiography, performed during the first of her attacks, had been entirely within normal limits.

Case 73   A 9-year-old girl with attacks of classical migraine since the age of 3. One of her attacks, at the age of 5, had been followed by an ophthalmoplegia of many weeks' duration. Two brothers, both parents, and other close relatives were subject to classical migraine, but none had experienced ophthalmoplegic symptoms.

Case 99   A 44-year-old engineer who has had repeated attacks of ophthalmoplegic migraine since the age of 19. The pain is invariably left-sided, and of excruciating severity, and (in the patient's words) "it doesn't stop until the eye is completely out" (i.e. until there is total paralysis of the third, fourth and sixth nerves on this side). There was at first a slow but complete resolution of ophthalmoplegia after each attack, within a couple of weeks; but then an increasing residual deficit. He has tried virtually every medication (ergotamine, Inderal, Dilantin, calcium-channel blockers, etc.), as well as biofeedback, chiropraxy and acupuncture—and has found all of them useless. When he gets an attack he self-medicates it with injections of DHE 45 and steroids; and if he is lucky, it will die down, and not go on to a total ophthalmoplegia. He has had "every test"—angiograms, brain scans—but no angioma or aneurysm has ever shown up. When examined, some five hours after the start of an attack, he had a grossly dilated, unreactive pupil on the left, and deficits of medial, upward and downward gaze, only lateral gaze being full and unaffected. He fears he will end up with a "useless" left eye. He also describes a strange, unstable state at the start of many attacks: "fluctuations of hot and cold . . . my body goes into wild fluctuations . . . oscillations with a period of ten to fifteen minutes, getting wider . . . positive feedback, I guess."

PSEUDO-MIGRAINE

The diagnosis of migraine is usually made on the basis of a clinical history, supported where possible by observation of the patient during an attack. It is usually good sense to perform a few basic investigations (skull X-rays, EEG, etc.), although these may be expected to be within normal limits in the vast majority, say 99 per cent, of all cases. Certain clinical features, such as the apparent onset of migraines late in life, are *ipso facto* suspicious of organic pathology, and must be investigated with unusual care. It is particularly important, in cases of classical migraine, to question the patient carefully regarding the usual locations and qualities of the aura. We have already stressed that most migraine patients experience, at one time or another, auras referred to either or both sides of the visual fields or body-surface. Invariable unilaterality of the aura is a suspicious symptom, and constitutes grounds for detailed investigation of the patient. The following case-history is instructive in this regard:

Case 26   A 57-year-old woman who gave a history of having had "classical migraines" since the age of 16. She would generally experience 6 or 7 attacks a year, and there had been no recent change in this frequency. A careful interrogation revealed certain unusual features in her auras. Both scotomata and paraesthesiae were *invariably* confined to the right side of the visual field and body—the patient was emphatic that they had never occurred on the other side. Further, her paraesthesiae had on occasion remained unchanged and static for three hours, without showing any Jacksonian march. (It was pointed out, in the last chapter, that a single "sweep" of scotoma or paraesthesia normally takes 20 to 40 minutes.) In view of this minor but important divergence from the usual picture, further investigation was undertaken.

Skull X-rays showed a calcified mass in the left posterior hemisphere. Electroencephalography indicated a slow-wave focus, and brain-scan, an increased isotope-uptake in this region. Angiography revealed a massive parieto-occipital angioma in the left hemisphere.

Although it is not our intention to enter into the "differential diagnosis" of vascular headaches—a subject very adequately treated in many textbooks—we may emphasise, by means of a case-history, that conditions other than cerebral tumours, malformations or aneurysms may occasionally mimic migraines, or be mistaken for them:

Case 48   A 57-year-old woman developed a persistent and severe throbbing headache located in the left temple and eye. Her local physician diagnosed this as an "atypical migraine," although the patient had never previously suffered from headaches, and prescribed ergot drugs and tranquillisers for the patient. Since her symptoms failed to settle under this regimen, he referred her to me for further investigation. On examination, I found a tender and indurated left temporal artery, early papillitis and some diminution of central visual acuity. A sedimentation-rate was at once procured, and found to be 110 mm/hour (Westergren), and the presumptive diagnosis of "temporal arteritis" was made. The patient was at once placed on massive doses of prednisone, and the headache remitted within two days. There was, however, some permanent loss of visual acuity.

Case 50   A 50-year-old woman with occasional attacks of mild classical migraine—faint fortifications for a few minutes at most, sometimes followed by a vascular headache. Recently, however, she had a very different attack: she awoke with "flashing lights all over . . . shimmering lights . . . arcs of lighting," and a throbbing left-sided headache. She presumed this was another of her migraines. The visual phenomena, however, did not clear as they usually did in a few minutes, but continued all day, and all the next day too. Towards the end of this second day they became more complex in character; she seemed to see, in the upper part of the visual field to the right, "a writhing form . . . like a Monarch caterpillar, black and yellow, its cilia glistening," and then "incandescent yellow lights, like a Broadway sign, going up and down." She still considered herself, and was considered by her doctor, at this time, to be having an unusually severe and protracted migraine. Other hallucinations appeared the next day: "The bathtub seemed to be crawling with ants, there were cobwebs covering the walls and ceiling . . . people seemed to have lattices on their faces." Perceptual and agnosic problems appeared: "My husband's legs looked short, distorted . . . like some sort of trick mirror . . . everyone in the market looked grotesque—parts of their faces were gone." And, on the ninth day, she found she could see nothing to the right. At this time she was found to be hemianopic, and to have suffered a stroke involving the left occipital lobe. In this rather tragic case, the existence of genuine classical migraine attacks at first deflected attention from the possibility of a much more serious, apoplectic "pseudo-migraine."

PERMANENT NEUROLOGICAL OR VASCULAR DAMAGE
FROM MIGRAINE

Many patients and some physicians entertain considerable apprehension regarding the likelihood of permanent residual damage from migraine, an apprehension fanned by rare but dramatic case-reports (which may be reproduced or distorted in the popular press).

Many of these case-reports have probably inculpated migraine as a cause for cerebrovascular accidents, while failing to take into account the possibilities of concomitant hypertension, vascular pathology or co-incidence. There *are*, however, a number of case-reports (the subject has been reviewed by Dunning (1942) and Bruyn (1972), among others) in which the relation of vascular mishaps to attacks of migraine cannot be doubted. The term "complicated migraine" is sometimes used for such attacks in which neurological deficits lasting twenty-four hours or more occur in consequence of cerebral, retinal, or brainstem infarction. Such strokes or infarctions have even occurred in young people without de-monstrable cerebrovascular disease—the role of edema of the arterial wall, diminished blood flow and increased coagulability of blood have been postulated by various authors (Rascol *et al.*, 1979).

Nevertheless, it cannot be stated too strongly that such permanent residues are *surpassingly rare*. My own experience, no less than a perusal of the literature, has assured me of this: I have interrogated and exam-ined more than twelve hundred patients with migraine, and none of them has ever experienced any permanent damage from a migraine. For all its miseries, migraine is an essentially benign and reversible condition, and it is imperative to reassure all patients of this.

FIVE

The Structure of Migraine

We have now surveyed the major patterns of migraine, in all their bewildering variety and heterogeneity. We must pause, at this point, to take stock, and to simplify. A clear-cut definition of migraine retreats before us as we advance into the subject, but we are equipped now to formulate a number of general statements, and to trace the basic design or *structure* of migraine, as this underlies its innumerable clinical expressions and permutations.

We have observed that all migraines are composed of many symptoms (and physiological alterations) proceeding in unison: at each and every moment the structure of migraine is *composite*. Thus, a common migraine is fabricated of many components surrounding the cardinal and defining symptom of headache. Migraine equivalents are composed of essentially similar components aggregated and emphasised in other ways. The structure of migraine aura is similarly composite. Given the components a, b, c . . . we may encounter innumerable combinations and permutations of these: a plus b, a plus c, a plus b plus c, b plus c . . . etc.

Beneath these variable and disjunctive components, we may recognise the occurrence of other, relatively stable features, occurring in constant conjunction: these constitute, as it were, the *core* of the migraine structure. It is in the middle range—between the vegetative disturbances and the cortical disturbances—that the *essential* features of migraine may be found: alterations of conscious level, of muscular tonus, of sensory vigilance, etc. We may subsume these under a single term: they represent disorders of *arousal*. In extremely severe attacks, the degree of arousal occurring in the earlier or prodromal stages of the migraine may proceed to agitation or even frenzy, while the ensuing stages may be marked by a subsidence into lethargy or even stupor. In milder attacks the disorders of arousal may be overshadowed by the presence of pain or other florid symptoms, and thus be overlooked by patient and physician. Disorders of arousal, mild or severe, appear to be invariable features of all migraines.

Each stage in the course of a migraine is marked by the concurrence of symptoms at *different functional levels,* in particular the concurrence of physical and of emotional symptoms. These cannot be described in terms of one another: each level must be described by a language appropriate to it. Thus migraine is conspicuously a psychophysiological event, and requires for its understanding a sort of mental diplopia (to adopt Jackson's term) and a double language. The most primitive symptoms of migraine are both physical *and* emotional: thus *nausea,* for example, is both a sensation and a "state of mind" (the literal and figurative uses of the word nausea are of equal antiquity); nausea is in the region where the separateness of sensations and emotions has not yet been established. More complex symptoms have become dichotomised, so to speak, so that we may recognise, at every stage throughout an attack, a constant concomitance and paralleling of physical and emotional symptoms. We may, for example, portray the sequence of a typical (prototype) migraine in terms of the following five stages:

(1) The initial *excitement* or excitation of an attack (provided either externally by a provocative stimulus, or internally by an aura), in which the emotional aspects may be experienced as rage, elation, etc., and the physiological aspects as sensory hyperacusis, scintillating scotomata, paraesthesiae, etc.

(2) A state of *engorgement* (sometimes termed the prodrome, sometimes simply the earlier stages of an attack), characterised by the occurrence of visceral distension and stasis, vascular dilatation, faecal retention, fluid retention, muscular tension, etc., and, concurrently with these symptoms, feelings of emotional tension, anxiety, restlessness, irritability, etc.

(3) A state of *prostration* (frequently isolated by medical observation, and termed the "attack proper"), in which the affective experience is one of apathy, depression, and retreat, while its physical concomitants

are experienced as nausea, malaise, drowsiness, faintness, muscular slackness and weakness, etc.

(4) The state of recovery or *resolution*, which may be achieved abruptly (crisis) or gradually (lysis). In the case of the former, there may occur a violent visceral ejaculation, such as vomiting or sneezing, or a sudden excess of emotion, or both together; in the case of the latter, a variety of secretory activities (diuresis, diaphoresis, involuntary weeping, etc.) are accompanied by a concurrent melting away, or catharsis, of the existing emotional symptoms.

(5) A stage of *rebound* (if the attack has been brief and compact), in which feelings of euphoria and renewed energy are accompanied by great physical well-being, increased muscular tonus and alertness: generalised arousal.

This remarkable synchronisation of affect and somatic symptoms allows us to define the psychophysiological state of a migraine, at any given time, in terms of mood and of autonomic status (or, more accurately, arousal or nervous "tuning": concepts considered fully in Chapter 11). Thus we can conveniently depict the typical course of a migraine on a "map" in which affect and arousal have been selected as co-ordinates (Figure 6).

We may comment very briefly on the type of relation which may exist between these somatic and emotional symptoms of a migraine, while deferring full consideration of this topic until much later (Chapter 13). When considering the problem of fluid retention in migraine attacks, we noted Wolff's conclusions, based on painstaking experiment, that fluid retention and vascular headache were concomitant but not causally related to each other; the same is largely true of concomitant emotional and somatic symptoms. Their concurrence, if it cannot be explained in terms of direct causality (the physical symptoms causing the emotional symptoms, or vice versa), must either be traced to a common antecedent cause, or to a symbolic linkage. No other possibilities exist.

We must return now to the general problem of categorising the migraine experience, and formulating more exactly its relation to idiopathic epilepsy, fainting, vagal attacks, acute affective disturbances, etc., with which we have repeatedly noted its affinities. The terms of this formulation, at this stage, can only be clinical ones.

We recognise a migraine as being constituted by certain symptoms of

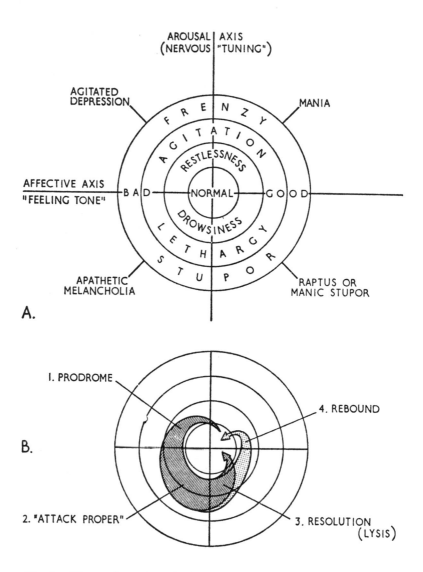

Fig. 6.   The configuration of migraine, in relation to mood and arousal

The psychophysiological shape or configuration of a prototypic migraine represented as a function of nervous "tuning" (degree of arousal) and affect. The contours of migraines and many other complex paroxysmal phenomena are conveniently inscribed on a map of this type.

a certain duration in a certain sequence. The structure of a migraine is extremely variable, but it is variable in only three ways. Firstly, the entire course of the attack is variable in *length*: the overall structure of a migraine may be condensed or extended (it is in this sense that Gowers speaks of vagal attacks as extended epilepsies): secondly, the course of an attack may be enacted at a variety of *levels* in the nervous system— from the level of cortical hallucinations to that of peripheral autonomic disturbances: thirdly, the symptoms at each level may present themselves in many different *combinations and permutations*. Therefore, instead of conceiving migraine as a very specific and stereotyped event, we must rather envisage a broad *region* encompassing the entire repertoire of migraine and migraine-like attacks; within this region, the migraine structure may be modulated in duration, in "vertical level" and in "collateral level," to use Jackson's terms.

The sequence of a full-fledged migraine (i.e. one which is not prematurely terminated, and of which the inaugural stages are recognised) has essentially two stages: a stage of excitation or arousal, followed by a protracted stage of inhibition or "derousal."

It is in these terms that we may first perceive the proximity of the migraine cycle to that of epilepsy, on the one hand, and to the more leisurely cycles of waking and sleep, on the other; the prominent affective components of migraines demand comparison, more remotely, with the excitatory and inhibitory phases of some psychoses. We have observed the occurrence of many transitional states between all of these: the occurrence of "migralepsies," insomniac and hypomanic states preceding migraines and epilepsies, dreamlike and nightmarish auras, apathetic depression during the inhibitory stage of migraine, the occurrence of somnolent and stuporous migraines, the inauguration of migraines during sleep, their abortion by brief sleep, and, finally, the long deep sleep which characteristically follows severe migraines and epilepsies. In all cases we may see the inhibitory states as morbid variations or caricatures of normal sleep, following upon inordinate excitations (migrainous prodromes and excitements, epileptic convulsions, psychotic agitations), as normal sleep succeeds the activities of the waking day. Gowers placed migraines, faints, sleep-disorders, etc., in the "borderland" of epilepsy; we can with equal justice reverse his words, and locate migraine and migraine-like reactions in the borderland of sleep.

It is important to observe that migraine is no more a suspension of all physical and mental activities than sleeping, or psychotic stupors; it is charged, on the contrary, with activities of an inward, private kind.

Inhibition at one level releases excitations at other levels. The diminution of motor activity and external ties during a migraine is matched by a great increase in internal activities, vegetative symptoms and their attendant, regressive affects—a paradoxical combination of inner violence and outer detachment—analogous to the dreaming of paradoxical sleep, or the concealed agitations and hallucinations of psychotic stupors.

Gowers, observing the gradual or sudden transformations of one type of migraine into another, or of migraines into epilepsies, fainting attacks, etc. concluded: ". . . We can perceive the mysterious relation, but we cannot explain it." We can do no more, at this stage, than point out that all such attacks share a certain formal resemblance in structure, merging into one another, and into the region of migraine. We cannot explore the "mysterious relation" any further without considering the *functions* of migraine and of other paroxysmal reactions which may take its place. We must move ahead, therefore, and learn when and why migraines occur.

PART II

The Occurrence of Migraine

Introduction

Many patients consider their migraines to occur "spontaneously" and without cause. Such a view leads, scientifically, to absurdity, emotionally, to fatalism, and therapeutically, to impotence. We must assume that all attacks of migraine have real and discoverable determinants, however difficult their elucidation may be.

The determinants of migraine are almost infinite in number, and may present themselves in many different combinations. We may simplify their discussion, as Willis did three centuries ago, by distinguishing predisposing, exciting and accessory causes of migraine. Thus among these Willis recognised the following determinants:

> An evil or weak constitution of the parts . . . sometimes innate and heredi-tary . . . an irritation in some distant member or viscera . . . changes of season, atmospheric states, the great aspects of the sun and moon, violent passions, and errors in diet . . .

We can never predict the occurrence of a migraine with certainty, but our inability to do so reflects only the limitations of our knowledge. It may indeed be certain that if conditions a, b, c, d . . . etc. are fulfilled, that a migraine will inevitably follow, but we are rarely if ever in possession of *all* the relevant knowledge. Thus we are reduced to speaking in terms of propensities and probabilities.

Chapter 6 is devoted to consideration of factors which predispose an individual to migraine, as far as these can be determined on clinical grounds. In Chapter 7 we discuss "idiopathic" migraine, attacks which tend to come periodically, or at irregular intervals, irrespective of the external circumstances of living; the exciting factors, in such cases, must be seen as internal ones related to inherent instabilities and periodicities in the nervous system. Chapter 8 is concerned with the many external circumstances—physical, physiological and emotional—which can excite migraine attacks in predisposed patients: such circumstances often bear an obvious one-to-one relationship to the occurrence of each attack. In Chapter 9 we explore the most important accessory cause of migraines, powerful emotional needs and stresses denied direct expression or resolution, which may force predisposed patients into a pattern of repeated migraines.

The Predisposition to Migraine

We are accustomed to think of any particular response as
either learned or innate, which is apt to be a source of
confusion in thinking about such things. . . . Is the response
inherited, or acquired? The answer is, Neither: either Yes or
No would be very misleading.

Hebb

If we say of X that he is an epileptic, we make two assertions, that he
has seizures, and that he has a propensity towards seizures. The latter
is considered to be inherent within him; we may label this inherent propensity an epileptic predisposition, diathesis or constitution. It may further be considered that his predisposition is not only inherent, but
immutable ("once an epileptic, always an epileptic"), and as such con-
demn him to a lifetime of caution, anti-convulsants, driving restrictions,
etc. A correlate of these assumptions may be the identification of pathognomonic "signs" of an epileptic constitution—epileptic stigmata.

These propositions are of great historical antiquity, and receive only
partial support from admissible data; such truth as they do contain is
clearly inflated by emotional bias. Similar assertions are frequently made
with regard to "schizophrenic predisposition," and these too must be,
and have been, subjected to the most critical scrutiny. These two examples may serve to introduce the subject of migraine predisposition which,
if it lacks the pejorative undertones of the commonly held opinions on
epileptic or schizophrenic predisposition, will reveal itself as even more
complex in its implications.

The notion of migraine predisposition rests on three groups of data:
first and foremost, studies on the familial incidence of migraine, and
subsidiary to this, studies designed to expose pathognomonic signs of
the diathesis, and to discover substrative "factors" or "traits" in migrainous and pre-migrainous populations. The basic assumption, of course,
is that migraine is a clearly-defined "disease" analogous, for example,

to sickle-cell disease which will occur in persons with sickle-cell trait, and only in such persons, when certain other conditions are fulfilled.

THE OVERALL INCIDENCE OF MIGRAINE

Headache is the commonest complaint which patients bring to physicians, and migraine is the commonest functional disorder by which patients are afflicted. Figures are only available on the incidence of migraine headache (cephalgic migraine), and these vary between estimates of 5 per cent and 20 per cent for its incidence in the general population. Balyeat (1933) found an incidence of 9.3 per cent in a population of almost 3,000 persons whom he interrogated. Lennox and Lennox (1960) found that migraine headache occurred in 6.3 per cent of medical students, nurses and non-epileptic patients whom they questioned. Fitz-Hugh's (1940) figure is as high as 22 per cent. Many further figures are cited and discussed in Wolff's monograph.

A general observation must be made concerning all such incidence figures. The terms of interrogation exclude many categories of patient and of migraine, e.g. those whose attacks are infrequent and unremembered, those whose attacks are mild and undiagnosed, and, not least, the many patients who experience attacks of migraine equivalent or isolated auras, and for this reason are not considered in the same frame of reference. We may assert that a substantial minority, perhaps one-tenth, of the population experience fairly common and readily-recognised cephalgic migraines. We may suspect that many more experience occasional or mild migraines, migraine equivalents, or migraine auras. Certain forms of migraine, it would seem, are much rarer. It has been stated that the incidence of classical migraine is not above 1 per cent in the general population (probably an underestimate); migrainous neuralgia is rarer still, and the hemiplegic and ophthalmoplegic forms of migraine are excessively rare, and are unlikely to be seen in a lifetime of practice by the average general physician.

FAMILIAL OCCURRENCE AND INHERITANCE OF MIGRAINE

It has long been held, and with good reason, that migraine has a strong tendency to run in certain families, and there are innumerable clinical and statistical studies which substantiate this fact. Lennox (1941), reviewing a massive population of patients with migraine (headache), noted that 61 per cent of them described a parent as having been affected with migraine, whereas only 11 per cent of a control group reported close familial involvement. Friedman has estimated that 65 per cent of migraine sufferers seen in a headache clinic give a family history of migraine. The *fact* of frequent familial incidence is indisputable; the interpretation of this fact is far from clear.

The most ambitious and the most sophisticated of these comparative statistical studies is that of Goodell, Lewontin, and Wolff (1954). These workers selected for study 119 patients with "severe headaches recurring usually over many years," and submitted all of these to close interrogation with regard to the incidence of migraine headaches in other members of their families (no distinction was made, for the purposes of this enquiry, between classical and common migraine). It was found, in a comparison of the offspring in these migrainous families, that 28.6 per cent of those with neither parent affected had migraine, 44.2 per cent of those with one migrainous parent had migraine, and 69.2 per cent of those with both parents affected had migraine. Goodell *et al.*, comparing the observed with the expected incidence in the 832 offspring considered, concluded that "there is less than one chance in a thousand that such deviations [from the expected incidence] would occur if the assumption of no inheritance were true . . . Furthermore, it is reasonable to assume that migraine is due to a recessive gene whose penetrance is approximately 70 per cent."

We must regard this conclusion as highly suspect and even absurd, despite the thoroughness and elegance of the study. There are at least three hidden assumptions of considerable dubiety, the first relating to sampling, the second to the homogeneity of the population studied, and the third, the most important, to the necessarily ambiguous interpretation of any study of this type. Firstly, only patients with severe, recurrent, long-standing migraine headache were studied, and interrogation concerning affected relatives was similarly framed in terms of these criteria. It is clear, therefore, that if mild or unremembered or infrequent attacks of migraine headache had occurred, or if migraine equivalent or migraine aura had instead been present, the figures of incidence might be very different from the ones obtained. Secondly, it is assumed, wholly without justification, that the population considered was genetically homogeneous with regard to migraine, i.e. that all migraines considered, whether of classical, common, or any other type, were genetically equivalent for purposes of the study. Thirdly, and most crucially, *familial incidence does not necessarily imply inheritance.* A family is not only a source of

genes but an environmental circumstance of enormous potency.[28] Goodell *et al.* are not unaware of this reservation but they do not take it
seriously. It must, however, be taken extremely seriously in view of the
evidence (to be discussed in later chapters) that migraine reactions are
readily adopted, learned, and emulated within the family environment.
A rigorous genetic study would have to concern itself with offspring of
migrainous parents reared by non-migrainous foster-parents, or, ideally,
with the incidence of migraine in identical twins separated at birth. No
method less stringent is adequate to distinguish the effects of "nature"
versus "nurture" in a reaction as complex and multiply-determined as
migraine. Without such controls, statistical studies of migraine (as of
schizophrenia) cannot claim to do more than quantify what one already
knows, that migraine tends to be commoner in certain families. They
cannot establish any genetic basis, let alone so elementary (and inher-
ently improbable) a basis as a single gene with partial penetrance.

If the ambiguities of sampling and symptom-variability are reduced,
and if particularly rare forms of migraine are studied, the likelihood of
a hereditary basis may be more plausibly stated. Thus classical migraine
is, roughly, ten times rarer than common migraine, yet tends to show a
more dramatic familial occurrence. Hemiplegic migraine, which can
hardly be overlooked or forgotten, tends to remain "true to type," and
is exceedingly rare in the general population, is almost always found in
the context of heavy familial involvement (Whitty, 1953).[29]

The matter is of more than academic importance, for if a patient
regards himself as "doomed" to a lifetime of migraine in view of a sinister family background of the disorder, and his physician takes an
equally fatalistic view of the matter, the chances of any therapeutic intervention are much reduced. Lennox and Lennox, usually most reasonable, write "Persons with migraine should think twice before marrying
one whose own or whose family history is positive for this disorder."
This statement, in view of the degree of doubt concerning genetic factors,
and the overwhelming importance of environmental factors, is little short
of monstrous.

[28] An instructive example of "pseudo-heredity" in the determination of complex psychophysiological reactions is Friedman's finding that not only 65 per cent of migraine
patients, but 40 per cent of patients with tension-headaches, give a family history of their
respective symptoms. It has never been suggested (nor is it likely to be suggested) that
tension-headaches have a genetic basis, but clearly they are adopted in households where
this is the family "style."
[29] While revising the proofs of this book, I have had occasion to see a patient with
hemiplegic migraine who has four siblings, a parent, an uncle and a first cousin similarly
affected.

SIGNS OF THE MIGRAINOUS CONSTITUTION

We will coalesce, for purposes of discussion, the two other grounds on which the notion of a specific migrainous predisposition is based—the clinical observation of "signs," and the experimental observation of "factors," supposedly diagnostic of migraineurs. Our discussion will do little more than allude to such signs and factors at this stage, for we reserve until later (Chapters 10 and 11) a detailed critique of current experimental work on the subject.

We understand by the term sign, in this context, a clinical characteristic which is highly correlated with the tendency to migraine, and which therefore occurs with exceptional frequency in most migraine patients and many of their relatives. Some such signs will be regarded as an integral part of the migraine constitution, and other signs may have a fortuitous but exceptionally common linkage with the tendency to migraine. The concealed assumption, in all cases, is that there is a unitary genetic basis—Wolff speaks of a "stock factor"—underlying migraine. Thus, to cite a particularly fantastic example of an alleged migrainous trait:

> Further evidence of the stock factor in migraine [writes Wolff] is reported by Erik Ask-Upmark, who made the interesting observation that out of 36 patients subject to migraine headache attacks, 9 had inverted nipples, as compared with 65 persons who were not subject to migraine, in whom there was only one instance of inverted nipples.

The majority of such observations, or theories, envisage a constitutional type with particular physical and emotional characteristics as especially or uniquely prone to migraine. Thus Tourraine and Draper (1934) speak of a "characteristic constitutional type" in which the skull shows acromegaloid traits, the intelligence is outstanding, but the emotional make-up is retarded. Alvarez (1959) discerns as prime characteristics of migrainous women:

> a small trim body with firm breasts. Usually these women dress well and move quickly. 95 per cent had a quick eager mind and much social attractiveness . . . Some 28 per cent were red-headed, and many had luxuriant hair . . . These women age well.

Greppi (1955) claims to perceive a migraine "ground," a particular psychophysiological constellation very common among, and peculiar to, sufferers from migraine:

... There is a certain delicacy or grace ... there are signs which indicate the development of an early intelligence and sensibility, of a critical and self-controlled temperament.

These accounts exemplify the "romantic" view of migrainous constitution. It is of more than historical interest that so many authors, from antiquity to the present day, are concerned to present so flattering a picture of the migraineur. Perhaps one may connect this tendency with the fact that most writers on migraine suffer from migraine. At all events, such descriptions are greatly at odds with the traditional accounts of epileptics and the epileptic constitution, with their menacing undertones of hereditary "taint" and constitutional "stigmata."

It is frequently stated that migraines are peculiar to a specific "migraine personality," which is usually portrayed as obsessive, rigid, driving, perfectionistic, etc. The adequacy of this concept may be measured by the clinical finding of exceedingly varied emotional backgrounds in migraine patients (see Chapter 9), and will receive critical discussion at a later stage (Chapter 13).

Some authors have stated that migraine patients may be placed in one or other of the four traditional psychophysiological categories (either Hippocratic or Pavlovian terms may be employed), a supposition which acquaintance with a handful of migraine patients should dispel. There is, however, some evidence that different styles of migraine may be commoner in particular constitutional types, as du Bois Reymond realised a century ago. Thus patients prone to "red" migraines tend to be overtly excitable and to flush with anger (they are, in Pavlov's terms, "strong excitable types," or "sympathotonic"), while other patients prone to "white" migraines tend to pallor, fainting, and withdrawal reactions in the face to emotional stimuli (being "weak inhibitory types" or "vagotonic"). But no general statement on the subject is applicable to migraine patients in their entirety.

Other workers have suggested that the tendency to migraine may be indicated by a variety of physiological parameters: a particular sensibility to passive motion, heat, exhaustion, and depressant drugs (e.g. alcohol and reserpine); exaggerated cardiovascular reflexes (e.g. pathological carotid sinus sensitivity); anatomical or functional "microcirculatory disorder"; the prevalence of slow-wave cerebral dysrhythmias; and a variety of metabolic and chemical dysfunctions. We can do no more, at the present stage, than state that none of these factors have been shown to be of critical relevance to migraine patients as an overall group, although certain of them may show consistent variations in particular sub-groups of migraine sufferers.

MIGRAINE DIATHESIS AND OTHER DISORDERS

The notion that there may exist, and the search for, other disorders correlated and connected with migraine diathesis is no more than a logical extension of the considerations already raised, but there are a variety of specific issues which demand separate consideration. The area is one of doubt and dispute, partly on questions of fact, partly on questions of interpretation (particularly the interpretation of statistical correlations) and, not least, on questions of nomenclature and semantics.

Opinions on the most basic issues range very widely. Critchley (1963), our foremost authority on the subject, states:

> . . . in early childhood, a migrainous constitution may manifest itself in the form of infantile eczema; a little later as travel sickness. At a slightly older age it can show itself as recurrent spells of vomiting . . . Are migraine victims more or less likely to develop peptic ulcers, coronary disease, rheumatoid arthritis, or colitis? My clinical impression . . . is that there exists a sort of negative correlation. Lifelong migraine seems to confer a sort of protection against the subsequent development of other stress disorders.

Graham and Wolff, on the other hand, see migraine populations as exceptionally prone to a variety of other disorders. Thus Graham (1952), tabulating the ills of 46 migraine patients, found that over half suffered from motion-sickness, more than a third from allergic manifestations, and a third from additional, muscle-contraction headaches. Further, their family histories were heavily weighted with epilepsy (10 per cent), allergies (30 per cent), arthritis (29 per cent), hypertension (60 per cent), cerebrovascular accidents (40 per cent), and "nervous breakdowns" (34 per cent).

Wolff (1963) approaching the question from the opposite end found complaints of headache (vascular or muscle-contraction) especially frequent in sufferers from functional heart disease, essential hypertension, vasomotor rhinitis, upper respiratory infections, hayfever and asthma, gastro-intestinal dysfunctions (duodenal ulcer, etc.) and "psychoneuroses." How are we to reconcile Critchley's image of migraineurs as privileged sufferers, enjoying a sort of immunity against other disorders, with the pessimistic vision of Graham and Wolff who portray them as laden with innumerable ills? And if such negative and positive correlations indeed exist, how shall we interpret them?

Before embarking on any general discussion, we must enquire more minutely into the evidence which is available concerning the correlation of migraine with specific disorders. There is general agreement that a history of motion-sickness, cyclic vomiting, or bilious attacks, in the earlier years of life is exceptionally common among migraine sufferers, although such tendencies and attacks are "replaced" by the adult migraines, for the most part rather rarely continuing their original intensity throughout life. Provided any statement correlating motion-sickness and migraine is a purely statistical one based on a large population, it cannot be gainsaid. If, however, one departs from a statistical approach and concerns oneself only with individual case-histories, it is at once obvious that many patients with migraine (especially those with classical migraine) never experienced motion-sickness or visceral eruptions in their earlier years, and may, indeed, have been exceptionally resistant even to stimuli which produce nausea in a majority of the population; conversely, it is obvious that many children who suffer (enjoy?) cyclic vomiting, motion-sickness and bilious attacks never develop "adult" migraines later in their lives.

The facts—or, rather, the quoted figures, with their attendant sources of error—are less clear concerning the correlation of migraine with hypertension, allergies, epilepsy, etc., and we will do no more than cite a handful of investigations from the many hundreds which burden the literature. Gardner, Mountain and Hines (1940) found migraine five times more frequent in a hypertensive population than in a control group without hypertension. These authors display a proper reserve in interpreting their data, accepting as equally admissible the hypothesis of a common genetic factor and that of other shared factors (e.g. the prevalence of chronic inhibited rage amongst hypertensives and migraineurs). Balyeat (1933) was so struck with the incidence of allergic reactions in migraine patients and their families, that he took correlation for identity, and claimed that migraine *was* allergic in nature in many cases, a view which has since commanded an astonishing following, despite the fact that Wolff, and others, have shown in critical experiments that migraine is almost never allergic in origin. Lennox and Lennox (1960) have long been concerned with the taboo topic of constitutional relationships between migraine and epilepsy. They find (from a study of over 2,000 epileptics) that 23.9 per cent of these have a family history of migraine, a figure substantially in excess of such family histories secured from their control group. They conclude that migraine and epilepsy have not only a common "constitutional" basis, but a related genetic basis.

MIGRAINE IN RELATION TO AGE

Constitutional disorders usually manifest themselves relatively early in life. We must enquire whether this is true of migraine. Critchley (1933), in an early paper on the subject, stated: "A person is either afflicted with migrainous diathesis from an early age, or he is completely spared. He is unlikely to acquire the malady in adulthood . . ." There are many figures in the literature which would seem to contradict this supposition. Lennox and Lennox (1960), studying 300 patients with migraine, noted that 37.9 per cent had their inaugural attack in the third decade or later.

My own experience (with 1,200 migraine patients, the majority adult) has provided abundant confirmation of the frequency of late-onset migraines, and has further indicated the necessity of breaking down the overall group into smaller, clinically-homogeneous subgroups before any meaningful statement can be made. *Classical migraine* has perhaps the greatest propensity to present in youth or early adult life, but I have seen a dozen cases in which an initial attack occurred after the age of forty; the distinctiveness and severity of classical migraines are such that prior attacks would be unlikely to escape the memory. Onset in the middle years is far more frequent in the case of *common migraines*, and of these I have seen at least sixty cases presenting after the age of forty, and perhaps a fifth of these presenting after the age of fifty; this clinical pattern is particularly seen in women who may become the victims of migraine during or after the menopause. *Migrainous neuralgia*, above all, is notorious for its capacity to come on in later life; I have had one patient who experienced an initial "cluster" at the age of 98, and many cases of onset in the mid-seventies have been recorded in the literature. There is indisputably a general tendency for migraine to present early in life and dwindle in frequency in the later years, *ceteris paribus*, but this is a rule with frequent and important exceptions.

The concept of migraine diathesis carries the implication that migraine is, in some fashion, latent within the individual, until it is provoked to manifest itself. The following case-history illustrates how migraine may remain dormant for the greater part of a lifetime, only springing into action, so to speak, given an extraordinary environmental provocation:

Case 15   This patient, a 75-year-old woman, presented herself with the complaint of severe and frequent classical migraines. She had been experiencing
two to three attacks a week, each preceded by unmistakable fortification-figures and paraesthesiae. Her attacks had come on immediately following the
tragic death of her husband in a car accident. She admitted to being intensely
depressed and to entertaining suicidal thoughts. I asked her whether she had
ever had similar attacks before, and she replied that she had had exactly
similar attacks in childhood, but had not experienced one of these, to her
knowledge, for 52 years prior to her current paroxysm. Over the course of
some weeks the patient's depression lifted, with the combined influences of
time, psychotherapy, and anti-depressant drugs. She "became herself" once
more, and her classical migraines disappeared into the limbo where they had
been dormant for half a century.

A further case-history emphasises, even more forcefully, that a migraine diathesis (granting its reality) may remain latent and unsuspected
until late in life:

Case 38   This patient was a 62-year-old woman who had suffered from headaches of overwhelming severity for four months. The first, indeed, was so
alarming that her husband, a physician, at once procured her admission to
hospital. The suspicion of a sub-arachnoid haemorrhage or intracranial lesion
was entertained, but all investigations were negative, and after three days the
attack subsided. A month later she suffered a similar attack, and a month
after this a third attack. At this stage I saw her in consultation. I questioned
the patient, a very intelligent and reliable witness, and she professed herself
certain that she had never experienced any symptoms resembling her current
periodic attacks. Struck by their monthly occurrence, I enquired whether she
had been placed on any drugs recently, and she at once mentioned that her
gynaecologist had placed her on a hormone preparation, four months before,
to be taken cyclically (the drug was a contraceptive oestrogen-progestogen
preparation prescribed for post-menopausal symptoms). A comparison of
dates revealed that each attack had occurred in the week intervening between
the cycles of hormone-administration. I advised her to try the effects of omitting the hormone. She did so, and experienced no further attacks.

GENERAL DISCUSSION AND CONCLUSIONS

This chapter, necessarily, has been one of statement and counter-state-
ment, of doubts, hesitations, and qualifications. We must now, in conclusion, consider the reasons for doubt which apply to statistical studies
on migraine predisposition, and the legitimate meanings which can still
be given to this concept.

Our first comments must bear on the *validity of sampling*. If statements concerning the frequency of this or that trait in a population are to be of any value or interest, the population must be a relatively homogeneous one. Such statements with reference to migraine are based on the assumption that migraine is a single disorder with a unitary basis. They present to us a variant of that fiction—the average man: the average migraineur is shown as a hypertensive perfectionist with one inverted nipple, multiple allergies, a background of motion-sickness, two-fifths of a peptic ulcer, and a first cousin with epilepsy. Actual clinical experience soon persuades anyone who works with migrainous patients that they are an exceedingly heterogeneous group. Some have classical migraines, some common: some have striking family histories, many have no family histories; some have allergies, some do not; some react to particular drugs, some do not; some are sensitive to alcohol or passive motion, some are not; some outgrow their attacks at a youthful age, others start them at a later age; some have red migraines and some white; some have prominent visceral components, and others chiefly cephalgic components; some are hyperactive, some are lethargic; some are obsessional, others are sloppy; some are brilliant, and some are simpletons . . . In short, migraine patients are as remarkable for their diversity as any other section of the population. Such heterogeneity of the population and the symptoms under survey may invalidate and render meaningless any statistical survey, and demand, for investigative purposes, that the clinical material be broken down into smaller and more homogeneous groups. If the data are disparate, they must not be put together for purposes of comparison. We cannot reconcile Critchley's clinical impression of negative correlation between migraine and other disorders with the positive correlations claimed by Graham, Wolff and others. What we must do is to question the value of any and all such general statements. It is clear to the observant physician (and Critchley has fully conceded this in his many clinical publications) that *some* migraine patients remain strikingly faithful to their migraines, apparently finding in these an adequate outlet and expression of whatever nervous instability or stress is driving them; other patients exhibit protean and sudden transformations from one migraine equivalent to another, or from migraine to asthma, faints, etc.; and a third group seem to have a wide-open psychosomatic maw, and embrace any and every functional disorder they can. In some the image of functional disease is fixed and held from an early stage of life, moored to something unchanging in physical reactivity or emotional demand; in others, continually modulated emotional stresses may play upon a xylophonic reactivity an endless series of illness variations.

Our second concern must be with the *validity of interpretation* of statistical correlations. Let us assume that a particular study has skirted sampling errors and emerged with a correlation coefficient, a figure denoting the coincidence of two factors, *a* and *b*. It may be inferred that *a* causes *b*, that *b* causes *a*, or that both share a common cause. All such inferences, particularly the last, are to be found in the literature on migraine predisposition: thus Balyeat sees allergy as causing migraine, some authors see migraine as causing or favouring cerebrovascular accidents, and a majority of workers hold to the hypothesis of a shared diathesis—Wolff's "stock factor"—which can express itself as migraine or as many other disorders. None of these inferences can be justified on statistical grounds alone. A correlation is no more than a figure of coincidence, and in itself implies no logical connection between the phenomena studied. If a particular group of patients show high incidence of both migraine and hypertension, there may be a dozen reasons for this, and the reasons for their hypertension have no necessary connection with the reasons for their migraine. The high incidence of allergic reactions in migraine patients is very generally conceded, but Balyeat's theory of an allergic causation of migraines is demonstrably in error. We have, in such a case, to fall back upon considerations of biological strategy and analogy, and simply say that allergic and migrainous reactions may serve similar purposes in the organism (see Chapter 12) and thus alternate or coexist as equivalent physiological options.

Our final concern is with the *validity of terms* which have been employed in this area: predisposition, diathesis, constitutional susceptibilities, stock factors, etc. We may accept, with some reservations, that a relatively specific predisposition may exist and be transmitted in cases of hemiplegic migraine and in many, though far from all, cases of classical migraine; but these entities are rare, and constitute less than one-tenth of the overall migraine population. We must express the strongest doubts as to whether there exists any specific predisposition to common migraine, let alone a universal "migraine diathesis." How then shall we explain the apparent limitation of migraine to a section of the population, and its emphasis in certain families?

We can accept no terms except the most vague and general ones at the present time. It seems clear that many migraine patients are distinguished by *something* which is present in greater degree than normal.

The repertoire of this something is very wide—has not Critchley said that it may manifest itself, in the earlier years, as infantile eczema, motion-sickness, and recurrent spells of vomiting? And to this short list we must add all the varieties of migraine which were considered in Part I of this book, and beyond these the many other paroxysmal reactions—faints, vagal attacks, etc.—with which migraines may coalesce or alternate. It is in these terms—of a multiply-determined reaction, with innumerable variations of form and apparently endless plasticity—that the concept of migrainous diathesis must be used, if it is to retain any meaning at all. Moreover, this something permits an infinite number of gradations so that the migraine population, far from being clearly defined and set apart, merges into the general population at every point. Everyone, every organism, must be considered to have the potential for reactions *qualitatively* akin to migraine (see Chapter 12), but this potential is exalted, as it were, and made specific in a particular fraction of the population.[30] The facile assumption of a "migraine diathesis" as something simple, specific, unitary, quantifiable, or reducible to elementary genetics explains nothing, answers nothing, and begs every question; worse still, it obscures the elucidation of the true determining factors of migraine—in the individual and in his environment—by the use of a contentless phrase. Certainly there is something in a migraine patient which makes him more liable to his attacks, but the definition of this something, this predisposition, will demand our exploration of a much wider field of reference than the genetic and statistical considerations which have been considered in this chapter.

If we hope to understand or treat a patient with migraine, we are likely to find the circumstances of his life-history to be of the greatest importance in having determined and shaped his symptoms; when we have exhaustively explored and weighed such environmental factors, we may legitimately speculate upon the possibilities of constitutional or hereditary factors. Painstaking exploration of clinical histories is indispensable if we are to avoid the temptations of purely theoretical concepts —migraine "diathesis," migraine "stock factor," single-gene inheri-

---

[30] "At one end of the series stand those extreme cases of whom one can say: These people would have fallen ill whatever happened, whatever they experienced . . . At the other end stand cases which call forth the opposite verdict—they would undoubtedly have escaped illness if life had not put such and such burdens on them. In the intermediate cases in the series, more or less of the disposing factor . . . is combined with more or less of the injurious impositions of life" (Freud, 1920, p. 356).

tance, etc.—which may be no more than fictions. We must adapt the words with which Freud closed a famous case-history:

> I am aware that expression has been given in many quarters to thoughts . . . which emphasise the hereditary, phylogenetically acquired factor . . . I am of the opinion that people have been far too ready to find room for them and ascribe importance to them . . . I consider that they are only admissible when one strictly observes the correct order of precedence, and, after forcing one's way through the strata of what has been acquired by the individual, comes at last upon traces of what has been inherited.

SEVEN

Periodic and Paroxysmal Migraines

MIGRAINE AND OTHER BIOLOGICAL CYCLES

Equilibrium in biological systems is achieved only by the continuous balancing of opposite forces. Frequently it is maintained homeostatically, by continuous small adjustments to a dynamic system. At other times, its achievement depends on profound alterations of the system occurring at intervals, cyclically or sporadically. Some of these cycles are universal, like the alternation of sleeping and waking, while others are manifest in only a fraction of the population, as with cycles of epilepsy, psychosis, and migraine. In all of these cases, the tendency to cycling is inherent in the nervous system, although the innate periodicity may be accessible to a variety of external influences. We will speak, therefore, of "periodic migraine" in considering attacks which occur at fairly regular intervals, *irrespective of the mode of life*, and of "paroxysmal migraines" in regard to apparently spontaneous attacks which occur at irregular or widely-separated intervals.

Periodicity, in this sense, may mark the pattern of any form of migraine, but is peculiarly characteristic of classical migraines and of cluster headache. In the case of common migraine and migraine equivalents, an inherent periodicity is less common, and the clinical pattern of attacks tends to be far more dependent on the external or emotional circumstances of the patient.

DURATION BETWEEN ATTACKS

The length of time between successive attacks of classical migraine is usually somewhere between 2 and 10 weeks, individual patients generally adhering fairly closely to their own time-patterns. Liveing cites the following figures:

> ... [of 35 patients with periodic migraine] in 9 cases the attacks returned once in a fortnight, and in 12 once a month; while intervals of 2 to 3 months prevailed in 7. The remaining 7 comprised exceptionally long or short periods.

Comparable figures were found by Klee (1968) in his series of 150 carefully-documented cases, 33 per cent of patients having migraines at intervals of less than 1 month, 20 per cent of patients having migraines at intervals of 4 to 8 weeks, 26 per cent at intervals of 8 to 12 weeks, and the remaining 21 per cent at intervals of 3 months or more. My own experience of the incidence-patterns of classical migraine is in accordance with these findings. It must be stressed, however, that crude incidence-figures of this type may be ambiguous or even meaningless, unless care has been taken to exclude the effects of periodically-recurring external or emotional circumstances provocative of migraines: we will later make reference to some determinants of a "pseudo-periodicity" of this type.

The grouping of common migraines, if the effects of adventitious circumstances can be excluded, tends to be more closely packed than that of classical migraines. A number of severely affected patients may have two or more attacks weekly, a frequency which would be most unusual in the case of classical migraine. We may note, in passing, that very frequent periodic common migraines show a striking tendency towards nocturnal occurrence. Patients who experience periodic common migraines only once a month (as in du Bois Reymond's case, quoted at the start of the first chapter) may often account themselves relatively lucky. Often but not always, for there appears to be a tendency towards a reciprocal relation between the frequency and the severity of such attacks, widely-spaced attacks being correspondingly more severe. One of Liveing's patients expressed this concisely, and with a certain moral undertone, writing:

> I have long ceased to care for longer intervals; I know that I have a *certain quantity of suffering* which I must go through, however it is broken up or divided, and I would as soon have it regularly as not.[31]

[31]Similar sentiments are often expressed by patients with manic-depressive cycles. Such cycles represent not only physiological and chemical alterations in the body, but *moral cycles* also, with exemption from the harsher dictates of conscience during periods of elation, and an exaggeration of conscience in the self-hating, self-accusing periods of de-

The same point is brought out in Klee's careful statistical study. Thus, one may envisage the overall severity of migraine, in many patients, as the product of severity and frequency of attacks, and the "certain quantity of suffering" of which Liveing's patient speaks as a *volume* of migraine divisible into various aliquots.

We may also consider cluster headache as a form of periodic migraine, provided that we regard the entire cluster (which may comprise a hundred individual attacks of migrainous neuralgia) as a single monstrous attack of migraine. The interval between clusters is far longer than that between common and classical migraines: an average interval might be a year, and the range of intervals will lie between three months and five years. Some clusters, it may be added, occur at annual intervals almost to the day.

Bizarre patterns of intermittency are sometimes seen, as in the following case, unique in my experience, which shows periodic clustering of common migraines:

Case 52   A 55-year-old man of serene disposition who has experienced annual "sieges" of common migraine for 19 years. For a period of 4 to 6 weeks, he is utterly incapacitated by almost daily attacks of great severity and considerable duration (12 to 20 hours). These attacks are characterised by bilateral vascular headache, intense nausea, repeated vomiting, and many other autonomic symptoms, viz. in no sense resemble attacks of migrainous neuralgia. The siege begins and ends suddenly, for no apparent reason, and the patient is wholly exempt from migraine for the remainder of the year.

The most irregular patterns of occurrence are seen in some cases of classical migraine, and especially of isolated migraine auras. I have had a number of such patients who may have gone for 6, 12 or 30 months without an attack, only to have a sudden "bad period" with three or four attacks in quick succession (such headaches are not uncommon in some epileptics).

IMMUNITY BETWEEN ATTACKS

There is, characteristically, a time of absolute immunity to further attack following every severe attack of periodic migraine, as du Bois Reymond has reminded us:[32]

---

pression. The depression is often felt to be payment for the mania, as a vicious migraine may be anticipated after a protracted exemption from pain.

[32] Perhaps the most dramatic example of post-ictal immunity is seen with reference to cluster headache. During the cluster, patients may be exquisitely sensitive to the taking of alcohol; following the cluster, they can immediately take quantities of alcohol without

. . . For a certain period after the attack I can expose myself with impunity to influences which before would have infallibly produced an attack.

The immunity diminishes by degrees, and the likelihood of the next attack increases commensurately. Following the termination of absolute immunity, gross provocations may elicit a (somewhat premature) attack. As the relative immunity grows less, more and more trifling stimuli may suffice to detonate the impending attack. Finally, when the attack is "due" (or a little overdue), it *will* occur, explosively, whether or not there is any provocation.

Essentially similar cycles of sensitivity and immunity to attack are seen in many cases of idiopathic epilepsy and asthma. In each case, on a different time-scale, one must envisage the same form of graduated refractoriness and sudden discharge which is characteristic of all biological cycles, from the millisecond intermittency of nerve-impulses to the annual sheddings of leaves and skins.

APPROACH OF THE ATTACK

Periodic migraines, more clearly than others, especially if they are severe and infrequent, tend to have clear-cut prodromal symptoms, restlessness, irritability, constipation, water retention, etc., before common or classical migraines, and sometimes a peculiar form of burning or local discomfort before the onset of a cluster attack (as in Case 7). Patients with extremely infrequent severe attacks may experience other forms of physiological premonition for some days before the actual attack, as tiny seismic disturbances may signal the approach of a major earthquake. Thus one patient (Case 16), who experienced attacks of classical migraine every year or two, observed luminous spots darting across his visual field for two to three days before each attack. Other patients may suffer from myoclonic jerks, chiefly at night, for a day or two before each rare attack, a symptom which is shared by some epileptics.

PSEUDO-PERIODICITY

We have set apart periodic migraines, somewhat arbitrarily, as expressions of an inherent cyclical process in the nervous system. In practice,

---

ill-effects. The approach of a subsequent cluster may be signalled, before any spontaneous attacks of pain, by the recurrence of alcohol-sensitivity and mild alcohol-induced attacks.

we may encounter considerable difficulty in demarcating the effects of innate neuronal periodicity from those of other internal cycles (physiological or emotional) or of undiscovered external cycles. We may demonstrate these ambiguities by a few clinical examples.

A colleague of mine, who suffers from migrainous neuralgia, affirms that his attacks wake him at exactly 3 o'clock every morning, and that, if necessary, he could set his watch by this. Shall we ascribe such attacks to some idiosyncratic Circadian cycle in his nervous system, to some occult physiological cycle elsewhere in the body, to the chiming of a distant clock causing a migrainous conditioned reflex, or to some dark childhood memory (the witnessing of a primal scene) associated with this dangerous hour? A patient of mine (Case 10), who has been subject for many years to monthly attacks of classical migraine, occasionally replaced by abdominal migraine or violent mood-disturbance, insisted that his attacks always coincided with a full moon, and produced a remarkable diary in support of this. When he gave me his history, I recalled the old words of Willis, about ". . . the great aspects of the sun and moon" as determinants of migraine. The patient appeared obsessed by his lunar migraines, but whether the moon caused the migraine, and the migraine the obsession, or whether the obsession caused the migraine, I could not distinguish. An uncanny periodicity may also characterise "anniversary migraines" which are analogous to anniversary neuroses. I think, in this context, of one patient, a nun, who professed to have a classical migraine every Good Friday, a contemporary version of Easter stigmata. Personal anniversaries—of birthdays, marriages, disasters and traumas, etc.—not infrequently determine strictly periodic attacks of migraine, or of other functional illnesses.

One of the recurring themes of this book is that migraines are enacted at many simultaneous levels, and that their machinery, similarly, may be set in motion at any or every level. Although the precipitant of periodic, idiopathic migraines is, by definition, a neuronal one, we must allow that equally effective trigger-mechanisms may exist at many other levels, from local segmental reflexes which have assumed a tic-like sensitivity, to recurrent stimuli at the highest level, in the forms of obsessive expectations, recapitulative phantasies, etc. Whether the clockwork is originally at a cellular level (as in allergic reactions), at a molecular level, at the level of cerebral periodicities, or at the level of motive and emotion, may subsequently become irrelevant, for the periodicity of the attacks may finally become immanent and *entrenched* at every functional level. Such considerations suggest themselves with particular force in the interpretation of menstrual migraines, in which it is most useful to regard the migraine, not as a response to a single isolated "factor," but as a reflector of many simultaneous periodicities—of hormone level, of fundamental physiological and biological periodicities, *and* of concurrent moods and motives. Any one of these, one may suspect, may on occasion perpetuate the periodic pattern, as is implied in the following history:

Case 74   This 68-year-old woman had experienced menstrual migraines, and no others, since the age of 21. Her menopause, 30 years later, made no difference to the pattern, her attacks continuing to occur at 28- to 30-day intervals.

CONCLUSIONS

The forms of migraine considered in this chapter illustrate, *par excellence*, the Willisian notion of "idiopathy," sudden explosions set off in a charged and waiting nervous system. Liveing's term "nerve-storms" is an incomparable metaphor, for one cannot avoid visualising the slow gathering of forces and tensions in the nervous system, the sudden breaking of an electrical storm, the ensuing serenity and clear skies.

In attacks of this type, the entire migraine—from the first coruscation of the aura, or first intimation of prodromal excitation, to the last echoes following the resolution of the attack—presents itself as an integral unit; it is, so to speak, preformed and complete, with an irresistible tendency to move through its course until it dies away and permits the establishment of a new (if temporary) physiological equilibrium. Periodic and paroxysmal migraines are difficult to avert and difficult to abort, but in return promise an ensuing immunity of substantial length. They also tend, in their symptoms and styles, to be the most stereotyped of all migraines, the least tailored to circumstantial considerations, and the least flavoured with emotional undertones and strategies. They are *precipitated*, abruptly and completely, from physiological solution, in a manner reminiscent of a sudden crystallisation from a supersaturated solution. They mark the climax and ending of a physiological season; the attack is *dehisced*, like the bursting of ripe fruit, so that the cycle may start into motion again.

POSTSCRIPT (1992)

Willis's notion of "explosion," Liveing's of "nerve-storms," Gowers's of "convulsiveness"—all of these are images of instability, criticality, singularity, images of intensely critical states or configurations in the nervous system, points at which the slightest stimulus can have a catastrophic effect. The idea of such states or points was first given general expression by Clark Maxwell in the 1870s. After describing the explosion of gun cotton, he goes on to say:

> In all such cases there is one common circumstance—the system has a quantity of potential energy, which is capable of being transformed into motion, but which cannot begin to be so transformed till the system has reached a certain configuration, to attain which requires an expenditure of work, which in certain cases may be infinitesimally small, and in general bears no definite proportion to the energy developed in consequence thereof. For example, the rock loosed by frost and balanced on a singular point of the mountain-side, the little spark which kindles the great forest. . . . Every existence above a certain rank has its singular points. . . . At these points, influences whose physical magnitude is too small to be taken account of . . . may produce results of the greatest importance.

Similar considerations were forced on me when I asked patients to keep calendars and diaries of their migraines. Such calendars might, indeed, reveal particular (and often unsuspected) *causes* of migraines (as discussed in Chapter 8) but, as often, would fail in this regard, and reveal that the situation was not a cause-and-effect one, but rather one of *provocation*—the setting-off of attacks, at a certain point, by stimuli which, at other times, would be ineffective and trifling. Infinitesimal events, events of no importance in themselves, could precipitate attacks, could become momentous, once the system reached "a certain configuration," a Maxwellian "singular point." Thus, there ceases to be a linear relation between stimulus and response, and we can no longer speak in terms of cause and effect—the behaviour of the system becomes nonlinear, once it has passed a critical point. But if we can no longer establish a fixed relation to particular causes, this does not mean that attacks are occurring at random, but rather that one must look at the behaviour, the geometry in time, of the entire, very complex "dynamical" system. We have already intimated (in the postscript to Chapter 1), that it may be important to look at the evolution of individual attacks in terms of their overall dynamics as complex systems—and the same is true, and even more striking, with the occurrence of attacks, "the spacetime continuum," as Dr. Gooddy puts it, "which the patient with migraine both suffers and creates."

EIGHT

Circumstantial Migraine

We will be concerned, in this chapter, with the consideration of circumstances which tend to provoke attacks of migraine. We will confine our terms of reference to *acute, transient states* which, as such, may elicit a single attack of migraine, while deferring discussion of chronic circumstantial provocation to the following chapter. Our data are culled, for the most part, from the observations of reliable patients who have learned to watch the occurrence of their own attacks, to keep diaries, and act as impartial observers of their own propensities. These data are supplemented, here and there, by experimental observations made under controlled conditions. We must reiterate, yet again, that one cannot hope to establish a one-to-one relation between circumstance and attack; there is at most a general tendency between the two.

The circumstances which we have to consider are so various and so numerous, that some form of preliminary classification is necessary as an aid to exposition. The categories adopted are purely informal and pretend to no rigour. I have taken the liberty of employing the vernacular, here and there, in the interests of greater vividness.

AROUSAL MIGRAINES

This term denotes the occurrence of migraines in circumstances which activate, arouse, annoy, and jangle the organism.[33] Among such circumstances we may recognise the following: light, noise, smells, inclement

[33] A similar miscellany of arousing circumstances may provoke many analogous reactions as, for example, hayfever. As Sydney Smith remarked of himself in this connection:

climate, exercise, excitement, violent emotion, somatic pain, and the action of certain drugs. We should also include in this category, as *intrinsic* excitations liable to be followed by a migraine reaction, the arousal of migrainous prodromes and auras. This list makes no pretence of being complete.

LIGHT AND NOISE

There are many patients who insist that glaring light and blaring noise are liable to give them a migraine. Emphasis is usually laid upon the intensity and duration of the provocative circumstance, upon its unbearability, upon the annoyance which precedes the attack, and the explicit wish to terminate the experience and find quiet and modest illumination. A number of patients in this class enter one's consulting-room wearing dark glasses, and not a few of them have learned the word "photophobic." Crowded summer-beaches with sunlight beating down upon the ocean, and machine-shops blazing with unshielded lights, are common grounds of complaint. Other patients claim specific intolerance of films and television.

With regard to the last of these, the question of *flickering light* as a highly-specific provocative circumstance must be considered. The presumed mechanism of reaction in such cases is a special one, and will be discussed separately later in this chapter.

SMELLS

We have noted the occasional occurrence of olfactory hallucinations in migraine aura, and the rather common enhancement, distortion and intolerance of smells which may occur *during* a migraine: both of these, no doubt, are responsible for a number of spurious or misleading histories which would otherwise seem to inculpate smells as a provocative circumstance. Yet there do exist, additional to these, reliable patients who appear to have developed, or possess innately, a specific sensitivity to certain smells (tar is often mentioned), or a general sensitivity to "bad" smells. Such histories are particularly common in the colourful older literature. Liveing, for example, cites the case of the following patient:

"The membrane is so irritable, that light, dust, contradiction, an absurd remark, the sight of a dissenter, anything, sets me asneezing."

. . . a distinguished member of the Academy, and a hospital physician, who cannot take part in a post-mortem examination without being instantly seized by vomiting and an attack of migraine. The same thing happens if by any chance they omit thoroughly to ventilate the wards which are under his care before his visit.[34]

INCLEMENT WEATHER

Any or all climatic extremes, it would seem, may occasion an attack of migraine in suitably predisposed patients, or be blamed for doing so. Storms and winds are the classical examples, and there are a number of patients who claim a sort of meteorological clairvoyance, and avow that they can predict the approach of the Hamsin or Santa Ana, or of impending thunder, from the migraines they suffer at such times. A colleague of mine tells me that her Swiss childhood was marred, at certain times, by migraines which occurred during the annual south-westerly gales which blow across Zürich, and that she never suffered attacks at any other time.

Other patients, less exotic in their reactions, tend to have repeated migraines in very hot or humid weather. Here the provocative circumstances should perhaps be construed differently, as likely to induce listlessness and prostrated states which favour the appearance of migraine.

EXERCISE—EXCITEMENT—EMOTION

Violent exercise (which must in its nature include elements of both physiological and psychological excitement) is often mentioned as a unique occasion of migraine by younger patients. Characteristically, the attack comes on shortly *after* the exercise, very rarely during it. We may recall a patient cited earlier (Case 25, p. 104) whose classical-cum-facioplegic attacks would come after a violently competitive cross-country race, and at no other time.

Violent emotions exceed all other acute circumstances in their capacity to provoke migraine reactions, and in many patients—especially sufferers from classical migraine—are responsible for the vast majority of all attacks experienced. Liveing writes: "It does not seem to matter much what the character of the emotion is, provided it be strongly felt."

[34] We must make an observation, in this context, which may be applied willy-nilly to many of the odder and more idiosyncratic circumstances sometimes held responsible for migraine attacks, viz. that a true organic sensitivity may be mimicked by what Liveing would call a "pathological habit," namely a conditioned reflex. We may remember such patients with "rose-fever" who start to sneeze if presented with a paper rose.

I think, however, that we can be more specific: we find, in practice, that sudden *rage* is the commonest precipitant, although *fright* (panic) may be equally potent in younger patients. Sudden *elation* (as at a moment of triumph or unexpected good fortune) may have the same effect.

Such reactions have a paradoxical quality, in that they tend to *arrest* a person in mid-excitement, or immediately following the peak of excitement. There are a variety of clinical parallels, some of which can serve as "alternatives" to the migraine reaction: we must particularly note the extremely acute reactions of narcolepsy and cataplexy (which frequently occur in response to rage, orgasm, or hilarious excitement), the reactions of "fainting" (vasovagal syncope) and "swooning" (hysterical stupor) in response to a sudden emotional "shock"—pleasant or unpleasant—and, in more pathological contexts, the reactions of "freezing" (as exhibited by Parkinsonian patients) and "blocking" (as exhibited by schizophrenic patients). Nor are reactions of this type confined to human beings: we will find reference to a variety of biological analogues and homologues in Chapter 11.

It should be observed that the provocative emotions in all cases would be ranked as "kinetic" in James Joyce's terminology: they arouse the organism and tend in their normal course to lead to action (fight, flight, jumping for joy, laughing, etc.). They may be contrasted with the "static" emotions (dread, horror, pity, awe, etc.) which are expressed in stillness and silence, and slowly abate, after many hours, by lysis or catharsis. It is exceedingly rare for such static emotions to ignite a migraine.

We may recognise here two *styles* of dissipating tension or emotion: the ejaculation (whether this be verbal, somatic or visceral) which suddenly dissipates a state of tension; and a slow leaking-away, a lysis, which accomplishes the same end more gradually: laughter versus tears, the spark versus the corposant.

Other forms of psychophysiological excitement may be mentioned briefly. A few patients are unfortunate enough to experience migraines immediately following *orgasm: vide* Case 2 and Case 55 (p. 101, p. 170).

Finally, as we have already intimated, the entire cycle of excitation: inhibition may become integral and internalised, an aura or prodrome acting as provocation for a migraine.

PAIN

Somatic pain (from muscle and skin) tends to provoke and arouse; visceral pain (from viscera, vessels, etc.) tends to have the opposite effect, to produce nausea, passivity, etc. Both may induce migraines, although by different mechanisms. Perhaps the commonest example of the former in action is provided by the occurrence of an acute (muscle) injury in an active man, who, aroused, enraged and thwarted by the pain, develops a migraine superimposed upon his other problems. The effects of visceral pain will be considered subsequently.

The question of *drug-actions* in relation to migraine will be relegated to a separate discussion later in this chapter.

SLUMP MIGRAINES AND CRASH-REACTIONS

These neologisms denote the occurrence of migraines in circumstances of exhaustion, prostration, sedation, passivity, sleep, etc. Many of these circumstances are normally and physiologically associated with states of pleasant satiety and consummation, delectable drowsiness and lassitude, and healing sleep. But let the physiological reaction be more intense, let it assume an unpleasing affective tone, and we see a *slump-reaction* of one type or another. Slump-reactions thus represent exaggerations and travesties of peaceful and restful states.

EATING AND FASTING

A hearty meal is followed by pleasant feelings of satisfaction and con-summation, a little doziness, and the active, but inconspicuous, processes of digestion, etc. A closer scrutiny will reveal a multiplicity of post-pran-dial reactions:

> The picture has been presented of parasympathetic activity in an old man sleeping after dinner. His heart-rate is slow, his breathing noisy because of bronchial constriction; his pupils are small; drops of saliva may run out of the corner of his mouth. A stethoscope applied to his abdomen will reveal much intestinal activity. (Burn, 1963)

This description provides an unappetising, almost a Swiftian, dissection of a dear old man enjoying his after-dinner nap.

Now consider these same physiological reactions amplified, distorted, and rendered symptomatic. We may recognise three slump-syndromes in this regard: "Indigestion," "Dumping syndrome," and "Post-prandial migraine." We may say, if we wish, that the first is "due" to an over-loaded stomach, and the second to acute hypoglycaemia—although both contentions are questionable. Phenomenologically, however, they all rep-

resent parodies, or pathological, variations of normal post-prandial torpor and vegetative state.

We must also consider certain pathological reactions to *fasting*. When
some hours have elapsed since a meal, the "normal" reaction is to become somewhat restless and wonder when dinner is due, viz. appetitive
activity and arousal. If no meal is forthcoming and the fast extended,
there will sooner or later supervene symptoms of prostration or collapse.
In a few patients the blood-sugar will fail to be maintained after x hours
of fasting. And a small but definite proportion of patients are liable to
migraine reactions under these circumstances.

Case 54   This 47-year-old woman experienced 3 to 5 common migraines a
month with no immediately discernible cause for these. She was instructed to
keep a diary, in the hope that this might uncover some provocative circumstance not previously attended to. Her diary revealed, on her next clinic visit,
that her attacks tended to come if she missed breakfast. An extended glucose
tolerance-test was undertaken, which revealed a 5-hour blood-sugar of 44 mg
per cent. At this point the patient was pale, sweating, and complaining of
headache. Further tests established the diagnosis of "functional hypoglycaemia." The patient was instructed to make a point of having breakfast, and to
keep sugared orange-juice on her bedside table. Thereafter, she was virtually
free of attacks.

HOT WEATHER AND FEVER

Normal reactions to hot weather include lassitude and sweating; when
fever is present, malaise and vascular headache may be added to these
symptoms. A number of migraine patients show over-reaction to thermal
stimuli, and tend to get attacks in association with hot weather or fevers.
Thus an attack of mild "flu," or a febrile "cold" which would be trivial
to a majority of people, may become the occasion of an incapacitating
migraine in predisposed patients.

PASSIVE MOTION

Gentle passive motion is normally soothing and soporific—hence a baby
may be rocked to sleep. In a certain portion of the population, however,
the response to passive motion (or direct vestibular stimulation) is inordinate and intolerable—such people may suffer from intense "motion-
sickness" in childhood (with nausea, vomiting, pallor, cold sweating,
etc.) or thereafter; if vascular headache is present in addition to the above

symptoms, a motion migraine will result. Exaggerated responses to vestibular stimulation is perhaps the commonest, and certainly one of the
most incapacitating, idiosyncrasies of many migraine patients, and as
such they may be shut off from many of the simpler pleasures in life:
swings in childhood, roller-coasters in adolescence, and travelling by bus,
train, ship or plane at all times. It is important to note that *passivity* and
passive stimulation are essential in these reactions; many patients who
are extravagantly prone to motion-sickness are perfectly able to drive
their own cars, or pilot their own boats and planes.

EXHAUSTION

A hard day's work normally leads to a delicious tiredness, but may, in
predisposed patients, determine a pathological variant of this, namely
exhaustion, incipient collapse, and sometimes migraine. There may be a
similar incapacity to tolerate a loss of sleep which would readily be borne
by the majority of the population. Such sleep-deprivation is very likely
to provoke a migraine or migranoid reaction in predisposed patients,
and not infrequently other allied reactions discussed in Chapter 5, particularly narcolepsy. Other factors, e.g. illness, diarrhoea, fasting, etc.,
may summate with an otherwise inconsiderable fatigue or sleep-deficit
to a crucial level of exhaustion, at which point a slump-reaction is likely
to occur. Thus Parry (a sufferer from isolated visual auras) noted of
himself that:

> Violent fatigue, more especially when accompanied by from 8 to 10 hours'
> fasting . . . sometimes brings them on . . . so too has the exhaustion following
> a smart attack of diarrhoea.

DRUG-REACTIONS

We have already touched on the subject of drug-reactions in relation to
migraine in various contexts, e.g. in allusion to "hangovers," abnormal
reserpine-reactions, etc. These too must be construed as exaggerations
and perversions of normal physiological responses. Anyone is likely to
feel sleepy, or slightly ill, after many drinks, but intense nausea, or a
common migraine, or an attack of migrainous neuralgia after a single
drink is excessive, and represents the abnormal reactivity many migraine
patients must learn to accept in themselves, whether they choose to compromise with this predisposition, defy it, or "take a chance" on it. Simi-

larly "hangovers," when florid, represent a pathological reactivity, and are not infrequently the harbinger, or first sign, of a future migraine candidate.

There are an immense number of depressant drugs besides alcohol, some of which are notoriously unsafe for certain patients. The most infamous of these is perhaps *reserpine*, which may be used, in a variety of proprietary preparations, to control hypertension. Reserpine may provoke not only migraine, but many other allied reactions, e.g. stupor, narcolepsy, shock, (psychological) depression, and Parkinsonian akinesia.

The uses and abuses of the *amphetamines* must also be noted in this context. Amphetamines cause a powerful arousal of central and peripheral nervous activity, which is liable to be followed by a commensurate "slump" as their action wears off. We have already seen that some patients may make spontaneous comparisons of the excitatory and inhibitory phases of their auras with amphetamine action(s) (*vide* Cases 67, p. 67 and 69, p. 85), and we will later have occasion to speak of the therapeutic uses of the amphetamines in migraine (Part IV). Our concern at this stage is with the liability to migraine, and other allied reactions, in the "let-down" period after heavy amphetamine dosage. The following case-history is instructive:

Case 43   This 23-year-old patient had been subject to one or two common migraines a month since the age of 19. Eight weeks before she consulted me, her condition had taken a sudden change for the worse. She described herself as now experiencing daily migraines, which at first were confluent with one another ("migraine status"). Other very recent symptoms included intense tiredness, frequent narcolepsies, persistent lacrimation, diarrhoea, and depression. I was initially at a loss to explain this sudden and mysterious change in her state, and wondered whether some emotional tragedy had occurred of which she was reluctant to speak. On her second visit, she admitted that she had been addicted to Ritalin, and had been taking no less than 1,600 mg daily for over a year. When she stopped taking the drug abruptly, she experienced the above monstrous withdrawal syndrome of a depressive, slumped, parasympathetic "status."

"LET-DOWN" SITUATIONS

It is common knowledge that migraines tend to come "after the event," whatever the "event" is. Thus, patients often complain of experiencing migraines after an examination, a childbirth, a business triumph, a holiday, etc. An important recurrent pattern of this type is exemplified by "weekend migraines" (sometimes alternating with weekend depressions, diarrhoea, "colds," etc.), during the slump-period which follows a hectic week. Such propensities will be discussed in greater detail in Chapter 9, and in Part III.

NOCTURNAL MIGRAINE

It is often a matter of astonishment to patients that they should sometimes be woken from sleep by a migraine, and their astonishment may only be increased when they are assured that an association between sleep and migraine is not merely common, but to be expected.

We may distinguish several varieties of nocturnal migraine on the basis of careful histories: there are attacks which come at the dead of night, jerking patients from the deepest sleep; there are attacks which tend to come at dawn, intruding on an uneasy half-waking slumber; there are attacks coalesced with dreams (the most reliable histories are obtained from some patients with classical migraine, who wake in the second or headache stage with a clear memory of dream-images and scotomatous figures mixed together); and there are attacks associated with nightmares (night-terrors and somnambulisms).[35]

Attacks of migrainous neuralgia, *par excellence*, tend to wake patients from the deepest layers of sleep. The onset of such attacks is extremely acute, yet those who experience nocturnal attacks are never able to recollect any dreams from the time of their onset.

Classical migraine is sometimes nocturnal, and common migraine is very frequently so; I have notes of more than forty severely-affected patients whose many attacks were *exclusively* nocturnal. Many such patients assert that they dream more, or more vividly, on nights when they suffer migraines, and all-night electroencephalographic studies performed on some such patients have shown an apparent increase in the amount of paradoxical (rapid eye-movement, or dreaming) sleep associated with their attacks (Dr. J. Dexter, 1968: personal communication).

Exceptionally clear histories are given by nightmare-prone patients

---

[35] It is not uncommon for patients to dream of an aura, or to experience, either frank or camouflaged, the entry of aura phenomena into the flow of dreams, and it is always important to enquire whether patients have such dream-auras. I describe a personal experience of such a dream-aura in *A Leg to Stand On* (pp. 95–101), and have discussed the general subject in "Neurological Dreams," *MD Magazine*, February 1991.

regarding the frequent linking together of the nightmare experience and subsequent migraine symptoms (see Case 75, for example). The fact of the association is clearer than its interpretation; it is difficult to assert whether the dreaming or nightmare experience causes a migraine, is caused by a migraine, or simply shows a number of clinical and physiological similarities to the migraine experience.

Nor indeed are these interpretations mutually exclusive. We have cited a number of case-histories illustrating the occurrence of "dreamy states," delirious states and "daymares" as components of migraine auras, and one may question whether in some cases of very constant conjunction between nightmares and classical migraines, the former is not itself the chief or sole manifestation of an aura.

Equally plausibly, one may conceive the intense emotional and physiological excitation of the dreaming (and especially the nightmare) state to provide an adequate arousal stimulus for migraines in predisposed subjects. One can do no more, at the present time, than note the undoubted affinity of migraines to occur during sleep, and to be associated, in particular, with restless and dreaming sleep.

RESONANCE MIGRAINE

We must consider under this head one important, highly-specific, if somewhat rare, form of circumstantial migraine, viz. the elicitation of a scintillating scotoma by flickering light of certain frequencies, patterned visual stimuli of specific type, and even certain visual images and memories.[36]

Flickering light from any source—emitted from a fluorescent or television-tube, reflected from cinema-screens or metallic surfaces, etc.—may elicit the *immediate* appearance of a scintillating scotoma with a scintillation-rate identical with the frequency of the provocative stimulus. The use of a stroboscope demonstrates that only flicker-frequencies in a narrow band (between 8 to 12 stimuli per second) are effective in provoking the scintillating scotoma. The same frequency-band has also been shown to be most effective in provoking photo-myoclonic jerking or true photo-epilepsy in predisposed patients.

I have received accurate descriptions of such photogenic scotomata

---

[36] A charming example of an aural response to visually-patterned and intermittent stimulation is provided by a case-history cited in Liveing, in which the patient's attacks were evoked by the sight of falling snow, and no other circumstance.

from several patients, one of the most interesting of these being a nurse who also exhibited photo-myoclonus and photo-epilepsy as alternative responses to flickering light.

Visual fixation on appropriate patterns may similarly serve as flicker-stimuli. Several descriptions of this are provided by Liveing:

> ... M. Piorry says of himself ... that he can produce the phenomenon of the luminous vibratory circle at will by strongly fixing the sight, or reading.

Reference is also made to a patient whose attacks had occasionally been brought on by looking at a striped wallpaper or a striped dress. We must recognise the closest analogy between these phenomena and those of photo-epilepsy and reading-epilepsy. In the case of the former, for example, a moving patterned stimulus may be provided by rapidly waving the fingers before the eyes, or—in one published case—bobbing up and down before a Venetian blind.

The analogy may be pressed even further. Penfield and Perot (1963), in a massive review of their epileptic patients, describe the "psychical precipitation" of attacks in some patients by vivid visualisation of the circumstances of the original (primal) attack. Similarly it is noted by Liveing that Sir John Herschel "a sufferer from purely visual megrim states ... that an attack was produced in him by allowing the mind to dwell on the description of the appearances."

We are forced to seek an explanation for two facts: the *immediacy* of the scotomatous response, and its numerically-precise *synchronisation* with the flicker-stimulus. The most economical conjecture is that such phenomena are due to a quantitative attunement, or *resonance* within the nervous system, following the impact of appropriate stimuli.[37] The provocative stimuli are not necessarily visual—the very word "resonance" is suggestive of sound! Intolerance of noise (phonophobia) is an almost universal feature of the irritability characteristic of many migraines, but what needs emphasis here is the *peculiarly* aggravating, or provocative power of *sounds of certain frequencies*.

We live in an increasingly assaultive and noisy environment, and one may obtain the clearest histories of the provocative effects of this in some migraineurs. Some patients are immediately affected by the sound of

---

[37] Since drafting the original manuscript, I was fortunate enough to be given the detailed case-history quoted in Chapter 3 (Case 75), in which migrainous paraesthesiae, in company with other symptoms of an aura, were apparently evoked by resonance to an oscillatory tactile stimulus of appropriate frequency.

pneumatic drills—and speak of the rapid, repetitive chattering of these as being peculiarly provocative of migraines—not just their intensity, but the *chatter* of their noise. The combination of high intensity with insistent repetition makes the beat of loud rock music migrainogenic to some patients, a phenomenon analogous to musicogenic epilepsy.

That it is not the intensity of the sound as such; nor some particular hated timbre, but, very specifically, its *frequency* that is intolerable, may be tested experimentally in a clinical laboratory, monitoring the patient's brain waves by EEG. One may find, in these circumstances, that it is only *particular frequencies* of flashing light or banging noise which cause gross disturbance in the brain wave patterns, *driving* these first, in synchrony with the stimulus, and then *kindling* a severe, paroxysmal cerebral response.

In striking contrast, pleasant, melodious and truly musical stimuli rapidly restore constancy and rhythmicity to the brain waves, and can terminate the paroxysmal response, both clinically and electrically. We may see very clearly how the *wrong* sound, or "anti-music," is pathogenic and migrainogenic; while the *right* sound—proper music—is truly tranquillising, and immediately restores cerebral health. These effects are striking, and quite fundamental, and put one in mind of Novalis's aphorism: "Every disease is a musical problem; every cure is a musical solution."

A similar response—first "driving," then "kindling" (to use key words in the electroencephalographic parlance)—may be evoked by *tactile stimuli.* A nice example of this was given in Chapter 3 (Case 75), where the intense vibrato of a motorbike was provocative of a migraine.

MIGRAINES PROVOKED BY VISUAL FIELD DISTORTIONS

As migraines may be evoked by unusual rhythms and disturbances in *time,* so may they be provoked by odd symmetries or asymmetries in *space.* The following history from a gifted observer (Case 90) indicates this strange spatial sensitivity or vulnerability in some patients:

> As some of my migraines start with disturbances in my visual field, so some may be *provoked* by unexpected twists and oddities which suddenly strike me. A button may be done up askew in a coat. The whole coat looks askew and bothers me oddly. Then this skew in the coat *becomes* a skew or twist in my vision, sets off a local distortion in my visual field, which may then spread until it engulfs the greater part of the visual field. Or it may be some-

thing askew in a face—like a tic, or a grimace, or a spasm—some asymmetry. Once it was set off by seeing a man with Bell's Palsy. The perception is momentary, but it can set off a spatial disturbance that lasts for several minutes.

Klee speaks of strange forms of "metamorphopsia"—distortion of contours, eccentric misplacements within the visual field, micropsia, macropsia, and the like—as occurring in severe migraine auras (see p. 75), but does not discuss the *induction* of visual auras, in some patients, by the altered or unexpected appearances of things. The migraineur—like the artist—may be singularly sensitive to any "transformations," deformations, or divergences from the expected. They may induce for him a spreading topological deformation, a whole topsy-turvy, Escher-like, world of strange distortion. Once this is *recognised* by the patient, it ceases to be a bewilderment or terror, and can become—as perhaps it was for Escher—a stimulus to the creative imagination.

MISCELLANEOUS CIRCUMSTANTIAL MIGRAINES

We have by no means exhausted our listing of the circumstances under which migraines tend to occur, but we face serious difficulties in attempting to categorise what remains. We must deal with the following topics: migraine in relation to food and dyspepsia; in relation to the bowels, especially constipation; in relation to menstrual periods, and hormones; and in relation to allergies. We will conclude with a brief consideration of "sympathetic" migraine, in relation to the above concomitances and certain other aspects of the attack itself.

FOOD, MIGRAINE, AND THE STOMACH

There is a sizeable proportion of patients who, feeling ill ("bilious" or "dyspeptic") during or before the headache, ascribe all their attacks to "something I ate." In saying this, they unwittingly echo a long and ancient tradition of thought. This tradition may be exemplified by the following passage taken from Tissot's *Treatise*:

> . . . All patients remark that their stomachs are not as comfortable as usual on the approach of an attack; that if they are careful over them the attacks are not so frequent; and that if they take anything which deranges the stomach the attacks are more frequent and severe.
>
> Persons who suffer from migraine and stomach derangement feel the migraine diminish in proportion as the stomach recovers itself . . . Almost invariably, on the instant the stomach discharges its contents, the pains cease . . .

Plates

Most of the following paintings have been done by nonprofessional artists as depictions of visual phenomena they have experienced in migraine auras. They are attempts at literal reproductions of the phenomena; they are not meant to be symbolic (although some symbolism may be present too). (All photos courtesy British Migraine Association and Boehringer Ingelheim Ltd., except Plate 3B, courtesy Dr. Ronald K. Siegel, and Plate 8, courtesy Dr. Ralph M. Siegel.)

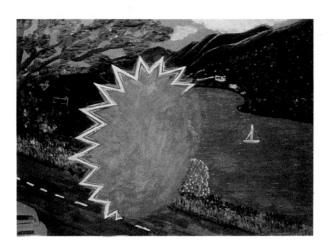

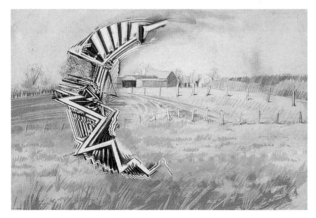

Plate 1A.   A classical zigzag fortification pattern—its brilliance, in life, is as dazzling as a white surface in the noonday sun, and the edge is in continual scintillation.

Plate 1B.   This migraine fortification shows characteristic angles and lines, both fine and coarse.

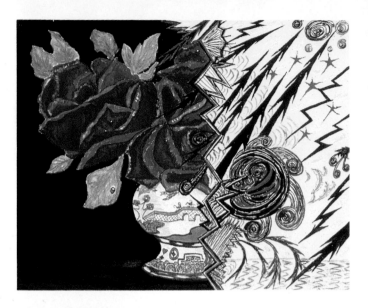

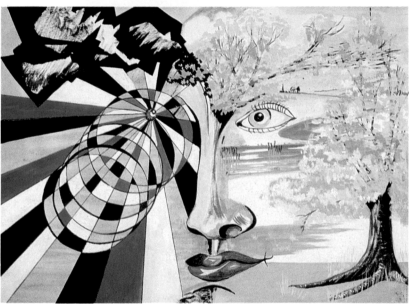

Plate 2A.   In this still-life of roses, half the image is replaced by migrainous zigzags, stars, and whorls—the latter often concentric and spiral. The other half of the image is normal.

Plate 2B.   Half of this image is replaced by a geometrical hallucination consisting essentially of a radial form with colored spokes, and a spiral or helix. Some sharp-edged fragmentation may be seen above these. The right-hand side of the image is normal.

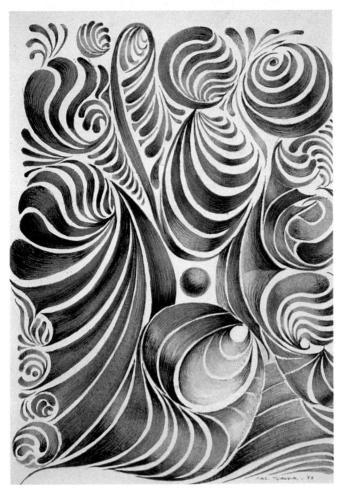

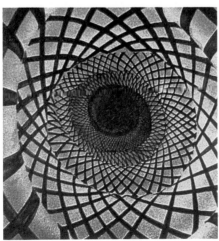

Plate 3A. This painting, by a migraine patient, shows scrolls across the visual field.

Plate 3B. A "tunnel" hallucination seen during intoxication by cannabis; similar forms may be seen in migraine aura.

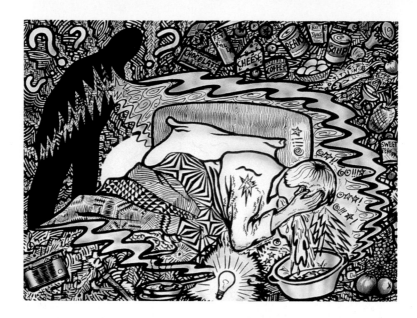

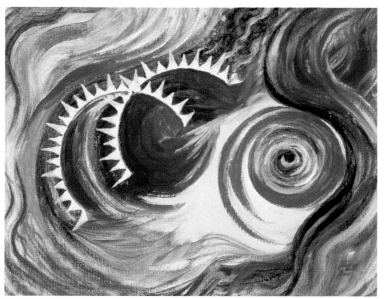

Plate 4A.   This migrainous patient shows himself vomiting in a world reduced to fortifications, lattices, swirls and zigzags, bursting out over the entire visual field. The dark shadow bending over him may be a phantom image.

Plate 4B.   "All the interior of the fortification, so to speak, was boiling and rolling around in a most wonderful manner, as if it was some thick liquid all alive."

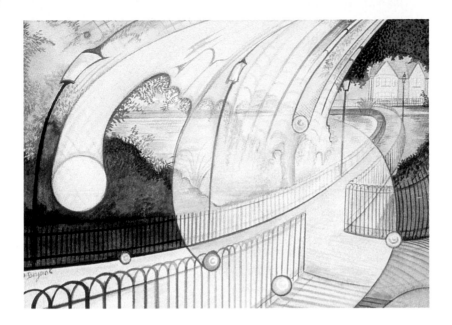

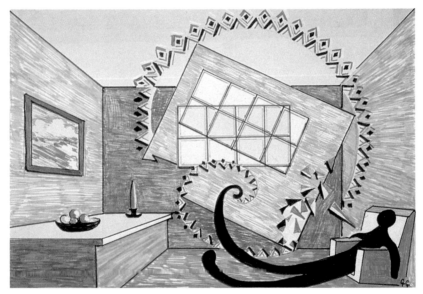

Plate 5A. A topological misperception or hallucination in which objects in one half of the visual field are distorted into curves. This patient experienced a dynamic disturbance with a sense of violent forces, blowing or pulling objects out of shape.

Plate 5B. In addition to migrainous fortifications, and bizarre tiltings, this painting shows a haptic spiral hallucination of the legs.

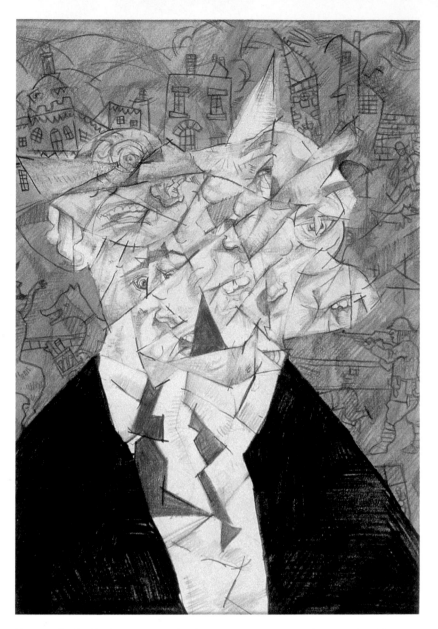

Plate 6.   In this fascinating example of mosaic vision, an entire face is replaced by disjointed, sharp-edged planes and polygons, as in a Cubist painting.

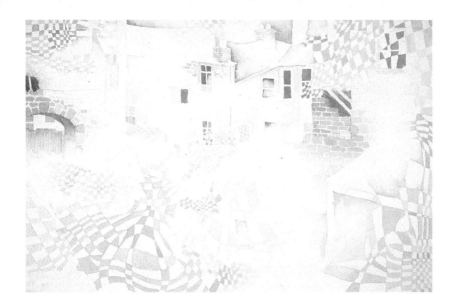

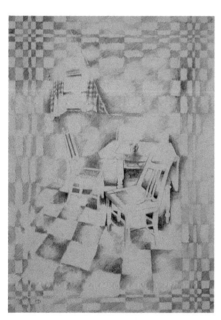

Plates 7A, 7B. These two paintings show the appearance of both plane and curved rectangular lattices with varied spatial scales, which partially replace the image. In the actual hallucination, these lattices would be rapidly shifting.

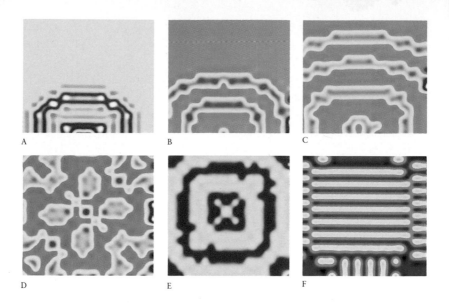

A B C

D E F

Plates 8A–8F. Some computer simulations of migraine aura on a neural network:
A–C) solitary spreading wave (simulated "scotoma"); D) symmetrical axial pattern
(simulated "lattice" or "web" constants); E) concentric wave pattern (simulated "tunnel"
or "funnel" constants); F) "rolls" (corresponding to radial or spiral form constants).

Tissot's conclusions from his observations we will hold back till the end of this chapter. Some of these clinical observations cannot be doubted; the difficulties lie in their interpretation. That gastric disorder may be *associated* with migraine or headache, does not necessarily indicate that it is its cause.

The matter can be (and has in the past been) argued to and fro interminably. For myself, I regard any concomitant or antecedent "stomach derangement" as an integral part of the migraine composite. Further, though I cannot gainsay the observations of a patient who insists that his migraines come after eating ham or chocolate, and under no other circumstances, I must regard the interpretation of this empirical fact as exceptionally tricky. I am not convinced that a migraine can ever be ascribed to a specific food-sensitivity, and I would suspect any association of the two to the establishment of a conditioned-reflex.

"CHINESE RESTAURANT SYNDROME" AND OTHER MIGRAINOGENIC FOOD

Experience since the first edition of this book has made clear that there *can be* specific food reactions, and that these may have a clearly defined chemical mechanism.

The phrase "Chinese restaurant syndrome" has become very familiar (though very distressing to Chinese restaurants!). Many persons, and an especially high proportion of migraineurs may show severe reactions to Chinese meals. In milder cases, there is just a feeling of malaise, with some shivering, pallor, borborygmus and nausea; in more severe cases there may be absolute prostration, with severe visceral and vascular upset (including a typical vascular headache), a confused and even delirious mental state and considerable faintness, if not actual "fainting." It is clear that such reactions come in the "borderlands" of migraine, and resemble the "migranoid reactions," the vasovagal attacks, the nitritoid crises, and so on described in Chapter 2. It is evident that one is seeing a parasympathetic or "vagotonic" response—and one to which migraineurs are especially prone. It is not every Chinese meal (most fortunately!) which provokes this—and there was a delay of several years in recognising that there was, indeed, a syndrome, because of its erratic and unpredictable occurrence. It took several years to incriminate the pathogenic factor—and when this was done it was found to be monosodium glutamate (MSG), very widely used as a food-additive for the enhancement of flavors, and by no means confined to Chinese restaurants (MSG, indeed, is not "natural" at all—and even in soy sauce is an artificial addition). A certain conflict of interests has arisen—as with so many potentially toxic additives: for MSG is uniquely useful as a flavor enhancer, and a majority of people will tolerate it well enough. However, with increased consciousness of its toxic potential, its use is less widespread and gross than it was before the syndrome was recognised about ten years ago.

Some migraineurs may find that there are certain other foods to which they are particularly sensitive—this is commonly remarked of strong *cheese*. Cheese (and several other foods) had indeed been regarded, back in the fifties, as carrying a specific danger for certain groups of patients— namely those receiving antidepressant drugs of the monoamine oxidase (MAO) inhibitor type: in such patients cheese and other foods might provoke a sudden and dangerous rise in blood-pressure, and other autonomic effects—and it was partly for this reason that these drugs, extraordinarily affective as they were as antidepressants, gave way to the much safer, but (on the whole) less potent "tricyclics." The pathogenic factor here is *amines* of various sorts, especially *tyramine*, but others as well, which innocuous in themselves may activate (or be activated by) other chemical substances to produce stronger disturbances in the chemical control-systems of the brain, especially those concerned with autonomic control. Although migraineurs are not at *dangerous* risk (like patients taking MAO-inhibitors), they tend to have less latitude than the nonmigraineur.

One should make such a statement only to qualify it; it is not all migraineurs who show MSG intolerance, cheese intolerance, and so forth, but only *some*: and sometimes, indeed, for only some of the time. Such specificity and selectivity suggest that not all migraineurs are the same; that there may, for example, be several different subgroups, who may be distinguished on the basis of differing brain chemistries, so that some are upset (or helped) by a food substance or drug to which other migraineurs are more or less indifferent. Such considerations of chemical specificity, which are of no less practical than theoretical importance, will be further discussed in the latter sections of this book.

THE BOWELS AND MIGRAINE

As some patients favour a gastric theory, so others are convinced of the intestinal origin of migraine, and have been moved to this conclusion by noting the association of their own migraines with disturbances of the bowel, particularly antecedent constipation. Here again, as with the question of stomach derangement and migraine, they are the unconscious heirs of a long tradition of belief. One may be given extraordinarily persuasive case-histories, such as the following:

Case 4   A highly-intelligent, not obviously moralistic or superstitious man of 28 who has suffered from migrainous neuralgia since childhood. He averages 4 to 6 attacks a month; there has never been either clustering or remission of attacks. This patient is emphatic that each attack is preceded by two or three days of constipation. For the remainder of the month, his bowels are regular and he is free from attacks. All the usual therapeutic approaches to migrainous neuralgia were tried and failed. Finally, with some embarrassment, I placed the patient on regular laxatives. He went an unprecedented period of three months without either constipation or migraines.

What shall we say? That the constipation is, in fact, an integral portion of the migraine—its prodrome: that the stuffed bowel produces a factor which may lead to migraine (*vide* serotonin theories, Chapter 11); or that a conditioned reflex has been set in motion? Any of these might be the case; the likelihood is, migraine being so over-determined a reaction, that *all* of them are the case.

MIGRAINE IN RELATION TO MENSTRUAL PERIODS AND HORMONES

We have already alluded (Chapter 2) to the invariable occurrence of autonomic and affective disturbances at the menses, and the occurrence of outspoken menstrual migraines, at least occasionally, in 10 to 20 per cent of all women during their reproductive periods. I have seen about 500 women with common migraines, and I would estimate that one-third of these experience menstrual migraines *in addition* to other attacks. I have notes of more than 50 patients who experience migraines *exclusively* at the menstrual periods. In contrast to these figures, the occurrence of classical migraine shows very much less tendency to be coupled with menstrual periods: of a total of 50 female patients with classical migraine, for example, only four have mentioned their occurrence at the menses, and none has experienced attacks confined to this time. Migrainous neuralgia is rare in women, and when it does occur appears to follow its own rhythm rather than the menstrual cycle.

Observations regarding the frequency of migraine at different times of the female life have been made since antiquity, and provide us with evidence of considerable consistency if questionable interpretation. We have emphasised the frequency of menstrual migraine, but we must note that attacks are by no means invariably pre-menstrual; a large minority of women experience attacks during and after the menstrual flow. We must note also that menstrual migraines although they usually cease at the menopause, may in some cases continue to occur with the same periodicity after the menopause (see Case 74). Much less common than menstrual migraines, but distinctive when they occur, are attacks experienced in the middle of the menstrual cycle, and presumed to be concomitant with ovulation. Common migraine is relatively rare before the onset of menstruation; classical migraine, however, shows no such restriction, and has frequently been recorded in early childhood. Very dramatic is the remission of migraine which may occur during pregnancy, characteristically during the latter half or last trimester of pregnancy; 80 to 90 per cent of all women with common migraine are likely to experience such a remission during their first pregnancy, and a smaller number will secure relief in subsequent pregnancies; remission is much less striking in cases of classical migraine (but see Case 11). Patients who have been exempt from migraine during the latter part of pregnancy not infrequently experience an exceptionally severe post-partum migraine one or two weeks after delivery. Finally, a matter of great contemporary concern, there are the varied and controversial effects of different hormone preparations—especially oral contraceptives—upon the severity and frequency of migraine attacks.

The subject is one of peculiar complexity, for the major changes in female reproductive function must be considered at so many levels: there are local changes in the uterus, etc., there are specific hormonal changes, there are very general physiological changes (at puberty, at the menses, at the menopause), and, finally, there are important psychological concomitants of all these changes. Which of these, we must enquire, carries the greatest weight in determining patterns of migraine throughout life?

Classical physiology viewed menstrual migraines as a form of hysteria: thus Willis and Whytt envisaged these migraines as being generated by local changes in the uterus, their symptoms being radiated throughout the body by a direct organ-to-organ transmission or "sympathy." This notion of "uterine megrim" was still very generally held in the middle of the last century. Liveing considered all such theories of local origin in great detail, and found them inadequate to cover the known facts, concluding:

> It is . . . to a widespread periodic excitation of the nervous system, and not to any mere uterine, or cerebral or general plethora pending the [menstrual] discharge, that I trace the manifestations of certain morbid tendencies on the part of the system, whether in the form of hysteria, megrim, epilepsy, or insanity, at these particular periods.

But Liveing knew nothing of hormones, and perhaps underestimated the ability of general physiological disturbances or psychological factors to modify a widespread periodic excitation of the nervous system.

It should not be difficult, one would imagine, to dissect out the role of hormonal influences, as opposed to other determinants, by observing the effect of purified hormonal preparations upon the severity and frequency of migraine attacks. There is, indeed, a vast literature on this topic, relating both to the effects of various hormone contraceptives on migraine patterns, and the effects of administering a variety of purified hormone preparations—androgens, oestrogens, progestogens, gonadotrophins, etc.

The vastness of this literature (which has been repeatedly and carefully reviewed) is a measure of the difficulty which has been encountered in coming to any clear conclusions. Thus, it was postulated, from the occurrence of ovulatory and pre-menstrual migraines, that these attacks were precipitated, respectively, by raised levels of oestrogen and by relatively sudden diminutions of circulating progestogens. Experience with current oral contraceptives has neither confirmed nor refuted this surmise: some contraceptives seemingly aggravate migraine, others appear to mitigate it, and yet others to have no effect upon migraine patterns; these varying effects have not been adequately correlated with the precise composition of the contraceptive used. Dramatic results have been claimed from the therapeutic use of androgens, oestrogens, progestogens and gonadotrophins in the treatment of migraine: all such studies, however, have represented "straight" trials of the hormone, with the notorious ambiguities which must attach to all such uncontrolled studies, particularly in regard to migraine which is infinitely placebo-sensitive (see Chapter 15). One must deplore the publicity which often attaches to such studies, and the subsequent touting of unproven or even dangerous hormone preparations as cures for migraine.

The number of carefully-controlled, double-blind trials of simple purified hormone preparations is exceedingly small. One may cite the recent study published by Bradley et al. (1968) concerning the effects of a fluorinated progesterone (Demigran) on migraine patients. Bradley et al.

found *no* significant effects upon the severity or frequency of migraine, save in the special case of menstrual attacks, which appeared to be slightly milder during Demigran administration.

There is a startling contrast between the modest or negative findings of such controlled studies and the spectacular results which have been claimed on the basis of "straight" trials of various hormone preparations. The entire subject is urgently in need of experimental clarification; certainly there is no strong evidence, at the present time, that any existing hormone preparation has *specific* (as opposed to placebo) therapeutic effects upon the occurrence of migraine.

One encounters, in practice, many case-histories which suggest that other factors—particularly the patient's needs and expectations—may play an important part in determining the occurrence or disappearance of menstrual migraines, the remission of migraines during pregnancy, etc. The following case-history may be considered:

Case 31   A 32-year-old Catholic woman with severe menstrual migraines. She had had four children, the last of which required an exchange-transfusion, in view of an Rh-incompatibility between the patient and her husband. Further pregnancies were considered undesirable, but the patient was constrained by her religious persuasions from taking any contraceptive measures. A gynaecologist was consulted, who informed the patient that she had "abnormally high levels of oestrogen" which were the cause of her menstrual migraines. He said that he would prescribe *for this* a hormone preparation (Ortho-Novum); he added that Ortho-Novum also happened to be a contraceptive, but its employment, in her case, was purely therapeutic, and only incidentally contraceptive. The patient's scruples were overcome by this assurance, and she consented to take the hormone. Her menstrual migraines vanished, and a year later had not returned.

This history is quoted, of course, for its ambiguity, not its simplicity. The effects of the hormone-preparation were clear, but the interpretation of its effects are far from clear. It would seem eminently possible, in this case, that the patient, justifiably and chronically terrified of further pregnancies, was restored to emotional calm by the knowledge of the pill's contraceptive power, and that *this* was the crucial factor in curing her migraines. One sees many cases of menstrual migraine, indeed, which respond excellently to psychotherapy and this alone, suggesting that hormonal influences are at most a *co-determinant* of such migraine patterns. There is also considerable evidence that the remission of migraines during pregnancy is at least as dependent upon the patient's state of mind and attitudes to pregnancy as upon any alterations in hormonal balance (see, for example, Case 56, p. 169).

We must conclude, therefore, that although menstruation, the menopause, and pregnancy, may have a profound effect in determining the patterns of migraine in certain patients, the mechanism of their action is uncertain, and is probably to be ascribed to multiple concomitant causes rather than the specific effects of hormonal changes.

ALLERGIES AND MIGRAINE

We have already observed the high incidence of allergic reactions in migraine patients, and the postulate (put forward by Balyeat and many others) that migraines, when they occur in patients with multiple allergies, are themselves to be regarded as allergic reactions. But statistical correlation *per se* implies nothing beyond the fact of concomitance: it does not imply any logical or causal connection between the two phenomena which are being correlated.

But the belief that migraine may be allergic in basis is widespread, and many migraine patients, after migrating from one doctor to another, finally place themselves in the hands of an allergist. This is likely to be followed by the elaborate ritual of testing for "sensitivities," and following this, by a series of impressive rules and prohibitions—avoiding dusts and pollens, changing the bed linen, exiling the cat, eliminating all sorts of delectables from the diet, etc. This solemn regimen will be reinforced by frequent injections, designed to "desensitise" the patient. Not infrequently, a therapeutic triumph is achieved, or claimed.[38]

But neither statistical correlation nor therapeutic magic is evidence for an allergic basis. It is necessary, as with hormone-trials, to investigate the matter with rigorous controls and techniques, as has been done by Wolff and many other workers (see Wolff, 1963), and such stringent approaches have indicated the extreme rarity of an allergic basis for migraines; less than one per cent of all migraine attacks are explicable in terms of allergic sensitivities or mechanisms.

The frequent coexistence of migrainous and allergic reactions in many patients, and their occasional capacity to "replace" each other in response to particular provocative circumstances, is nevertheless remark-

---

[38]There is, of course, a strong *moral* undertone to such regimens, as is true of so many successful ways of treating migraine. Sydney Smith, who suffered from hayfever, stresses the ascetic nature of his treatment: ". . . I am taking all proper care of myself, which care consists in eating nothing that I like, and doing nothing that I wish."

able, and requires explanation. We can only intimate our belief, at this stage, that migraine and allergic reactions are biologically *analogous*, and though fundamentally different in nature (allergic reactions representing local cellular sensitivities, and migrainous reactions complex cerebral responses) may be employed in similar ways by a patient. This is essentially the conclusion reached by Wolff who has suggested that ". . . the allergic disturbances and the migraine headache [may be] separate and independent manifestations of difficulty in adaptation."

SELF-PERPETUATION OF MIGRAINES

We cannot leave the subject of circumstantial migraines without asking ourselves two questions—questions which appear simple even to absurdity when formulated, but which are difficult to answer without bringing up concepts of a radical and even paradoxical kind. Firstly, we must ask, why do migraines last *so long*? We remarked in the last chapter that periodic (idiopathic) attacks usually moved through a compact predetermined course, and are over; circumstantial migraines, on the contrary, have a tendency to prolong themselves, often for day after day, long past the original provocative circumstances. Secondly, we must ask, is it possible for one symptom or component of a migraine to have a *direct* action upon another one?

We spoke, in the Historical Introduction, of the ancient "sympathetic" theories of migraine which dominated thinking for so many centuries, and we must now wonder whether any fragments of truth could have been caught up in the general framework of these theories, and, if so, whether they may be of relevance to the two questions we have asked. The theory postulated a peripheral origin of migraines (". . . an irritation in some distant member or viscera"—Willis), followed by a direct internal propagation of the symptoms (by "sympathy" or "consensus"), so that—in the words of Tissot—one part could suffer for another.

Discussion of the basis and mechanisms of migraine still lie far ahead of us, and we raise the spectre of "sympathy" not to explain the initiation of migraine attacks (which is a central process), but in relation to the maintenance of attacks already started, and the profound effects which individual symptoms may have on the total attack. Thus, it has always been known that vomiting may rapidly terminate the *entire* migraine attack. An even more commonplace observation is that a simple analgesic (e.g. aspirin) may serve not only to mitigate a migraine headache, but to disperse the *entire* attack. Conversely, it is common knowledge that aggravating a single symptom (as unpleasant smells may increase nausea) may, in turn, aggravate the *entire* attack.

These elementary observations are astonishing in their implications: for they imply that the entire migraine may be perpetuated by one or another of its own symptoms. In short, that a *migraine can become a response to itself.* Given the initial provocation, the original impetus, one may envisage that the subsequent continuance of many migraines may arise in this fashion from a series of self-perpetuating internal drives—a positive feed-back—so that the entire reaction is bound within its own circularity. These are terms in which one is compelled to think, when faced with the problem of migraines immensely outlasting their provocative circumstances, and protracted beyond any reasonable adaptive (or emotional) function: migraines as self-perpetuating, as fusing stimulus and response, as being held, so to speak, in a corridor of mutually interacting symptoms.[39]

The role of such self-perpetuating mechanisms may be of particular significance in migraine in view of the fact that *local* tissue-changes may occur and prolong individual symptoms (e.g. the train of changes which Wolff has demonstrated following dilatation of extracranial arteries); the persistence of an individual symptom, in this way, may cause the entire attack to persevere.

We must accept, then, that individual symptoms of a migraine can *drive* each other, or indeed the whole attack. Such driving may well be mediated by central reflex-arcs, but could also be understood in terms of purely peripheral mechanisms, on the supposition of direct action ("sympathy") between one viscus and another, or rather—putting the old doctrine in modern terms—between one autonomic plexus and another[40] (see Chapter 11).

CONCLUSIONS

The type of attack we have considered in this chapter must be viewed as radically different from periodic and paroxysmal migraines. The latter

---

[39] There are innumerable examples of such self-perpetuating symptoms, in which there is a reverberation of stimulus and response, or a maintained opposition between them—a sort of physiological echoing. A familiar example is Parkinsonian tremor (reverberation) and Parkinsonian rigidity (maintained opposition). In all such cases one must think—as in the perpetuation of a migraine—of *inertia* and *momentum.*

[40] A familiar example of such a peripheral autonomic interaction is the gastrocolic reflex—emptying of the bowel in response to filling of the stomach. This universal post-breakfast reflex is apparently not mediated by central mechanisms at all, but by a direct signalling from stomach to colon, a "sympathy" between these two parts of the gut.

gather force and impend in the nervous system; they are set off when they are "due," frequently by trivial or inoffensive stimuli which simply serve to detonate the attack; they run their fixed courses, and are followed by calm. They must be seen as idiopathic events, related primarily to the periodicities of the nervous system. Circumstantial migraines, in contrast, are only elicited by certain *types* of stimulus, and tend to show a significant relation, in their duration and severity, to the strength of this stimulus: thus they are, in essence, graded responses to graded stimuli. The circumstances evocative of these migraines are not trivial or inoffensive; they represent, at least potentially, major disturbances or disruptions or nervous activity. Thus, circumstantial migraines must be viewed not only as neuronal events, but as *reactions* which have a definite function in relation to their provocative circumstances.

We have seen that there are two forms of stimulus which are particularly prone to evoke migrainous reactions in predisposed individuals: inordinate excitations or arousals, and inordinate inhibitions or slumps. Within certain "allowable" limits (which vary greatly from person to person), the nervous system maintains itself in a region of equilibrium, homeostatically, by means of continuous, minor, insensible adjustments; beyond these limits, it may be forced to react by sudden, major, symptomatic adjustments.

Thus, excessive arousal (in the form of sensory bombardment, violent exercise, rage, etc.) tends to be followed by a reaction of prolonged recoil—an arousal migraine; conversely, excessive inhibition (in the form of exhaustion, response to passive motion, etc.) tends to lead, beyond a critical point, to a protracted slump-reaction—a slump migraine. In both cases we must envisage a protective function as being carried out by the migraine reaction, a warning to avoid particular circumstances which cannot be tolerated—excessive noise and light, exhaustion, over-sleeping, over-eating, passive motion, etc.

Beyond a certain point, we have noted, the migraine may achieve a momentum of its own, and be protracted far beyond what would seem to be any reasonable adaptive function. In such cases, we have postulated, the migraine may be perpetuated as a paradoxical response to itself, a physiological vicious circle.

We have had to consider one type of circumstantial migraine which cannot be fitted into either of the above categories, notably the attacks of aura or classical migraine which may be elicited by flickering light or visualisation of a scotoma. We have been compelled to postulate that innate resonance-mechanisms form the substrate of such migraines, as is also the case with photogenic epilepsy or photo-myoclonus.

Finally, we have had to postulate that migraine, in its capacity as a reaction, is readily amenable to conditioning, and that it may thus become secondarily linked to an enormous variety of idiosyncratic circumstances in the life-history of the individual. Only in this way can we explain bizarre linkings of circumstance and response which seem to defy any possible physiological sense. The final lengths to which such conditioning may go can lead to a singular situation, in which the occurrence of migraine will be linked to the patient's expectation of its occurrence (a familiar analogy to this is seen in the precipitation of an allergic response, an attack of "rose-fever," if the patient is shown a paper-rose). If this occurs, the patient may become trapped in a circularity of expectations and symptoms, caught in a sort of complicity with himself. A consequence of this, and of the relation between suggestible patients and speculative physicians, is that virtually any theory of migraine may come to generate the data on which it is based.[41] Cause and effect can become inextricably tangled: as Gibbon has observed, in another connection, ". . . the prediction, as is usual, contributed to its own accomplishment."

[41] The history of hysteria provides many familiar examples of such a merging between expectations and symptoms. Thus Charcot's depiction of hysteria was responsible for the frequent occurrence of the symptoms he depicted. With his death, and the changing of medical expectations, the forms of hysteria changed in turn.

NINE

Situational Migraine

There are apparently two essentially different causes [of
illness], an inner one, *causa interna*, which the man
contributes of himself, and an outer one, *causa externa*,
which springs from his environment. And accepting this
clear distinction, we have thrown ourselves with raging force
upon the external causes . . . And the *causa interna*, that we
have forgotten. Why? Because it is not pleasant to look
within ourselves . . .

Groddeck

As one receives the history from a migraine patient, the pattern of his
attacks is gradually clarified. It may be obvious, within minutes of first
seeing the patient, that he suffers periodic migraines which display an
innate rhythmicity irrespective of his mode of life, or that he has attacks
which are clearly coupled with one or more of the provocative circumstances considered in the last chapter. But there will remain a third group
of patients—a large group—who suffer from repeated and unremitting
attacks for no reason which is immediately apparent. Such patients, habitual migraineurs, may have experienced as many as five attacks weekly
for many years, and they are, therefore, the most cruelly incapacitated
of all migraine sufferers.

Faced with this afflicted group, one must infer that there exists some
chronic situation which "drives" their attacks, some goad which may be
physiological or psychological, intrinsic or extrinsic. A small minority
of these patients seem to suffer from an intrinsic physiological stimulus
to migraine. We may recognise in this category those patients who have
had extremely frequent classical migraines or migraine auras from earliest childhood, and who not uncommonly come from a family background heavily weighted with classical migraine. These rare patients (I
have not seen more than half a dozen in my entire experience) appear
to have some innate cerebral instability or irritability analogous to severe
idiopathic epilepsy. Patients with incessant attacks of migrainous neuralgia, not broken into clusters as is usually the case, may also be the

victims of some innate physiological mechanism, and in these one may conceive of some tic-like mechanism, of more peripheral location, analogous to that of trigeminal neuralgia. In a few patients one may discover the importance of certain extrinsic physiological stimuli (e.g. reserpine or hormone medication, the habitual use of alcohol or amphetamines, a particular sensitivity to environmental temperature or illumination, etc.), and be able to exclude these with happy results.

These possibilities will be considered and given a fair hearing by the physician, but by degrees it will be borne in upon him that the vast majority of patients with incessant unremitting migraines are not the victims of such physiological stimuli or sensitivities, but are caught in a malignant emotional "bind" of one sort or another, and *this*, he will come to suspect, is the driving-force behind their migraines. Sometimes the emotional stresses, reactions, conflicts, etc. are exposed and plainly in view, so that their existence and possible relevance to the migraine may be evident to both patient and physician. In other patients, the emotional substrates will be hidden and buried, so that their exposure (if this is deemed therapeutic) will be time-consuming and painful, challenging to the utmost the insight and the emotional resources of both patient and physician.

A proportion of patients (perhaps an especially high proportion among sufferers from habitual migraine) and a number of physicians doubt or deny that migraine can be a psychosomatic illness, and commit themselves to an endless search for physiological aetiologies and pharmacological treatments. Physicians who are prepared to think in terms of psychosomatic mechanisms have studied their patients in either of two ways. The first method of study is to investigate features of the patient's personality and life-situation as far as these are accessible in ordinary medical practice; such methods, necessarily, provide a relatively superficial picture of the patient's problems, but have the advantage that great numbers of patients may be submitted to observation (a classic among such studies was Wolff's investigation of 46 migraine patients).

The second method of study is a psycho-analytic one, and possible only in the very protracted and special conditions of an analysis; here the patient is studied in immense depth, but such investigations have the disadvantage that only a handful of patients are submitted to observation (a classic among such psycho-analytic studies is that of Fromm-Reichmann).

These two groups of investigators tend to use different languages, and their conclusions may therefore be difficult to compare. Furthermore, they are concerned with different aspects of the patient's emotional being, the first group being concerned with the overall features of overt personality, and the analysts with unconscious and often deeply-hidden emotional transactions in the psyche. There has been, nevertheless, a considerable unanimity of opinion with regard to the types of patient, and types of emotional posture, that may be seen in relation to habitual migraine. Wolff (1963) has delineated the features of the "migraine personality" in greater detail than all his predecessors. Migraineurs are portrayed by Wolff as ambitious, successful, perfectionistic, rigid, orderly, cautious, and emotionally-constipated, driven therefore, from time to time, to outbursts and breakdowns which must assume an indirect, somatic form. Fromm-Reichmann (1937) is also able to arrive at a clear-cut conclusion: migraine, she states, is a physical expression of unconscious hostility against consciously beloved persons.

My own method of study has been more akin to Wolff's, and has allowed me to interview many hundreds of migraine patients. In a number of cases (including those presented in this chapter) I have been able to see patients twice a month for prolonged periods, and thus to gain some insight into problems which would not have been apparent on a single interview, or even half a dozen interviews. I have not had the opportunity, and I have lacked the skills, for protracted depth-analysis of my patients.

During the early days of practice with migraine patients, and fresh from the literature on the subject, I tried to recognise, in every patient with habitual migraine that I saw, Wolff's stereotype of the "migraine personality," or Fromm-Reichmann's subtler qualities of ambivalence and repressed hostility. I was forced to the conclusion, by degrees, that neither of these generalisations had relevance to more than a proportion of the patients I saw. On the contrary, patients with severe habitual migraine seemed to me so various in their emotional pathologies and predicaments, that I despaired of putting them in a single category, unless I played Procrustes.

There is persuasive evidence that chronic emotional needs of a particular type characterise, for example, the majority of patients with peptic ulcers (see Alexander and French, 1948), but the analogy between such a psychosomatic disorder and habitual migraine is difficult to maintain. It appears, on the contrary, that migraines may be summoned to serve an endless variety of emotional ends. As migraines may assume a remarkable diversity of forms, so they may carry as various a load of emotional implications. If they are the commonest of psychosomatic reactions, it is because they are the most versatile.

CASE-HISTORIES

Case 76   This 43-year-old woman, a nun, had been subject to frequent common migraines and stuporous migraine equivalents since the age of 17, when she entered the religious life. Eleven months of each year were spent in the convent, and during these 11 months the patient would suffer two or three attacks of migraine, or migraine equivalent, weekly. She received one month of holiday annually, and during this she would rarely have even one attack.

Comment: This patient was an energetic, well-integrated if somewhat impatient person, a woman of strong practical ability who enjoyed exercise and fresh air, conversation and the theatre. Her strong sense of duty and altruism had been a main factor in directing her into the religious life. The claustrophobic conditions of convent life, the dearth of opportunities for physical and social activity, and above all the restriction of frank emotional expression, appeared to be main factors in driving this patient to somatic expression. Irritability, anger, sulking, etc., were not permissible in the convent, but migraine was. Given freedom from restrictions and impediments, she immediately lost the need for her attacks.

Case 78   This case was a 55-year-old woman with thrice-weekly attacks of common migraine. When questioned about her personal life, she admitted to constant anxiety concerning her husband, a diabetic prone to frequent and frightening insulin-reactions.

Her husband, a depressive with strong sado-masochistic traits, confessed, when interviewed alone, that he "guessed" how much insulin to take, and felt it "unnecessary" to test his urine for sugar. He was persuaded, with some difficulty, to place himself under competent medical care, and forthwith ceased to experience further insulin-reactions. With their disappearance, his wife became virtually exempt from migraine, and in a six-month follow-up had suffered only two attacks.

Comment: This patient had been living in a chronic anxiety-state, almost wholly bound up with her husband's illness. It might also be speculated that she wished to "join him" in a pattern of recurrent illness. With his liberation from illness her level of anxiety at once declined, and her migraines turned from habitual to occasional.

Case 79   A 46-year-old woman with three highly-intelligent, demanding, "difficult" and excessively-loved adolescent children. This patient had experienced very occasional migraines prior to the adolescence of her children, but had been subject to two or more attacks weekly since their entering their stormy puberties. Expressions of affection and maternal solicitude alternated with outbreaks of irritability. Each summer the loved but difficult children were despatched to youth-camps, and for three months the patient would be relieved of her anxieties, her irritability, and her migraine.

Comment: This situation, a common one in many parents, especially mothers, whom I have seen, is perhaps the best example of Fromm-Reichmann's theory.

Case 80   A 42-year-old woman with exceedingly frequent, and at times "almost continuous" migraine attacks, who complained that half of her waking hours were spent suffering, and a third of them in bed.
      When questioned about her personal life, she smiled and maintained that everything was "beautiful," her husband "a perfect gentleman," and her children "lovely." She vehemently denied that there were any problems of any sort: "There is not a cloud in the sky," she would say; "I have nothing to complain of except this wretched migraine."
      Over the course of several months, in which other members of the family were seen, it became apparent that there were innumerable problems. The family was in debt and heavily mortgaged, the husband was impotent, and the eldest child was a "drop-out" from school and a juvenile delinquent.

Comment: Here we see a situation with some similarities to the last case, but altogether more serious and pathological. The patient displays hysterical denial and repression of all "bad" emotional feelings, and maintains a set of conscious attitudes wholly at variance with the realities of her position. She is, indeed, "split" into two selves; one portion of her consists of denial and bravado, the other is a split-off system inflicting illness upon itself, and suffering continually.

Case 81   This 55-year-old man had been a former inmate of Auschwitz. He had suffered about one attack of classical migraine a month from the age of 7 until his incarceration in Auschwitz. During his 6 years in the concentration camp—6 years during which his wife, parents, and all other close relatives were killed—he did not experience a single attack of migraine. He was "liberated" by the Allies in 1945, and the following year emigrated to the United States.
      Since this time, he has been chronically depressed, guilt-ridden, preoccupied with the deaths of all his relatives whom he feels he might have saved, and intermittently psychotic. During this time he has also experienced 6 to 10 attacks of classical migraine each month, attacks which are refractory to treatment, and accompanied by the intensest suffering.
      He is also considerably "accident-prone," and during the two years that I saw him managed to sustain a Colles fracture, a fracture-dislocation of one ankle, and a head-injury. Each of these injuries was followed by several weeks'

remission of his migraines. It is also of interest that on the three occasions in which he has been hospitalised for psychotic depressions during the past 20 years, he was free from migraines.

Comment: This tragic case-history illustrates several points of interest. The exemption from migraine during his years in a concentration camp is a feature which has been described to me by several other patients: all forms of psychosomatic illness, and also frank psychosis, were apparently extremely rare in such conditions, presumably because they would have been lethally mal-adaptive. Since this time he has been frankly and greatly depressed, and has fully conscious, constantly reiterated, feelings of self-accusation and wishes for self-punishment.

His migraines gratify and reinforce such feelings, being sadistically inflicted and masochistically suffered. Sometimes an "accident" will serve a similar function, and thus dispense for a while with the necessity of migraines. When his depression reaches psychotic intensity and he feels himself to be in the hell he deserves, his hallucinations and delusions similarly dispense with the relatively inconsiderable migraines.

Case 56   A 43-year-old woman who had suffered severe common migraines, usually two or three attacks a month, since childhood. She could recollect only 3 periods during which she had been exempt from attacks: during a severe illness (sub-acute bacterial endocarditis), when she was in hospital for 4 months; during her first 3 pregnancies, when she went more than 6 months without attacks (this was in dramatic contrast to her fourth, unwanted, pregnancy, when she not only continued to have migraines throughout the 9 months, but had more severe attacks than usual for her); finally, during a three-month period when she was mourning for her father to whom she had been deeply attached.

Comment: This is, as it were, a case-history in reverse, showing certain situations in which a patient found herself *free* from life-long migraines, and as such supplements the preceding case-history. Exemption from migraine during pregnancy is a very common experience, and has generally been ascribed to the physiological or hormonal changes occurring during pregnancy (*vide* Chapters 8 and 10). The above case-history suggests that psychological factors must also be taken into account: the four pregnancies were, one may presume, physiologically similar, but the last of them was unique in being undesired by the patient. Freedom from migraine (and many other psychosomatic symptoms) is often procured during severe illnesses, and one must wonder whether medical attention, social support and sympathy, in conjunction with release from many habitual stresses, are perhaps the "liberating" factors, rather than the illness *per se*. Mourning, in which the free expression of emotion receives social support and sympathy, may absolve a patient from migraine and similar symptoms, in distinction to depressive reactions which tend to aggravate these.

Case 82   A 40-year-old woman who, when first seen, was suffering from a severe migraine and accompanied by her husband who took it upon himself to provide the "history." This he did with sadistic relish, disguised as "scientific detachment." A statistician, he had gone to extraordinary lengths to note the dates of every attack his wife had experienced in the past four years, compared these with the dates of her menstrual periods, the vagaries of her diet, changes in the weather, etc. He had computed correlation coefficients for all these "factors." Much of his time was evidently spent ministering to his wife, for he served as her physician, and computed with equal care precisely what drugs she should receive in each attack. Both he and she emphasise the necessity of frequent ergotamine and pethidine (Demerol) injections.

Comment: This case-history is essentially one of a *folie à deux* between two people who are both symbiotically and destructively dependent upon one another. The sexual aspects of their marriage had long since foundered, but had been replaced, apparently, by a sado-masochistic intimacy revolving around the patient's migraines.

Case 84   This patient, a 44-year-old man, had been employed for many years by an uncle whom he loathed. The conditions of work were unpleasant, and were made worse by his employer's habitual sarcasms; the salary, however, was considerably in excess of what the patient might have earned in comparable work elsewhere, and this had made him reluctant to seek "outside" employment. He suffered from continual belching and frequent migraines, two or three attacks weekly, throughout his working year, but was free of these during his annual monthly vacation.

Comment: This patient was caught in a dilemma in which humiliating conditions of work had been "accepted" for financial reward. Caught in a situation of deeply resented bondage, he felt himself unable to improve his working-conditions, or seek employment elsewhere. Ostensibly mute and compliant, he expressed his rage in physiological terms, as continued eructations and migraines.

Case 55   This 42-year-old man had once aspired to the priesthood, but was frustrated in this ambition. He lived a querulous and joyless existence, masochistically bound to his domineering mother with whom he lived. Seven or eight times a year, desire would override guilt, and he would steal out of the house to seek sexual contact. Within five minutes of orgasm, a "terrible" migraine would come upon him, and rack him with pain for the ensuing three days.

Comment: This guilt-ridden Catholic had morbid fears of sexual intercourse, which he construed as a sin richly deserving of punishment. His migraines provided the requisite punishment, three days of cephalgic penance, after which he regained his physiological and moral equilibrium.

Case 62   A 55-year-old woman whose symptoms wore briefly described in Chapter 2. Unmarried, and the only daughter of parents who had always been demanding and possessive, and were now ageing and in poor health, she was compelled to work at two jobs, for a total of 14 hours daily, to support the household. She had no friends, no social life, and had never had any sexual experience. She felt it her "duty" to support her parents and to be with them whenever she was not working.

At one time, indeed, she had made pathetic efforts to establish an independent existence, but these had been foiled first by parental intervention, and subsequently by her own discomfort and guilt if she went out alone. In the past 10 years she had lost all choice in the matter, for she suffered severely from migraine, ulcerative colitis, and psoriasis, not concurrently, but in a never-ending cycle.

Comment: This pitiful case-history illustrates the sacrifice of a life, and the trapping of this patient at three concentric levels: an intolerable domestic reality, an intolerable neurotic conflict, and an intolerable circle of psychosomatic symptoms.

Case 83   A 35-year-old engineer, this patient had founded, and directed, a highly-successful "thought-tank," a group which offered computing and mathematical research-work for many industrial and governmental concerns. Brilliant and insatiably ambitious, this patient drove himself and his subordinates to ruthless extremes.

He worked incessantly every evening and all Saturday. He permitted himself no hobbies, no social life, and no children. Every Sunday morning he would wake with a severe migraine. Originally he had forced himself to work despite the headache, but for the past two years the attacks had been accompanied by such nausea and vomiting that he was incapacitated for the day.

Comment: Here we see a patient with such a hypertrophied "drive" that he would work a seven-day week, or even a 168-hour week, if it were humanly possible. But it is not humanly possible, and his human limits were enforced by regular Sunday migraines which acted as physiological Sabbaths. This patient is the only one in the above series who has a "migraine personality."

CONCLUSIONS

We have concluded that the majority of patients who experience very frequent, severe, and unremitting migraines, for which no obvious circumstantial antecedents can be traced, are reacting to chronically difficult, intolerable, and even frightful life-situations. In such patients we are able to observe or to infer powerful emotional stresses and needs, and to realise that these are driving recurrent attacks. Of this species of migraine, and no other, we may legitimately use the term "psychosomatic illness." Such illnesses represent (in Borges's magnificent phrase) "apparent desperations and secret assuagements." We have noted, in one case-history, the alternation of migraines with another form of somatic assuagement—repeated accidents—and we might have presented much evidence regarding the alternation or replacement of migraines with repeated minor viral illnesses (colds, upper respiratory infections, herpes, etc.) and allergic manifestations, which may also, apparently, be pressed into similar roles in the emotional economy.

We believe that migraine may be adopted as an expression of emotional stress and distress of many different types, and that it is impossible to fit all patients into the stereotype of the obsessive "migraine personality," or to find in all of them chronic repressed rage and hostility. Nor should one claim that all patients with habitual migraine are "neurotic" (except in so far as neurosis is the universal human condition), for in many cases—a matter which will receive full discussion in Chapter 13— the migraines may replace a neurotic structure, constituting an alternative to neurotic desperation and assuagement.

PART III

The Basis of Migraine

Introduction

We have surveyed the forms which migraine may take, and the conditions under which it may occur. The greater part of this information was available to Liveing, Gowers, and Hughlings Jackson a century ago, and these physicians, Liveing above all, used it to derive astonishing insights not only into the nature of migraine, but into the organisation of cerebral activities.

This classical method, the collection and use of clinical data, has been overshadowed or displaced, in many areas of medicine, by the refinement of experimental methods. Experiment dissects and simplifies, striving to achieve uniform conditions in each experiment, and exclusion of all variables save the one which has been selected for observation. The application of such methods to the elucidation of migraine has been less successful than in many other fields; nevertheless, there still exists a widespread expectation that the "cause" of migraine is about to be established at any moment by virtue of some dramatic technical "breakthrough."

The passion to pinpoint a single factor in the pathogenesis of migraines has led many investigators to make unreasonable extrapolations from their data, statements of the following type: Migraine is due to an acute microcirculatory disorder (Sicuteri); Migraine is due to an oxygen deficiency in a strategic area of the brain (Wolff); Migraine is due to a disturbance of blood serotonin, etc.

The search for a single causative factor—Factor X—is likely to be successful if the event being studied has a fixed form and fixed determinants. But the essence of migraine, as we have seen, lies in the variety of forms it may take and the variety of circumstances in which it may occur. Therefore, though one type of migraine may be associated with Factor X, and another with Factor Y, it seems impossible, on *prima facie* grounds, that all attacks of migraine could have the same aetiology.

But we now encounter a much more fundamental problem, which springs from the fact that migraine cannot be considered simply as an event in the nervous system which occurs spontaneously and without reason: the attack *cannot* be considered apart from its causes and effects. A physiological statement *cannot* enlighten us concerning the causes of migraine, or its importance as a reaction or item of behaviour. Thus a logical confusion is implicit in the very formulation of such a question as: What is the cause of migraine? For we require not one explanation or one type of explanation, but several types, each in its own logical province. We have to ask *two* questions: why migraine takes the form(s) it does, and why it occurs when it does. These two questions *cannot* be coalesced. This was very clearly realised by Liveing who, after disputing the vascular theories of migraine fashionable even in his own time, observes:

> No one thinks of a condition of hyperaemia or anaemia of the nervous centres as the necessary antecedent of a fit of sneezing, laughter, vomiting, or terror, or *imagines that such a hypothesis would assist our comprehension.*

For all of these are reactions to something, and they cannot be explained without reference to this. The same is true of migraine, of all migraines, even those which occur periodically and without apparent relation to external circumstances; for these must still be construed in relation to some inner event or cycle in the body. Moreover migraine is not simply a physiological process; it is a set of symptoms, so far as the patient is concerned, and therefore requires description in experiential terms.

Thus to explain migraine we need three sets of terms, three universes of discourse. *Firstly* we must describe it as a process or an event in the nervous system, and the terms of this description will be neurophysiological ones (or as close to these as we can get); *secondly*, we must describe migraine as a reaction, and the terms of this description will be reflexological or behavioural ones; *thirdly*, we must describe migraine as it intrudes into the world of experience, as particular symptoms to which a particular affect or symbolic value is usually attached—and the terms of this description will be psychological or existential ones.

It is impossible to make any adequate statement on the nature of migraine without considering it, simultaneously, as *process*, as *reaction*, and as *experience*. We may note, by way of analogy, that exactly the same considerations apply, as the same confusions have occurred, with regard to our understanding of such a psychophysiological event as a psychosis. This too demands description at these three levels. To assert that (all) psychoses are "due" to disorders of amine metabolism (or taraxein, or vitamin deficiency, etc.) is not only demonstrably erroneous, but meaningless, as are comparable statements about the genesis of migraine. Even if it were able to provide an exact neurophysiological description of, say, a catatonic psychosis, it would tell us nothing of its causes or content. For the majority of naturally-occurring psychoses are *about* something, and in response to something, and these emotional contents and causes cannot be put in physical terms.

Chapters 10 and 11 will be devoted to considerations of the physiological bases of migraine; we will first discuss current experimental evidence and theories on the mechanism of migraine (Chapter 10), and this will be followed by a general discussion of the *structure* of migraine, based both on clinical and experimental evidence. Chapters 12 and 13 will be concerned with the *strategic* aspects of migraine, formulated first in behavioural terms, and then in psychodynamic terms.

TEN

Physiological Mechanisms of Migraine

Those who do not understand history are condemned to repeat it.

Santayana

HISTORICAL INTRODUCTION

Liveing devotes a fifth of his masterpiece to the consideration of the many theories of migraine which already existed in his own time, before going on to advance his own highly original ideas. We must retrace a certain amount of this well-trodden ground, not out of an idle reverence for the past, but because many of the major theories which exist today were in circulation in Liveing's time, and his comments on them retain their relevance today. We cannot do better, therefore, than follow his exposition and criticism of theories which existed in his own time, after which we may consider Liveing's own theory of nerve-storms, and its tenability today. Liveing discusses:

(a) The Doctrine of Biliousness.

(b) Sympathetic and Eccentric Theories.

(c) Vascular Theories:
   1. Arterial cerebral hyperaemia.
   2. Passive venous congestion of the brain.
   3. Vasomotor hypotheses.

(d) The Theory of "nerve-storms."

The humoral and eccentric theories, although still maintained in covert form by innumerable sufferers from migraine, have chiefly historical importance, and as such were considered in the introduction to this volume.

Theories of cerebral plethora gained prominence in medieval times—
even in Willis's day blood-letting was a favourite treatment for migraine.
Vasomotor hypotheses arose shortly after the innervation and contrac-
tility of arteries had been demonstrated, and dominated mid-Victorian
thinking about the mechanism of migraine as they continue to dominate
thinking today.

Du Bois Reymond attributed migraine headache to arterial spasm
from sympathetic stimulation . . . "a Tetanus takes place in the muscular
coats of the vessels of the affected half of the head; in other words, a
Tetanus in the territory of the cervical portion of the Sympathetic"; *Möllendorff*'s theory is the converse of this . . . "a one-sided loss of power
in the vasomotor nerves governing the carotid artery, whereby a relaxation of the artery and a flow of arterial blood towards the brain are
established," a condition which he compares to the effects of section of
the cervical sympathetic ganglion in animals; *Latham*'s theory combined
the virtues of the two preceding ones:

> . . . first of all we have contraction of the vessels of the brain, and so dimin-
> ished supply of blood, produced by excited action of the sympathetic; and
> that the exhaustion of the sympathetic following on this excitement causes
> the dilatation of the vessels and the headache.

While du Bois Reymond and Möllendorff only undertook to explain
the immediate mechanism of migraine headache, Latham extended his
vasomotor theory to cover *all* aspects of the migraine attack, and ascribed the scotomata and other manifestations of the aura-stage to cerebral vasoconstriction and local anaemia. Liveing was prepared to accept
that the immediate cause of migrainous headache was due to dilatation
in extracranial arteries, but could not accept a vasomotor hypothesis as
adequate to explain the many other aspects of migraine attacks, notably
the many, varied, and frequently bilateral symptoms of migraine aura,
the widespread vegetative effects throughout the body, the typical sequence of symptoms in an attack, and the metamorphoses in format
which the attacks could show.

Gowers too delivered a trenchant attack on Latham's hypothesis:

> The peculiarities in the disturbance of migraine [he writes] are its special and
> often uniform features, deliberate course, and its limitation to sensory distur-
> bance. To explain them on the vasomotor hypothesis we must assume first,
> an initial spasm of the arteries in a small region of the brain; secondly, that
> the contraction always begins at the same place; and thirdly, that it can give

rise to a definite, uniform and very peculiar disturbance of function. *There is no evidence of truth of any one of these assumptions.*

. . . we are not justified in assuming that the state of the surface vessels is an indication of the condition of those of internal organs. If it were, inasmuch as the recognisable vasomotor spasm is bilateral in almost all cases, even when the sensory disturbance is unilateral, we must assume a general contraction of the vessels of the brain. A general contraction could only cause a local disturbance of function by virtue of a local change in the functional tendency of the nerve-cells. But if such local change is admitted, the need for the vaso-motor hypothesis disappears. Lastly, *that vasomotor spasm can cause a deliberate, uniform, and peculiar "discharge" is not only unproved, but in the highest degree improbable.*

It is thus evident that the acuter minds of the last century had already realised and articulated, with perfect clarity, the shortcomings of Latham's vasomotor hypothesis, and the fact that no theory of this type, however stretched, could *conceivably* account for the characteristics of the migraine attack in its entirety. Nevertheless, the notion of a vaso-constrictor origin of the migraine process is still widely and uncritically held today, and new variants of the theory, ingenious if absurd, are continually put forward (see, for example, Milner, 1958).

Liveing's dissatisfaction with these vasomotor theories led him to formulate his own powerful and versatile theory of "nerve-storms."

We may again follow Liveing in the stages by which he constructs his theory:

On this theory, then, the fundamental cause of all neuroses is to be found, not in any irritation of the visceral, or cutaneous periphery, nor in any disorder or irregularity of the circulation, but in a primary and often hereditary . . . disposition of the nervous system itself; this consists in a tendency to the irregular accumulation and discharge of nerve force . . . and the concentration of this tendency in particular localities . . . will mainly determine the character of the neurosis in question.

Liveing explicitly distinguishes the notion of nerve force from that of the accumulation of any *substance*. His conception is a purely physiological one:

. . . a gradually increasing instability of equilibrium in the nervous parts: when this reaches a certain point, the balance of forces is liable to be upset and the train of paroxysmal phenomena determined by causes in themselves totally inadequate to produce such effects—just as a mere scratch will shiver to dust a mass of unannealed glass . . .

He comes to this conclusion from a consideration of the enormous number of factors of different kinds which can precipitate an attack:

> . . . the impression may come from without, and be of the nature of an irritation of some peripheral nerve, visceral, muscular, or cutaneous; or it may reach the centres through the circulation . . . or it may descend from the higher centres of psychical activity . . .

So many exciting factors, yet the effect is the same: in every case the nervous system responds with a migraine. Therefore, the migraine is *implicit* in the cerebral repertoire. Its structure is, as it were, *pre-formed*.

Liveing recognises that a migraine can act as a *consummatory discharge*, following and terminating the build-up of a tension: thus he compares it with a sneeze, a voracious meal or an orgasm. Indeed, these discharges may be "equivalent," and are thus liable to metamorphoses among themselves: he instances the ability of a fit of sneezing suddenly to terminate, or replace a migraine (*vide* Case 66, p. 30); or the apprehension of sudden danger terminating an intense sea-sickness; sexual excitement provoking an asthma; or tickling an epilepsy.

Liveing is well aware that migraine, as other "neuroses" he considers, may be established and facilitated by "pathological habit" (viz. conditioning).

Finally Liveing comes to consider "The Anatomical Seat of Megrim." He observes that the manifestations of migraine are almost exclusively sensory, and infers that "the disorder is limited for the most part to the sensory tract and ganglia of the sensory nerves, from the optic thalamus above to the nucleus of the vagus below."

He perceives that the occurrence of emotional manifestations, and speech and memory disorders in an attack, entail ". . . an extension of the disorder to the hemispheric ganglia," and that the frequent *bilaterality* of visual and tactile hallucinations is most easily reconcilable with the hypothesis of a "centric origin." The dilatation of the temporal arteries, and the slowing and smallness of the pulse, are ascribed to a peripheral radiation of the attack, through the vagus and its presumed connections with the sympathetic ganglia.

SOME CURRENT THEORIES OF THE MIGRAINE MECHANISM

We may now turn our attention to the major theories of the migraine mechanism which dominate contemporary thinking. Theories of a peripheral origin of migraine retain a certain public currency, but have long ceased to be seriously considered. We may include among these theories that of an allergic origin of migraine, which commands a somewhat wider assent among physicians, but may be ruled out of court on a variety of grounds (see Chapters 5, 6, and 8). Migraine arises in the central nervous system as clearly as the earth is round. The central nervous system is an electrochemical machine nourished by blood. Serious investigations of migraine therefore concern themselves with the nourishment of the nervous system (vasomotor theories), the chemistry of the nervous system, and the electrical activity of the nervous system, endeavouring to find pathognomonic abnormalities which may be related to the course and origin of migraine attacks.

VASOMOTOR THEORIES OF MIGRAINE

We have seen that the notion of a two-stage sequence in the migraine mechanism—a phase of vasoconstriction due to sympathetic hyperactivity followed by one of vasodilatation due to sympathetic "exhaustion"—is of considerable antiquity. Latham's theory has had both a stimulating and a stultifying effect on later research, on the one hand inspiring Wolff's brilliant experimental studies of the immediate mechanism of migrainous headache, but on the other hand discouraging the formulation of any alternative suppositions regarding the genesis of the migraine attack *in its entirety.*

Wolff was able to show, in a variety of elegant ways, that the intensity of migraine headache is closely proportional to the dilatation of extracranial arteries, and could be diminished by the effects of manual compression, adrenaline, and ergotamine on the dilated arteries, or by centrifugation of the entire body. In the later stages of migraine headache, it was shown, dilatation of the offending artery or arteries might be followed by a train of *local* changes, with exudation of a polypeptide-rich fluid provocative of local pain, and finally, a sterile inflammatory reaction.

> . . . the fact that an almost pure vasoconstrictor agent, such as norepinephrine, promptly reverses all the painful aspects of migraine headache is further evidence that the genesis of this pain is vasodilatation . . . At the onset of the headache there is concomitant dilatation of the large arteries, arterioles, and metarterioles. The dilatation of the arterioles and metarterioles increases the capillary hydrostatic pressure. The elevated capillary hydrostatic pressure favours the accumulation of pain-threshold-lowering material in the subcutaneous tissue of the scalp . . . postulated as "headache stuff." Dilatation and

distension of large arteries coupled with accumulation of this pain-threshold-lowering stuff result in headache. (Wolff, 1963)

The techniques described, supplemented by direct observation of minute vessels in the bulbar conjunctive, have provided a definitive account of the mechanism of migraine headache. When, however, Wolff and his co-workers endeavoured to apply similar techniques to the investigation of the pre-headache symptoms, in particular the scotomata, their findings were altogether less consistent and impressive, and more in need of *ad hoc* hypotheses. Experiments were made concerning the action of vaso-active substances (amyl nitrite, and carbon-dioxide-rich mixtures) upon the duration of scotomatous field-defects. The results of these experiments have not lent themselves to consistent replication. Nevertheless, Wolff felt justified in postulating the *probable* existence of local cortical ischaemia as the basis of the scotomata:

> It is therefore postulated that the greatly increased amount of blood which is maximally saturated with oxygen (after breathing mixtures rich in carbon dioxide) corrects an underlying oxygen deficiency in a strategic area of the brain, where the impulses which set up the compensatory vascular dilatation of the migraine attack may originate . . . The pathophysiology of scotomata is intimately linked with cranial vasoconstriction . . . It is possible that more than the occipital cortex is involved in the ischaemia and that symptoms stem mainly from the occipital cortex because of higher metabolic requirements of this part of the hemisphere . . .

Wolff himself, invariably strict and careful in his thinking, phrased these notions as a hypothesis, or series of hypotheses, and conceded that there existed a number of facts difficult to reconcile with the ischaemic theory. Many subsequent workers, however, ignoring the qualified and tentative expression of Wolff's opinions, have taken the vasoconstrictor hypothesis as proven beyond dispute, almost as axiomatic. Thus Graham starts a review of migraine with the following statement:

> The immediate mechanism of the migraine attack has been related by Wolff and his co-workers to disordered behaviour of the cranial blood-vessels.

Bickerstaff, describing what appear to be neither more nor less than severe classical migraines in a group of patients, asserts that their symptoms represent transient dysfunction in the territory of supply of the basilar artery. Selby and Lance, similarly, do not hesitate to ascribe migrainous syncope in their patients to transient ischaemia of the brainstem reticular formation.

When hypotheses insensibly harden into assumptions, further enquiry is terminated and the subject becomes petrified: such has been the case, for some years, with regard to the vasoconstrictor theory of migraine aura. It is necessary, therefore, to re-open the subject, and submit every aspect of the theory to rigorous scrutiny. It is not only possible but it is necessary to advance many considerations against that Latham-Wolff theory.

Firstly, and most obviously, it has never been submitted to direct observation; the cortical blood-vessels have never been observed during the course of a migraine aura, and it is more than questionable as to whether the vessels of the bulbar conjunctive can afford a reliable model of the behaviour of intracranial vessels; changes in the latter, moreover, are *not* constantly observed during migraine aura. Secondly, there is not infrequently an overlap of aura and headache stages, or the recurrence of repeated auras *during* the headache (vasodilator) stage, an important clinical fact not acknowledged by Wolff, and impossible to reconcile with the two-stage theory. Indeed a polysymptomatic aura may exhibit, at one and the same time, both excitatory and inhibitory features. The variability of the aura, presenting now in one form and now another, is at variance with the special vulnerability of the occipital cortex postu-lated in the ischaemic theory. It is difficult or impossible to conceive how the "very peculiar disturbances of function" to which Gowers alludes— the characteristic shape and march of scotomata, the vibratory quality of scintillations and paraesthesiae, etc.—can be explained simply on the basis of ischaemia: such sensory hallucinations as may occur in an attack of basilar ischaemia, or during vertebral angiography, tend to be simple and transient, and lack all the special features of the migrainous scotoma. The undoubted effects which vaso-active agents sometimes have on the duration or intensity of the scotomata imply nothing of the nature of the underlying migrainous process, but show only the effects of summat-ing two neurophysiological alterations. The known effects of lowered cerebral perfusion-pressure, as in postural hypotension, is to produce faintness, dizziness, and sometimes a brief swarm of "spots before the eyes," etc., a clinical picture which is very different from that of a mi-graine aura.

Such objections could be multiplied and elaborated without end. We are forced to conclude that the evidence favouring a vasoconstrictor ori-gin of migraine is scanty, indirect, questionable in its interpretation, and in need of many *ad hoc* assumptions even to assume an appearance of plausibility. More cogently, it shows itself utterly inadequate to explain the rich complexity of the aura format with its many, elaborate and varied symptoms. The ischaemic hypothesis is attractive in view of its simplicity, but is, alas, altogether *too* simple to account for a migraine.

CHEMICAL THEORIES OF MIGRAINE

There exist a number of chemical theories of migraine, posing as ultra-modern in style and appeal, but generically derived from the humoral theories of the Greeks. Dramatic advances in understanding the chemical bases of certain neurological diseases, and in our knowledge of neuro-pharmacology, have fanned the hope that we may be about to discover a chemical basis for Parkinsonism, psychosis, migraine, etc. In the late fifties, for example, certain biological amines became a focus of intense interest: these years yielded Woolley's monograph on the serotonin the-ory of psychosis, Sicuteri's introduction of serotonin antagonists for the treatment of migraine, and, shortly afterwards, the dopamine theory of Parkinsonism. It would be difficult to find a more dramatic example of what was earlier termed "Factor X" thinking.

Chemical theories of migraine are suggested by the outstanding auto-nomic components of the attack. The obvious and common symptoms of migraine are vascular headache, dilatation of extracranial vessels, nau-sea, increased visceral and glandular activity, and on occasion minor autonomic signs such as bradycardia, miosis, hypotension, etc. In addi-tion to these peripheral vegetative disturbances, there are likely to exist a number of centrally-determined symptoms such as muscular hypo-tonia, drowsiness, depression, etc. We have noted that features clinically and physiologically the opposite of the above symptoms—visceral stasis and dilatation, evidences of physiological and psychological excitation, etc.—may precede and follow the major course of the attack.

It is obvious that the cardinal symptoms of migraine, if we set aside the prodromal and rebound stages, represent *an increase in parasympa-thetic tonus, a diminution in sympathetic tonus, or both.* The termination of attacks, spontaneously, by various forms of physiological or psycho-logical arousal, or, therapeutically, by parasympathetic inhibitors or sympathomimetic drugs, reinforces the notion that an excess of para-sympathetic activity is characteristic of the major, and latter, portions of a migraine attack.

Chemical theories of migraine were suggested by their originators in order to explain the transient but profound intensification of parasympathetic tonus during the attacks, and all neurohumours known to act at synaptic junctions in the parasympathetic system have been suggested, at one time or another, as primarily responsible for the genesis of migraine. Three such mediators may be instanced: histamine, acetylcholine, and 5-hydroxytryptamine, although only the last-named of these need be considered in any detail.

The histamine theory of migraine is associated with the name of Horton (1956), who considered that the distinctive variant of migraine described in Chapter 4 as "migrainous neuralgia" arose from a special form of histamine sensitivity. He stated that attacks might be evoked by injections of histamine in predisposed patients, that gastric acidity increased during the attacks, and that histamine "desensitisation" could avert the attacks. Horton's remarkable therapeutic successes with histamine desensitisation have been duplicated by few other workers, and apparently represent no more than a placebo effect, a consequence of intensive medical attention and emotional contact with an enthusiastic physician. More importantly, the vascular headache evoked by histamine lacks the unique characteristics of migrainous neuralgia. Thirdly, it has not been possible to demonstrate elevated levels of histamine in this or any other type of migraine.

The acetylcholine theory of migraine is associated with the name of Kunkle (1959), who has examined the levels of acetylcholine in the spinal fluid during attacks of migrainous neuralgia. Elevated levels were found in some but not all of the affected patients; Kunkle concluded that his results lent "considerable support" to the basic hypothesis. Kunkle's findings have not been duplicated, and the question of whether or not there exist elevated levels of acetylcholine locally, systemically, or in the spinal fluid, is still *sub judice*. The matter has been somewhat displaced from the attention of researchers by the rise of more fashionable serotonin theories.

The serotonin theory of migraine was launched by Sicuteri in company with the discovery of the therapeutic effects of methysergide, a potent serotonin-inhibitor, in the prophylaxis of migraine. Kimball and Friedman (1961) observed that a migraine or migraine-like attack could often be induced in migrainous patients by Serpasil, and the attacks thus induced could readily be dispersed by the intravenous infusion of 5-hydroxytryptamine. More sophisticated work has been performed by Lance *et al.* (1967), who undertook direct measurements of total plasma serotonin (TPS) before, during, and after migraine attacks, and has observed an abrupt fall of TPS at the onset of migraine headache in a

majority of subjects. It is known that the intracarotid injection of serotonin causes tonic constriction of extracranial arteries, and it is postulated by Lance *et al.* that an abrupt fall in levels of circulating serotonin
may lead to a painful distension of the extracranial vessels by a rebound
phenomenon.

In summary, therefore, we may say that evidence for systemic alterations of histamine in attacks of migraine may be discounted, that evidence for involvement of acetylcholine is questionable, and that evidence
for involvement of serotonin appears rather impressive, although the
work of Lance will require repetition and substantiation by other workers. But having said this, we are no nearer whatever to establishing a
chemical basis for migraine. Acceptance of a chemical basis would require evidence analogous to Koch's postulates of pathogenesis: we would
need to demonstrate appropriate changes of Factor X in every attack of
migraine studied, simulation of all possible migraine symptoms by the
administration of Factor X, and, finally, the *dependence* of the migraine
reaction upon Factor X. These conditions, patently, have not been met
by 5-hydroxytryptamine. On the one hand, the migranoid syndrome
induced in Serpasil or reserpine has only a partial resemblance to a full-
blown migraine; reserpine cannot evoke the manifestations of migraine
aura. Conversely, migraines may continue to occur with undiminished
frequency following a profound depression of systemic serotonin levels
by methysergide.

The crux of the matter lies in the danger of confusing cause and concomitance. It is possible, though unlikely, that the clinical and physiological phases of migraine are accompanied by commensurate changes
in the blood levels of one or more neurohumours (unlikely because the
characteristic parasympathetc activities which compose a migraine may
be very localised and sequestered); but the establishment of such a parallel, such a correlation, would tell us nothing concerning cause-and-
effect. It would be necessary to show that the altered levels of substance
X in the blood constituted a sufficient and necessary antecedent of the
migraine.

ELECTRICAL THEORIES

Migraine is a primary disturbance of brain-function, whatever secondary
mechanisms, local or humoral, may be involved in its clinical expression.
Direct examination of cerebral activity, in a benign condition like mi-

graine, is effectively limited to electroencephalographic (EEG) studies, and it is with these, and their interpretations, that we must now be concerned.

It is more than 30 years since the Gibbses first studied the EEG in migrainous patients (see Gibbs and Gibbs, 1941), and a large and inconclusive literature has grown up during this period. EEG abnormalities of many kinds have been described in connection with migraine—generalised slow-wave dysrhythmias, convulsive patterns, focal abnormalities, etc.—with remarkably little agreement as to the incidence or importance of such findings. We can note only a fraction of the published observations, and we will exclude from consideration, in particular, the gross EEG abnormalities seen during hemiplegic migraines, for such attacks clearly involve secondary mechanisms additional to the primary process of common or classical migraines (see Chapter 4).

Strauss and Selinsky (1941), in a pioneer study, observed slow (3 to 6 cycles per second) activity during hyperventilation in 9 out of 20 migrainous patients. Engel et al. (1945) recorded focal slow-wave abnormalities confined to the appropriate occipital leads during the occurrence of scotomata in two patients. Dow and Whitty (1947), in the first large-scale study, noted "generalised dysrhythmia" in 30 migraine patients, "symmetrical bilateral episodic activity" in 12, and "persistent focal abnormality" in 4 patients. Cohn (1949), investigating 83 patients with classical migraine, found that nearly half of them displayed an excessive amount of slow-wave activity between attacks; patients who exhibited such abnormalities were said to have "dysrhythmic migraines," and to profit from anticonvulsant therapy. Heyck (1956), in an authoritative study, observed non-specific, diffuse, slow-wave dysrhythmias in 13 out of 62, and focal abnormalities in 5 out of 62 migraine patients. Selby and Lance (1960) obtained inter-ictal records on 459 patients with migraine and allied vascular headaches; almost one-third of these were regarded as "abnormal," i.e. characterised by persistent or intermittent slow (4 to 7 cps) activity. Wave-and-spike patterns of convulsive type were recorded in two cases.

Recent work has attempted to determine whether any other patterns of EEG activity may be prominent in migraine. Whitehouse et al. (1967) have examined the recordings of 28 migrainous children and a similar number of matched controls for the incidence of so-called 14 and 6 cps positive spikes (a pattern first described by the Gibbses (1951), and considered by them as possible evidence of thalamic or hypothalamic epilepsy). They concluded that there was a definite though not dramatic excess of such positive spike patterns in the migrainous group. The pattern observed in one patient did not alter during the presence of a migraine attack. While fully aware of the uncertainties which surround the interpretation of 14 and 6 positive spikes, especially in children, Whitehouse *et al.* consider their findings, in conjunction with clinical evidence, as strongly suggestive of a primary autonomic disorder in the patients studied: ". . . it would be more satisfactory [they write] . . . to regard migraine as a primary disturbance in autonomic function with secondary vascular effects and with the possibility of explaining . . . humoral factors . . . as intermediary factors."

Dexter (1968), in a very recent unpublished study, has obtained all-night EEG recordings on patients suffering from nocturnal migraines. These patients were invariably in the stage of paradoxical (REM) sleep at the time they awoke with headache, but it was not possible, however, to predict the onset of attacks in such patients by the appearance of paradoxical sleep patterns in the EEG.

It is evident that these studies have failed to uncover any clear and consistent EEG abnormality peculiar to migraine. Lennox and Lennox (1960), summarising a twenty-year experience of such recordings, conclude that there is "nothing distinctive" in the tracings of migraine patients; one cannot, for example, diagnose migraine on the basis of an EEG record.

It has been impossible to define any EEG abnormality which bears a *specific* relation to migraine, as wave-and-spike patterns do to epilepsy. At most, there is a questionable statistical increase of slow-wave "dysrhythmias" beyond the 15 to 20 per cent incidence of these in non-migrainous populations (Gibbs and Gibbs, 1950). We must acknowledge, however, that there have been exceedingly few tracings obtained during the actual occurrence of migraine auras (as were those of Engel *et al.*), and none, apparently, during states of migrainous syncope, stupor, or coma. Thus the severest forms of migraine still remain a *terra incognita* to the electroencephalographer.

Why, we may wonder, have such studies achieved so little in comparison to the volumes of information we have concerning epilepsy? Several reasons suggest themselves. First, we have no reliable method of eliciting a migraine aura, in contrast to the ease of provoking seizure-activity; the migranoid reactions induced by reserpine, for example, have no aura component. Secondly, we cannot record from the exposed brain or use deep electrodes, as is justified in many cases of seizure-disorder. Thirdly, we cannot identify migraine or any migraine-like process in animals.

Lastly, and perhaps most importantly, the existing parameters of EEG recording, which are highly suitable for monitoring epileptic processes, may be entirely inappropriate for the study, or even the detection, of the migraine process.[42] We have already observed that the rate of spread of migrainous paraesthesiae, for example, is some hundreds of times slower than that of their epileptic counterparts, while the time-base of other migrainous processes, in turn, is much greater than that of the aura.

That *some* form of electrical disturbance accompanies the generation of a migraine can hardly be doubted, but the nature of this disturbance is still quite speculative. Lashley (1941), plotting his own scotomata (see Figure 3B), estimated that their enlargement corresponded to a wave of excitation moving across the visual cortex at a rate of about 3 mm per minute, followed by a wave of total inhibition. Milner (1957) remarks on the quantitative similarity of this rate of spread to that of "spreading depression," an electrotonic disturbance which may be induced in the exposed cerebral cortex, and which was originally described and investigated by Leão (1944). It has been impossible to monitor Leão's spreading depression by scalp-electrodes, or, more importantly, to demonstrate its occurrence in or relevance to any known physiological process. Further, as was emphasised in our discussion of the vasoconstrictor theories, clinical evidence indicates the occurrence of a widespread alteration of cortical function rather than any local process, ischaemic or depressive.

Lashley concluded, nearly thirty years ago, that "nothing is known of the actual nervous activity during the migraine," and this statement, regrettably, still holds true at the present time. Deep in the brainstem, as Liveing inferred, is the origin of the migrainous process, slow tonic changes of excitation and inhibition; but the detection of these changes, and the demonstration of their nature and cause, have completely eluded us, and may continue to do so for a number of years to come.

CONCLUSIONS

The last thirty years have witnessed an intensive search for vascular, chemical, and electrical disturbances occurring in relation to migraine

---

[42] Recently, working with my electroencephalographer, P. C. Carolan, I have had the extraordinary luck of monitoring the EEG in two patients—identical twin sisters—during the course of severe scotomatous migraine auras. In both cases we saw enormous slow-waves down in the delta range (1–3 Hz) confined to the occipital electrodes, which disappeared in a few minutes as the patients regained their vision.

attacks, and a proliferation of theories postulating such abnormalities as essential, fundamental mechanisms in the causation of attacks. This huge mass of research is documented in several thousand papers (Wolff's bibliography, compiled in 1960, and listing 1,095 references, represents only a selection of these), and we have done no more than comment on what appear to be, at the present time, the more important lines of investigation. We have altogether ignored certain fields of research—as that which searches for allergic factors in the causation of migraine—and certain sub-theories (e.g. the investigation of auto-immune mechanisms, and of possible mast-cell abnormalities, in relation to the serotonin hypothesis), as being of very doubtful relevance to the main physiological issues.

The immediate cause of migraine headache has been fully dissected by Wolff and his colleagues, and may be fully explained in terms of the dilatation of extracranial arteries and the release of local pain-producing factors. It is doubtful, however, if vasomotor mechanisms underlie other important aspects of the migraine attack, and it seems impossible that the symptoms of migraine aura, in particular, could be explained by considerations of local cortical ischaemia.

It is established that such substances as mecholyl, histamine, reserpine, etc. may produce clinical syndromes which have *some* resemblances to *some* migraine attacks, although such iatrogenic reactions lack many essential features of spontaneously-occurring attacks. There is some evidence, as yet insufficiently substantiated, that systemic humoral changes (e.g. of 5-hydroxytryptamine) may accompany some spontaneously-occurring attacks, but there is *no* evidence that such changes constitute the sufficient and necessary antecedent of all attacks. It seems exceedingly improbable that migraine could have any unitary metabolic basis, in view of its profound variations (and transformations) of clinical format, the almost instantaneous induction (and, on occasion, termination) of some migraine auras, and the tendency for migraine attacks to recur despite chemotherapy with potent blocking agents (e.g. methysergide, a serotonin-inhibitor).

We conclude that such vascular and humoral factors as have been discovered, and may be discovered in the future, can have at most a *partial* significance in the pathogenesis of migraine, as intermediary factors which are sometimes of relevance in some attacks. The vasomotor (Latham-Wolff) hypothesis can only be of limited utility, as was evident to Liveing a century ago (". . . No one . . . imagines that such a hypothesis would assist our comprehension . . ."), and the same is true of any chemical hypotheses. These *lack interest*, for they *cannot* cast light on the full complexity of the migraine problem.

> You'll reply that reality hasn't the least obligation to be interesting. And I'll answer you that reality may avoid that obligation but that hypotheses may not. (Borges)

Electrical studies do not lack interest, in this sense, for they are attempts to define a unique neurophysiological correlate of migraine. They have been completely unsuccessful, hitherto, but may be expected to achieve some success with increasing technical refinement. It seems certain, for example, that migraine aura must have reasonably distinctive physiological correlates. Whether we can hope to discover a unique migraine "process" in the nervous system, underlying every form of migraine, is another question, and one which will be discussed in the following chapter.

ELEVEN

The Physiological Organisation of Migraines

The four and twenty letters make no more variety of words
in divers languages, than melancholy conceits produce diversity of symptoms in several persons. They are irregular, obscure, various, so infinite, Proteus himself is not so
diverse . . .

Burton

The problem with migraine, as Robert Burton found with melancholy,
is the infinite variety of symptoms we are called upon to explain. We
must attempt to formulate a theory, or set of theories, altogether more
general than the simple mechanisms with which we were concerned in
the last chapter: general enough to cover every aspect of every type of
migraine, yet capable of specific application to any particular symptom.

We will start by considering the symptoms of migraine at different
functional levels, from the lowest to the highest, and the possible mechanisms underlying these symptoms. If these methods do not prove sufficient for the task, we will be compelled to adopt radically different
notions as to what is meant by a "function" or a "center" in neurophys-
iology, and to think in terms of dynamic organisation of functional systems, rather than in the traditional terms of fixed neural apparatus and
mechanisms.

We have seen that the vegetative symptoms of migraine represent
parasympathetic predominance, and we cannot fail to be struck by the
fact that the varying emphasis of different symptoms is matched by the
anatomical and functional configuration of the parasympathetic nervous
system. There exist anatomically discrete ganglionic plexuses in all the
major visceral, vascular, and glandular structures of the body, constituting the lowest level of neural representation of the inner or visceral body.
We may postulate that the existence of many such functionally discrete
plexuses can provide a physiological basis for a variety of distinct parasympathetic syndromes: that local neuronal activity in such plexuses,

once ignited by an initial discharge from the central nervous system, may persist—for minutes, hours, or days—as a functionally discrete, sequestered excitation. In the case of a patient with a protracted, localised, hemicrania, for example, we may visualise a relatively isolated disorder immured in a single perivascular plexus; in other cases, local neuronal excitations may be lodged in the mural plexuses of the stomach, the colon, the lacrimal glands, etc. The initial neuronal alteration may subsequently be reinforced by local tissue changes, e.g. the transudation and sterile inflammation which occurs in protracted vascular headaches, or other long-term changes which follow the initial neurogenic disturbance. The vegetative symptoms of migraine, at their last and lowest level, may be mediated, graded, and isolated, by virtue of the nerve-net configuration of the parasympathetic system. The "instructions" as to which format of attack, which migraine equivalent, will be selected is presumably determined by central mechanisms, although local differences of threshold, either innate or conditioned, may also play an auxiliary role. It is characteristic, however, that when one end-organ, or one local plexus, is removed from the system (as by surgical intervention), the migraine attacks will recur with a slightly altered format. This suggests that *fixed peripheral mechanisms are used as available, the central organisation of migraine being plastic and flexible.*

The term parasympathetic was originally employed, and is conveniently restricted, to denote peripheral structures and activities. It is clearly insufficient to speak of migraine as a parasympathetic attack, for all attacks have central, cerebral, components as well. Suitable concepts and terms are those devised by Hess, from his famous studies on central autonomic and diencephalic function (Hess, 1954). Hess uses the term "ergotropic" to denote the combination of peripheral sympathetic activity with central arousal, and the term "trophotropic" to denote the converse of this. These terms are not only physiological ones, but biological or organismal terms. Thus ergotropia denotes the tendency of an organism to direct itself to the outside world, to be active, to perform work, etc. for which it will be equipped by increased vigilance and sensory acuity, increased muscular tonus, increased sympathetic tonus, etc. Trophotropia denotes the tendency of an organism to direct itself inwards, to its domestic economy, for which it will be equipped by increased visceral and glandular activity, allied to relative inhibition of conscious level, sensory acuity, and muscular tone. Hess's terms recommend themselves as being outstandingly useful for our understanding of migraine attacks. It is evident that all of his criteria of trophotropia (increased parasympathetic tonus, diminution of arousal, hypersynchronisation of EEG, etc.) are met during the bulk of the migraine attack: the major part of a migraine, we may say, represents a *polymorphic trophotropic syndrome.*

The experimental elaboration of Hess's concepts, and their application to clinical problems, has been undertaken by many workers, among whom Gellhorn is pre-eminent. Thus it has been shown (see Gellhorn, 1967) that there exist—at all levels in the neuraxis—ergotropic and trophotropic systems which are anatomically, physiologically, and pharmacologically distinct. It has been shown that ergotropic and trophotropic activities are normally held in a reciprocal balance; this balance determines what Gellhorn has called the "tuning" of the nervous system at any given time. Thus, inhibition of the ergotropic system is associated with excitation of the trophotropic division, and vice versa. Typically, also, any marked change in autonomic tuning will be followed by a rebound-phenomenon in the opposite direction.

We may now translate the sequence of a common migraine into Hess's terms. The prodromal or inaugural symptoms are those of ergotropic predominance; the bulk of the attack represents a collapse into trophotropia; and the symptoms of the rebound are again ergotropic. Thus a common migraine may be envisaged as a three-stage paroxysm in slow motion, in which consistent and characteristic changes of nervous tuning occur. This notion roughly corresponds with Lennox's description of migraine as an "autonomic seizure." We cannot state the precise level of origin of the migraine process, and indeed suspect the question to be meaningless when put in this way, for ergotropic and trophotropic systems are represented, hierarchically, throughout the core of the neuraxis, from the (intermedio-lateral) spinal horns, to the brainstem reticular formation, to the hypothalamus, and ultimately in the mediobasal divisions of the cerebral cortex.

We may also identify a cycle of excitation and inhibition in the very condensed course of the migraine aura, the cycle of excitation (scintillating scotomata, paraesthesiae, excitement, diffuse sensory arousal, etc.) and inhibition (negative scotomata, anaesthesia, drowsiness, faintness, syncope, diffuse sensory inhibition, etc.), and, if it occurs, re-excitation taking only 30 to 40 minutes.

We arrive therefore at a picture of the migraine process similar to that which Liveing proposed a century ago: *a form of centrencephalic seizure, the activity of which is projected rostrally upon the cerebral hemispheres, and peripherally via the ramifications of the autonomic nervous system.*

We may picture the cortex as subjected to an ascending bombardment in the course of a migraine aura, to which it responds with secondary activities of its own: these secondary activities are multifocal (scintillating scotomata, paraesthesiae, etc.), set upon a background of diffuse cortical arousal. In analogous fashion, we may envisage peripheral autonomic plexuses as subject to a descending barrage, to which they respond with secondary, multifocal activities of their own. This picture of the migraine process is presented, schematically, in Figure 7.

It is obvious, however, that we will require further concepts and terms in order to describe the activations of the cerebral cortex during the course of a migraine aura. The visual hallucinations of migraine provide us with the clearest indications of these higher processes and their organisation.

We have observed (see Chapter 3) that there tends to be a *sequence* of visual hallucinations from the most elementary to the most complex type; this sequence is very similar to that which may occur in response to certain drugs (e.g. mescaline), sleep deprivation or sensory deprivation. Thus we may compare the migraine sequence to Hebb's (1954) account of visual hallucinations induced by sensory deprivation:

> It appears that the activity has a rather regular course of development from simple to complex. The first symptom is that the visual field, when the eyes are closed, changes from a dark to a light colour; next there are reports of dots, lines, or simple geometric patterns . . . the next step is seeing something like wall-paper patterns . . . Then come isolated objects, without background . . . finally, integrated scenes usually containing dream-like distortions.

The patterns and passage of the simplest migraine phosphenes across the visual field are reminiscent of the hallucinations of colour and abstract form (flickering lights, stars, wheels, discs, whirling bans, etc.) described by Penfield and Rasmussen as being evoked by direct stimulation of the exposed visual cortex (area 17).

The format of scintillating scotomata is apparently unique to the migraine process, and has not (yet) been simulated by any experimental procedure. Lashley (1941) has speculated that the characteristic microstructure of these scotomata (minutely angled, and coarser in the lower portions of the visual field as shown in Figure 3) is related to the underlying cytoarchitectonic pattern, or neuronal grain, of the primary visual cortex (coniocortex).

Lashley has also commented on the rate of spread of scotomata, and calculates that this would correspond to a wave of excitation moving

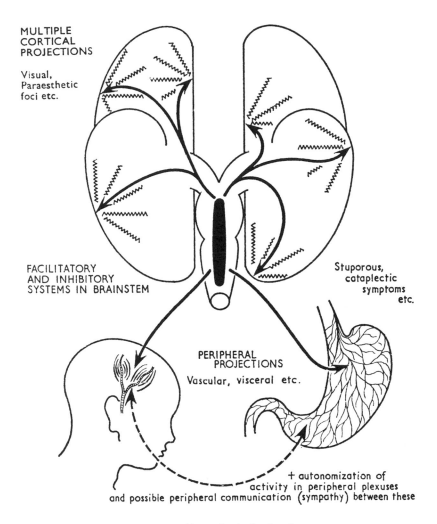

Fig. 7.   Scheme of hypothetical migraine process

Schematic representation of migraine process as a slow, cyclical, centrence-phalic seizure-activity, which is projected rostrally to the cerebral cortex, where it ignites the secondary processes of the migraine aura (scotomata, paraesthesiae, etc.), and caudally, to the ramifications of autonomic plexuses throughout the body. The process (in Gowers's words) is "... very mysterious ... there is a peculiar form of activity which seems to spread, like the ripples in a pond into which a stone is thrown ... in the region which the active ripple waves have passed, a state is left like molecular disturbance of the structures."

over the (primary) visual cortex at about 3 mm per minute, followed by a wave of total inhibition. He conceded that "nothing is known of the actual nervous activity" underlying this process, and does not commit himself, therefore, either to the theory of a locally initiated disturbance or a secondary one in response to excitation from infra-cortical levels.

It is not clear why the visual cortex should be more sensitive to stimulation than the corresponding areas of cutaneous-kinesthetic cortex (area 3) or auditory cortex (area 41); nor is it clear what fundamental process is reflected in the flicker-rate of scotomata or paraesthesiae (6 to 12 per second). It is, however, probably more than coincidental that these flicker-rates are of the same frequency as the alpha-rhythms, and of the frequencies of stroboscopic illumination most prone to cause photic driving of the EEG, photo-epilepsy, and photo-scotomata. One may suspect that this frequency is related to a fixed and finite rate of perceptual elaboration or scanning.

Following the occurrence of simple phosphenes and scintillating scotomata, there may ensue visual misperceptions and hallucinations of higher order: Lilliputian and Brobdignagian vision, various forms of visual agnosia, mosaic vision, and stereotyped (cinematic) sequences of visual images. It is experimentally established (Penfield and Rasmussen, 1950) that stimulation of the secondary or peripheral fields of the visual cortex may generate organised visual hallucinations arranged in a definite space-time sequence, and we may speculate that all the more complex visual hallucinations arise at this level (or higher). With regard to the phenomena of mosaic vision, and the varying size of mosaic perceived (see Figure 4), it is evident that we must postulate some form of functional schematisation *beyond* anatomically-fixed cytoarchitectonic patterns.

Konorski (1967) has put forward and substantiated a theory of perceptual or gnostic units (minimal perceptual structures) which may have relevance to the phenomena of mosaic vision. We have indicated that the latter starts as a barely perceptible graininess or minutely crystalline appearance, and passes through stages of increasingly coarse mosaic formation, till at last it results in visual agnosia. We may speculate that these symptoms represent the subjective experience of progressively enlarging gnostic units, which, normally invisible, obtrude themselves into consciousness as they enlarge, presenting themselves as polygonal units of increasing coarseness, until, finally, their size exceeds their information-content, at which point the recognition of objects will become difficult or impossible, as in a photograph with too coarse a grain.

The most complex sensory hallucinations of migraine aura take the form of synaesthesiae and other sensory interactions, and dream-like sequences involving sensory images of every modality, receptive and expressive aphasias, and general disorders of thought and behaviour.

We may speculate that this hierarchy of hallucinations in migraine auras is correlated with the successive activations of different cortical fields. The central cortical fields (e.g. area 17, in the visual cortex) are "distinguishable from the other fields by the 'coarseness' of their neuronal structure, which is adapted for the reception and return of intensive flows of excitation" (Luria, 1966). These central fields, especially those of the visual cortex, appear to be most sensitive to a rostrally-projected excitation, and their response is experienced as simple somatotopic hallucinations in the visual or tactile fields (scotomata and paraesthesiae); strong excitations may spread into the secondary sensory fields, and here give rise to agnosic deficits and more complex hallucinations of a single modality; in the most intense migraine auras the tertiary cortical fields may be activated—these are associated (in Luria's words) with "the most complex forms of integration of the conjoined activity of the visual, auditory, and kinaesthetic analysers," and their stimulation gives rise to disorganisation of the most general manifestations of cortical activity, i.e. to complex confusional states. Figure 8 depicts the areas of cortex occupied by primary, secondary and tertiary fields, and their overlapping and abutment on one another.

We see that the *range of disorder* is vast in migraines, going from elementary vegetative disturbances (with involvement of peripheral auto-

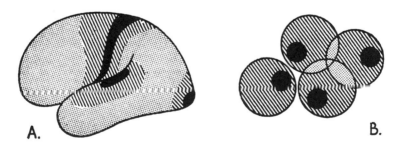

A.   B.

Fig. 8. Cortical fields in relation to migraine aura

Distribution and differentiation of primary (black), secondary (shaded) and tertiary (stippled) neuronal fields of cerebral cortex. Elementary sensory hallucinations (visual, tactile, auditory) are presumed to arise from excitation of the low-threshold primary fields, and more complex alterations of perceptual and integrative function from spread of intense excitation into secondary and tertiary fields (redrawn from Polyakov).

nomic plexuses), through disturbances of central arousal mechanisms, to a variety of cortical disturbances involving several orders of neuronal fields. This is the repertoire of migraine. We must now concern ourselves with the question of its variations and variability within this range. Thus common migraines show no symptoms of cortical involvement; isolated migraine auras show chiefly the symptoms of cortical involvement; classical migraines are conducted at several levels of involvement.

We must enquire into the physiological basis of the permutations and transformations which are so characteristic of migraine: the transitions from one migraine equivalent to another, from common to classical migraine, from migrainous neuralgias to common migraines, from migraines to epilepsies, faints, vagal attacks and all the other allied reactions which Gowers would place in the same borderland. *These* are the most difficult and fascinating aspects of migraine, and it is clear that they cannot even be approached unless certain radically different concepts of cerebral functioning are adopted. *It is impossible to explain the varying levels and transformations of migraine in terms of fixed neural mechanisms.*

This was clearly realised, a century ago, both by Liveing and by Hughlings Jackson; both arrived at similar answers, although Jackson's was far more carefully worked out. Liveing stated that ". . . the concentration of this tendency [nerve-force] in particular localities . . . will mainly determine the character of the neurosis in question." Jackson was compelled to forgo notions of anatomically unique centres and anatomically located functions, and intead visualised the nervous system as hierarchically-organised, as consisting of several levels at which every function was represented:

> I am supposing the nervous system to be a sensory-motor mechanism, from bottom to top; that every part of the nervous system represents impressions or movements, or both . . . The periphery is the real lowest level; but we shall speak of three levels of central evolution. (1) The lowest level consists of the anterior and posterior horns of the spinal cord . . . and of the homologues of these parts higher up . . . (2) The middle level consists of Ferrier's motor region, with the ganglia of the corpus striatum, and also of his sensory region. It represents all parts of the body doubly indirectly. (3) The highest level consists of highest motor centres (pre-frontal lobes) and of highest sensory centres (occipital lobes).

Thus, each function was conceived to have a complex "vertical" organisation: the localisation of a symptom could in no way be identified with the localisation of the particular function which was impaired. Different epilepsies demonstrated a hierarchic dissolution of function: thus, a *grand mal* was envisaged as a highest-level fit, and an attack of laryn-gospasm (laryngeal epilepsy or migraine) as a lowest-level fit. Jackson discussed migraine briefly, but was clearly only considering classical at-tacks when he wrote:

> I believe cases of migraine to be epilepsies (sensory epilepsies) . . . I think the sensory symptoms of the paroxysm are owing to a "discharging lesion" of convolutions evolved out of the optic thalamus, i.e. of "sensory middle cen-tres" . . . I believe the headache and vomiting to be post-paroxysmal.

Common migraines, with their predominantly vegetative symptoms, would be accounted forms of lowest-level fit, and migraine auras with complex hallucinations and dreamy states as highest-level fits. *All forms of migraine, in Jacksonian terms, share the same organisation, expressed through homologous mechanisms at different levels.*

Jackson was especially concerned, in his analysis of epilepsies, with the hierarchical representation of movement and motor functions within the nervous system, whereas we are concerned with the vertical organisa-tion of autonomic and sensory functions. The fact that these too are represented and re-represented at progressively higher levels in the neur-axis provides, as it were, another dimension of choice in the format of attacks. The migrainous sequence or syndrome may be expressed at the highest Jacksonian level (as a complex aura), the middle Jacksonian level (as an elementary aura, involving only the primary sensory fields of the cortex), or the lowest Jacksonian level (as a common migraine, or mi-graine equivalent). Jackson also speaks of collateral spread as well as vertical spread in the origin of epilepsies, the former referring to involve-ment of a contiguous area at the *same* functional level. The absence of an anatomically-defined "discharging focus" will mean that there is no restriction on such lateral spread: thus an aura emanating, for example, from the activation of primary sensory fields may involve or "choose" the visual or the tactile fields indiscriminately, while a lowest level com-mon migraine may involve any portion of the autonomic fields at brain-stem level, generating now a cephalgic attack, now an abdominal attack, now a precordial attack, with equal facility.

The verification and extension of Jackson's ideas on function and localisation within the nervous system has become the special concern of the post-Pavlovian reflexologists, and has entailed radical redefinition and rethinking of many basic doctrines (see Luria, 1966). Thus, accord-ing to this school, a function is, in fact, a functional system directed towards the performance of a particular biological task. The most sig-nificant feature of such a functional system is that it is based on a dynamic "constellation" of connections, situated at different levels in the nervous system, and that *these* may be freely substituted for one another or interchanged with the task itself remaining unchanged. Thus (in Luria's words) "such a system of functionally united components has a systematic, not a concrete, structure, in which the initial and final links of the system (the task and the effect) remain constant and unchanged, while the intermediate links (the means of performance of the task) may be modified within wide limits."

These considerations, discussed by Luria in reference to movement and motor tasks, recommend themselves as indispensable for the understanding of migraine and its transformations *as autonomic and psychosomatic tasks*. The task may be shaped by the necessity of neuronal discharge (in a periodic or paroxysmal migraine), or by physical or emotional need(s), as in circumstantial or situational attacks; the final link, the effects of the migraine, is the restoration of a physiological (or emotional) equilibrium. But the adaptive task has a systematic and not a concrete structure, *i.e. the actual mechanisms employed may be many, various, and inconstant*. There may be as many ways of concocting a migraine as of cooking an omelette. If one particular intermediate link, one mechanism, is eliminated, the whole system can be reorganised in order to restore the disturbed task.

Thus, as in motor or perceptual tasks, the particular mechanisms are subordinated to the overall strategy. This principle has great practical and therapeutic importance as well as theoretical interest. It means, for example, that *if migraine is necessary in the physiological or emotional economy of an individual, attacks will continue to occur, to be elaborated, whatever particular mechanisms are eliminated*. Excise one temporal artery, one end-organ, and another one will be pressed into use: endeavour to block attacks with, say, a serotonin-inhibitor, and attacks are likely to recur utilising a different intermediate mechanism.

Functional systems such as these (says Luria), complex in composition, *plastic in the variability of their elements*, and possessing the property of dynamic autoregulation, are apparently the rule in human activity.

RECAPITULATION

The migraine reaction is characterised, at lower functional levels, by protracted parasympathetic or trophotropic tonus, preceded and suc-

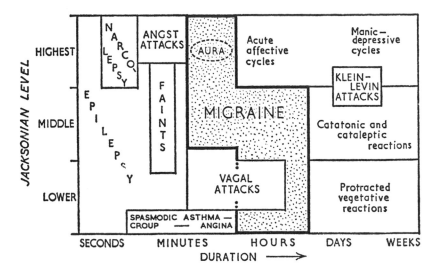

Fig. 9.   Migraine in relation to some allied disorders
    Migraine and neighbouring disorders are here represented in terms of time-base and neural (Jacksonian) level; either of these may be modulated—hence the metamorphoses to which migraine is prone. All of the disorders here represented are distinct and individual, but nevertheless have borderlands in which they merge into another.

ceeded by physiologically opposite states. At its higher functional levels, it is characterised by activation (and succeeding inhibition) of countless cortical fields, from the primary sensory areas to the most complex integrative areas. Migraine is considered as a form of centrencephalic paroxysm in slow-motion, in the case of the aura 20 to 200 times slower, and in the case of a common migraine some thousands of times slower, than their epileptic counterparts. It is also necessary to consider migraine as a complex adaptive task performed by a complex functional system, in which the means of performance (which are extremely variable) are subordinated to its ends.

    Migraine grades into a diffuse borderland of allied paroxysmal and adaptive reactions. We may represent this schematically by the use of two axes, the ordinate denoting the functional (Jacksonian) level, and the abscissa the duration of such reactions (Figure 9). Ideally, a third axis should also be present, indicating the varied syndromes of migraine and allied reactions at a given time-scale and functional level.

    For practical purposes (diagnostic and therapeutic) we can identify a majority of migraines as migraines and nothing else; theoretically, we may expect every variety of hybrid and transitional attack to occur, at levels where migraine becomes confluent with epilepsies, faints, vagal attacks, and other autonomic and affective crises.[43] From time to time, we encounter such hybrid and transitional attacks, which defeat (and, indeed, render meaningless) the business of differential diagnosis.

We must suspect that physiological boundaries are no more precise, in this context, than clinical boundaries, and that it may, therefore, be chimerical to search for a unique and pathognomonic "migraine process" in the nervous system. We cannot conceive that research will expose an underlying abnormality as crisp and concise as the spike-and-wave pattern of certain epilepsies. We must envisage instead a broad spectrum of nervous activities expressed at different functional levels and on different time-bases.

[43] We have been particularly concerned with the formal and clinical interrelationships of *brief* cerebral reactions and paroxysms. It is beyond the scope of this work to explore the affinities between these and certain *extended* reactions—especially affective and catatonic crises—although we have indicated in Figure 9 their presumed continuity with migraines, epilepsies, etc. The reader may be referred to Bleuler's descriptions of transitional crises in this borderland (the complement of Gowers's borderland), and his conclusion (*Dementia Praecox*, p. 178) that ". . . there is a continuous scale of transitions, from the true organic cerebral attack to the agitated states." A similar continuity may be traced with regard to inhibitory states: an exemplary case-history has been provided by Pierre Janet (1921), who describes in a patient the onset of "paroxysmal disorders of consciousness in the form of fainting spells more or less prolonged" culminating in a sleep-like disorder five years in duration.

TWELVE

Biological Approaches to Migraine

Preservative reflexes include the following groups: (1)
Reflexes concerned with assimilation of necessary materials.
(2) Reflexes concerned with excretion of waste and unused
materials—expiration, urination, defaecation. (3) Reflexes
concerned with recuperation (sleep). (4) Reflexes concerned
with preservation of progeny.

    Protective reflexes include: (1) Reflexes concerned with
the withdrawal of the whole body or any part from the
operation of a noxious or endangering stimulus. (2) Reflexes
concerned with the rejection of harmful agents from the
surface of, or inside, the body. (3) Reflexes concerned with
annihilating or disarming harmful agents.

Konorski, 1967

We have discussed some of the internal or physiological mechanisms of
migraines as these may lend themselves to the fabrication of the clinical
attack. We must now approach the problem from a different aspect, and
concern ourselves with the relation of the migraineur and his migraines
to the environment. The terms we will be compelled to use, in considering the biological origins and uses of migraine and migraine-like reactions, will be organismal ones: reflex, drive, and adaptation.

    It was stated earlier (Chapter 10) that we would hesitate to recognise
in animals anything which might be termed a "migraine," and that this,
amongst other factors, had limited the experimental investigation of the
subject. Must we then regard migraines as peculiar to our own species?
Speech is predominant in man, and certain very sophisticated reactions
(Darwin instances laughing, frowning and sneering) are exclusively
found in man, but these activities and reactions are not usefully compared to migraines. Migraine, in contrast to these, is a remarkably primitive reaction involving massive alterations of vegetative activity and of

general activity and behaviour. We have considered migraine, thus far, in chiefly experiential terms, as the symptoms of which a patient may complain, and at this level, obviously, we can derive no information from animals which may suffer but cannot express complaints. If we are to form any picture of the biological role(s) of migraine, and of its homo-logues and analogues in the animal world, we must instead concern our-selves with the *behaviour* of the migraine patient, and the circumstances to which this behaviour has relevance.

Let us then construct a stereotyped picture of migrainous behaviour. As the symptoms mount, the patient will go to his room and lie down; he will have the blinds drawn and the children hushed; he will tolerate no intrusions. The intensity of his symptoms will drive other thoughts from his mind; he may be sunk, if the attack is very severe, in a leaden, stuporous daze. He pulls the blanket over his head, excluding the outer world, and enveloping himself in the inner world of his symptoms. He says to the world: "Go away. Leave me alone. This is my migraine. Let me suffer in peace." At length, perhaps, he falls asleep. And when he wakes, it is all over, the migraine is done, its work is accomplished; there may be a post-migrainous surge of energy, almost literally a re-anima-tion. The essential terms of the attack are these: retreat from the outer world, regression, and, finally, recuperation.[44]

In somewhat less formal terms, the migraine reaction tends to be characterised by passivity, stillness and immobilisation; commerce with the outer world is minimal, while inner activities—particularly of secre-tory and expulsive type—are maximal. It is in *these* general terms that we may perceive the primary adaptive function of a migraine (whatever complex uses are subsequently superimposed), and in these terms that we may seek for parallel reactions both in the human and the animal world.

It is particularly as a Konorskian protective reflex that we envisage the primary role of migraine, as a withdrawal of the whole body from "the operation of a noxious or endangering stimulus," in short, as a *particular form of reaction to threat.* Concurrent with this role, and perhaps inseparable from it, is an offensive function (annihilating or

[44] Subsequent to the writing of this passage, I encountered Freud's comments on sleep: "Sleep [he writes] is a condition in which I refuse to have anything to do with the outer world and have withdrawn my interest from it. I go to sleep by retreating from the outside world and warding off the stimuli proceeding from it . . . I say to it as I fall asleep: 'Leave me in peace, for I want to sleep' . . . Thus the biological object of sleep seems to be recu-peration, its psychological characteristic the suspension of interest in the outer world" (Freud, 1920, p. 92).

disarming harmful agents) and an expulsive function, both of which would seem to be of particular relevance when the "harmful agent" is felt or symbolised as a harmful or hateful emotional situation. The recuperative aspects of migraines are most clearly seen in those attacks which follow protracted physical or emotional stress, and which mimic most closely the role of sleep. Thus "threat," in this context, is being used in its widest possible sense, as covering both acute and chronic situations, and both physical and emotional circumstances.

Response to threat, in the animal world, may take either or both of two fundamentally different forms. The form which is most familiar, and which springs immediately to mind, is the use of an active physical response, the fight-flight response, with its emotional correlates of rage or terror. The general mechanisms of this have been incomparably described by Cannon (1920) with respect to acute reactions, and by Selye (1946) in regard to sustained physiological reactions. The acute fight-flight picture is one of extreme arousal and sympathetic dominance: muscles tensed, deepened breathing, increased cardiac output, extreme sensory vigilance, every external faculty keyed to its highest pitch, and a reciprocal inhibition of internal (parasympathetically-driven) processes. The acute reaction induces and is reinforced by the secretion of adrenalin and other pressor amines, while the chronic reaction involves adrenocortical activity and a chain of chemical and tissue reactions secondary to this.

The fight-flight reaction is dramatic in the extreme, but it represents only half of biological reality. The other half is no less dramatic, but it is dramatic in a contrary style. *Its* characteristics are those of passivity and immobilization in response to threat. The antithesis between these two styles of reaction was memorably described by Darwin in his comparison of active fear (terror) and passive fear (dread). In the former, says Darwin, there is "the sudden and uncontrollable tendency to headlong flight." The picture of passive fear, as Darwin portrays it, is one of passivity and prostration, allied with increased splanchnic and glandular activity (". . . a strong tendency to yawn . . . death-like pallor . . . beads of sweat stand out on the skin. All of the muscles of the body are relaxed. Utter prostration soon follows. The intestines are affected. The sphincter muscles cease to act, and no longer retain the contents of the body . . ."). The general attitude is one of cringing, cowering, and sinking. If the passive reaction is more acute, there may be abrupt loss of postural tone or of consciousness. If the passive reaction is more protracted, the physiological changes are less dramatic, but still in the same direction.

We find throughout the animal world a repertoire of passive reactions at least as important, and considerably more variable, than the active responses to threat. All of them are characterised by immobilisation (with some inhibition of postural tone and arousal), usually in conjunction with increased secretory and splachnic activity. A handful of examples will suffice. A fearful dog (especially if it belongs to Pavlov's "weak inhibitory type") cowers, and may vomit and be incontinent of faeces; the hedgehog responds to threat by curling up; the jerbil by a sudden cataplectic loss of muscular tone; the opossum by a trance-like arrest or "sham death." The frightened horse may "freeze" and break into a cold sweat; the threatened skunk freezes and secretes profusely from modified sweat-glands (here the secretory response has assumed an offensive function); the menaced chameleon freezes and changes colour to mimic the environment through another variant of internal secretion. Even in the protozoa, we find active, predatory responses in some groups, and passive protective responses in others. It is clear that the passive response to threat has been utilised, from the start of life, as a biological alternative to active reactions. The passive reaction, indeed, is frequently superior to the active response in terms of survival value. Where the aroused animal faces (or flees) danger and threat, the inhibitory reaction enables it to *avert* these, to become, one way or another, less accessible to danger.

The human repertoire is particularly rich in such passive protective reactions many of which occur paradoxically (strictly speaking, in Pavlov's nomenclature, ultra-paradoxically) in the context of physical or emotional crisis. Among such relatively acute reactions we must rank narcolepsy and cataplexy, nervous "freezing" and "blocking," an enormous variety of Parkinsonian "crises," and fainting. On a somewhat more extended time-scale we see vaso-vagal attacks (as Gowers describes these) and, of course, migraines. We must also recognise as inhibitory protective reactions such states as "swooning" (hysterical stupor), and much more protracted depressive and catatonic stupors. Pathological sleeping (especially in its most baroque form of catalepsy) is the exemplar of the longer-lasting human inhibitory reactions, as is hibernation in the animal world.

The survival-value of passive reactions and inhibitory states is clearly apparent in the animal world, whereas it tends to be obscured or overshadowed in some of the more obviously pathological passive reactions in human behaviour. But we will find it impossible to comprehend the origin and perpetuation of such human reactions unless they are seen, first and foremost, as having biological survival-value. Paradox is implicit in the nature of such reactions; sleep and hibernation serve to protect the organism, but may also expose it to other vicissitudes. Inhibitory, parasympathetically-dominated states in man afford, in Alexander's seductive phrase, a "vegetative retreat," but the seclusion of retreat may become a psychophysiological imprisonment. The ultimate paradox is the simulation of death to avoid death, as we see in the "sham death" of the opossum, and, perhaps, some human sleeps and stupors.

This then is the hinterland of biological reactions from which we conceive migraines to have arisen in the course of evolution, and to have become, with the elaboration of human nervous systems and human needs, progressively differentiated and refined. Our image is of an "Ur-migraine,"[45] or archetype, a crude passive-protective-parasympathetic type of reaction of longer duration than the common freezing and stun reactions. Perhaps such primordial migraines—similar to the undifferentiated reactions considered in Chapter 2—were chiefly in response to a variety of physical threats: exhaustion, heat, illness, injury, pain, etc., and certain elemental and overwhelming emotional experiences, especially fear.

The development of large social units, and the cultural repressions inseparable from this, have doubtless necessitated, as they have permitted, a far greater variety of vegetative retreats and protracted passive reactions than were previously possible. These psychosomatic reactions, along with neurotic defences and reactions, represent the only alternatives in situations where direct action is neither permissible nor possible. We envisage that psychosomatic reactions, like neurotic defences, have become not only more necessary with the increasing complexity and repressiveness of civilised life, but also more versatile and sophisticated: thus, the simple protective reflexes we have discussed may evolve into the richly allusive, over-determined and protean migraines so common in present society.

Proceeding parallel with the elaboration of such strategic needs and uses has been the increasing complexity of the nervous system, and, in particular, the progressive encephalisation of integrative functions in the course of mammalian evolution. In relatively primitive mammals (opossums, hedgehogs, etc.) in which cortical development and control are rudimentary, cerebral reflexes must still be of relatively stereotyped form

---

[45] We do not imply that a particular man (or animal) once experienced an Ur-migraine, of which all subsequent migraines were descendants. The term is no more than a figment of logical history—like the notions of an *Urpflanze*, an *Urmensch* or a *lingua adamica* (see Rieff, 1959, pp. 225–228).

and little susceptible of conditioning. The elaboration of the cortical mantle permits the unfolding of more numerous, more various, and more easily-conditioned cerebral reflexes. The final differentiation of hierarchically-ordered neuronal fields in the human cortex (see Chapter 11 and Figure 8), we conceive, has permitted the development of the most complex and distinctive feature of migraines, the aura. The complexities of migraine aura (with its possibilities of complex sensory and integrative disturbances, aphasia, etc.) is, as it were, a testament and by-product of the unique differentiation of the human cortex, and could not conceivably occur in less complex nervous systems. We may recognise, in analogous fashion, the primordia of epilepsies and psychoses in more primitive mammals, and perhaps in non-mammalian vertebrates (abrupt convulsions and loss of consciousness; states of uncontrollable excitement and entrancement, etc.), but must perceive their most complex and individual characteristics—hallucinatory and ideational disturbances—as dependent on cortical development and differentiation, and above all the final elaboration of frontal and temporal lobes in our own species.

Thus to the question posed at the start of this chapter: Is migraine a uniquely human reaction?, we must answer yes and no. It makes no sense to regard migraine as a human invention. We must see it, rather, as having a most ancient lineage of biological precursors, as exemplifying a most primitive and generalised form of adaptive reaction which has been refined and differentiated by the unique possibilities of human nervous systems and the unique nature of human needs. The final shaping of the migraine reaction depends on the development of the individual in relation to his environment, and it is with this psychological determination and individuation of migraines that we will be concerned in the following chapter.

THIRTEEN

Psychological Approaches to Migraine

For this is the great error of our day . . . that physicians separate the soul from the body.

Plato

We were concerned in the last chapter with certain primitive reactions
which might throw some clue on the origin and differentiation of the
human migraine reaction. By speaking in terms of the entire organism
and its protective reflexes and tactics we were able to skirt the perennial
problems (or pseudo-problems) of mind-body "duality" and psychophysiological "conversion." But these neither tell us, nor are designed to
tell us, anything of the internal processes which underlie the behaviour;
they tell us nothing concerning the emotions or "state of mind" of the
reacting animal. Catatonic stupor in a human being can be a protective
tactic, and its adoption may be related, internally, to an appalling sense
of existential danger. We can provide a most detailed phenomenal description of catatonia without making any reference to the feelings of
the catatonic (as Bleuler did), but we cannot provide an *existential* description of the state without detailed analysis of the feelings and motives
of the patient. We take it as axiomatic that every attack of migraine has
tactical value to the person (the tactic may be a purely physiological one,
e.g. a homeostatic manoeuvre), but we will be particularly concerned,
in the present chapter, with the relation of migraines to the patient's
emotional being.

We made a somewhat arbitrary classification of migraines in the descriptive portion of this book, and we must now examine this classification more closely in so far as it may be related to the emotional economy
of an individual. "Periodic" migraines were portrayed as the expression
of some innate neuronal periodicity, and "circumstantial" migraines as

a response to highly specific, individual circumstances which might be physiological (exhaustion, etc.) or emotional (rage, fright, etc.). The fact that such attacks may have clearly-defined physical or physiological antecedents does not exclude the possibility that they may *also* have other functions or uses which may not be immediately apparent. In particular, any attack of migraine (and indeed any event in a person's existence) may be invested with an emotional significance over and above its literal significance. A periodically-recurring or physiologically-induced event may be pressed into service as a symbolic event. We may reinforce this point by considering the uses to which seizures may be put; certain children may discover that flickering light will induce a convulsion in them, and proceed from this discovery to repeated self-induction of seizures (e.g. by shaking a hand rapidly before the eyes, or jumping up and down before a Venetian blind); certain adults provoke seizures in themselves by deliberate or "accidental" omission of their medication. In such cases, the epilepsy has found a second use, a perverse employment, determined by complex and often unconscious motives in the patient. It is well established that "accident-proneness," which masquerades as a series of chance misfortunes, tends to be restricted to certain self-punitive and self-destructive individuals.

It is not suggested that all periodic and circumstantial migraines, or even a majority of them, are coupled in this manner to the motives of the individual. Many migraines occur, pass, constitute occasional inconveniences, and carry no special load of emotional implication. But the possibility of their serving other purposes, of many and various kinds, is always present.

The third pattern of migraines described—habitual or situational migraine—demands a much more complex frame of reference. We are here concerned, not with periodic or sporadic attacks which may or may not have some emotional significance, but with an unremitting, malignant illness, which is generated by (and itself may aggravate) chronic, severe, emotional stresses. The origins and primordia of migraine may be discerned, we have imagined, among simple protective reflexes and tactics. Circumstantial migraines may also be discussed in such terms, given the special reservations we have made. Habitual migraine cannot be usefully considered save as an expression of a major portion of the entire personality. Habitual migraine, like all psychosomatic illnesses, like hysteria, like neurosis, is among the most complex of human creations.

The terms which are necessary for its understanding are those which distinguish human beings, at least quantitatively, from other animals:

the complexity of mental and emotional structure, and the dominance of symbolism. We have motives and counter-motives which endure through our lives; these are organised and partitioned into sub-systems, the integrity and separation of which are maintained by all the mechanisms which Freud has delineated. Of particular importance in the determination of habitual migraine and other psychosomatic illnesses are those motives which serve no protective functions, save in the most paradoxical of senses—masochistic and self-destructive drives.

A comprehensive dissection of motives and symbolisms, as these may determine the pattern of habitual migraine in a patient, is not to be achieved except by depth-analysis. In a majority of cases, however, the major motivational determinants of migraines may be partly exposed (and subjected to some therapeutic intervention) without so intensive an exploration of the personality.

We have already indicated by a number of case-histories some of the motives which may generate habitual migraines (Chapter 9), and we will now venture to tabulate the major strategic roles which migraines may play in the economy of the individual. The list is incomplete and schematic, of necessity, and cannot do justice to the complexity and flux of the forces which are actually at work, and which tend to interact and combine with one another, so that many migraine attacks are as richly over-determined as dreams.

Biologically the simplest, and dynamically the most benign of migraines, are *recuperative*. These tend to occur, circumstantially, following prolonged physical or emotional activity, and habitually as the notorious "weekend" attacks. There is usually a rather sharp collapse from the preceding or provocative period of over-activity and tension, the phase of prostration may be profound and even stuporous, and it is followed, characteristically, by a post-migrainous rebound and sense of awakening and re-animation. Wolff has particularly concerned himself with attacks of this type, and their occurrence as "let down" phenomena in ruthlessly obsessive and driving personalities. Recuperative attacks have the closest biological analogy to sleep, and are clearly preservative reflexes in the Konorskian sense.

Allied to these, geared to environmental or emotional stress, but less benign in their pattern, are those migraines which are *regressive*. Like recuperative migraines, these afford (in Alexander's phrase) a "vegetative retreat"; but whereas recuperative attacks tend to be undertaken in privacy and solitude, like sleep, regressive attacks are marked by pitiful suffering, dependency-needs, and cries for help. In a word, they assume the characteristics not of sleep, but of illness. Severe ones, in family contexts, may radiate the tragic qualities of death-bed scenes. Regressive migraines are not infrequently found in the context of illness-prone or hypochondriacal personalities, and are often presented, to the physician, in the context of multiple physical complaints, real or imaginary. We have observed that their pattern may be less benign than that of recuperative migraines: we are here considering not the occasional regressive attacks which any migraineur may have, but an indulgence, a morbid welcoming, of such attacks with ever-increasing frequency, so that the patient slips, by degrees, into illness as a way of life ("that long disease, my life").[46]

An extremely important variant of such migraine patterns, and one which continues to show the primal protective role of the migraine reaction, are those attacks which we may term *encapsulative* and *dissociative*. There are a number of patients in whom periodic or sporadic migraines are experienced which seem to embed, and (in the oblique terms of a physiological drama) to enact and "work through" an accumulation of emotional stresses and conflicts. I have the impression that many menstrual migraines (and other allied menstrual syndromes) do exactly this, condensing, as it were, the stresses of the month into a few days of concentrated illness, and I have observed, in a number of patients, that curing them (depriving them) of such menstrual syndromes may be followed by a release of diffuse anxiety and neurotic conflict into the remainder of the month. Such migraines, in a word, may serve to *bind*, and thus circumscribe, painful chronic or recurrent feelings, a consideration which must be borne in mind before they are too zealously dispersed.

---

[46] It is possible, and perhaps important, to represent the recuperative and regressive functions of migraine in terms of libido-theory. We have depicted migraines in terms of retreat and turning-away from the external world, and have repeatedly likened it to sleep. We have also portrayed migraine as enveloping the sufferer in his symptoms, demanding and pre-empting his attention, like the symptoms of organic illness or hypochondria. Freud pictures sleep and suffering in the following terms: ". . . Sleep [he writes] is a condition in which all investments of objects, the libidinal as well as the egoistic, are abandoned and withdrawn into the ego. Does this not shed a new light upon the recuperation afforded by sleep . . . ? . . . In the sleeper the primal state of the libido-distribution is again reproduced, that of absolute narcissism, in which libido and ego-interests dwell together still, united and indistinguishable in the self-sufficient self." And of immersion in symptoms, he writes: ". . . Certain conditions—organic illness, painful accesses of stimulation, an inflammatory condition of an organ—have clearly the effect of loosening the libido from its attachment to objects. The libido which has thus been withdrawn attaches itself again to the ego in the form of a stronger investment of the diseased region of the body . . . This seems to lead to a possibility of understanding hypochondria, in which some organ, without being perceptibly diseased, becomes in a very similar way the subject of a solicitude on the part of the ego" (Freud, 1920, pp. 424–426).

More malignant than these, for the emotional substrates are more intense and much further removed from consciousness, and the migraines, correspondingly, are far more frequent, is that pattern of habitual migraine we have termed dissociative. In such cases (see Case 80, p. 168) the personality becomes sectioned, one part of it affirming a bland reaction or bravura wholly at odds with environmental and emotional reality, and another portion becoming autonomised as a circular sado-masochistic system devoted to the infliction and experiencing of suffering. Such cases, which are often of the greatest severity, may be peculiarly resistant to insight or treatment, for the migrainous portion of the personality (the migraine selflet) is likely to be insulated from the remainder of the personality by thick walls of repression and denial. The dynamics and mechanisms of this bear the closest analogy to those involved in the formation of hysterical symptoms, with the important difference that migraines are rooted in physiological reactivity, whereas hysterical symptoms (though intensely real) are fictions, neurologically, arising from a pathology of the imagination.

The last two categories of migraine pattern we must consider are distinguished by having acquired special strategic significances of a peculiarly hostile type. The first of these is the *aggressive* migraine, and it is with this type that Fromm-Reichmann (1937), Johnson (1948), and many other analysts have particularly concerned themselves. The emotional background is one of intense, chronic, repressed rage and hostility, and the function of the migraines is to provide some expression of what cannot be expressed, or even acknowledged, directly. Such migraines are implicit assaults or vengeful attacks, and tend to occur in situations of intense emotional ambivalence, i.e. in relation to individuals who are both loved and hated. Such indirect expressions of hatred are particularly seen in the interaction of the migrainous patient with parents, children, spouses, and employers, and revolve about the dynamic of demanded yet intolerable dependence or intimacy (see Cases 61, 62, 79, and 84). A particular form of this reaction is the *emulative* migraine, in which there exists an ambivalent and malignant identification with a migrainous parent; joining the parent in illness, competing with him, hoisting him with his own migrainous petard. It seems certain that many examples of familial occurrence of migraine (as of many other illnesses) require explanation in these terms, rather than in the simplistic terms of direct inheritance (see Chapter 6).

When the hostility is turned inwards, there is seen the last pattern of habitual migraine we must consider, repeated *self-punitive* attacks. Such patients are deeply masochistic, spiteful, chronically depressed, covertly paranoid, and sometimes overtly self-destructive (see Case 81). The migraine rarely suffices as an expression of the inner feelings, and is likely to be accompanied by other expressions of self-hatred. These patients, in many senses, are the most deeply pathological and deeply afflicted of all; they require, as desperately as they will resist, therapeutic intervention, but this (if it is allowed by the patient) is more likely to be successful than in cases of dissociative migraine with hysterical features.

There are, of course, innumerable special uses of migraine which may cut across the broad categories we have constructed. Particularly common, and sometimes the occasion of cruel misunderstanding or punishment, are those attacks which may occur in children forced to attend schools they detest: any form of functional illness—repeated attacks of migraine, of vomiting, or of diarrhoea, of asthma, or of hysterical symptoms—may serve to shield the child from some of the rigours and horrors of school life, while drawing attention to miseries which dare not, or cannot, be voiced directly.

Among famous figures who were finally liberated from intolerable conditions by such attacks must be mentioned Pope, who employed "megrim," and Gibbon, who had hysterical attacks. Gibbon later wrote of these: ". . . The violence and variety of my complaints . . . excused my frequent absence from Westminster School . . . a strange nervous affection (painful contractions of the legs, etc.) . . . my infirmities could not be reconciled with the hours and discipline of a public seminary . . . I secretly rejoiced in these infirmities, which delivered me from the exercises of the school and the society of my equals . . ." Finally, on his liberation from school and his entry to Oxford, Gibbon's symptoms ". . . most wonderfully vanished," and never returned.

We see that the emotional backgrounds of migraine may be many and various, and we would suspect that there must exist not simply *a* connection, but several types of connection, between the state-of-mind and the overt attack. We have already implied the probability of a major distinction in generative mechanisms by setting apart circumstantial from situational migraines. The former, we have seen, may be promptly and dramatically provoked by intense, passionate excitements—rage, terror, elation, sexual excitement, etc. The latter, in contrast, occur in the context of emotional tensions, drives, needs, etc., which are chronic and have been denied direct or adequate expression: here we have recognised aggressive, destructive and libidinous drives, anxious tensions, obsessive tensions, sadistic and masochistic needs, etc. We must further add that these chronic emotional needs and tensions are frequently repressed and remote from consciousness. Thus we might wonder, from the start, whether such circumstantial migraines are best considered as *reactions to* overwhelming emotion, and situational migraines as *expressions of* chronic, repressed, emotional drives.

We have presented our data, and we must advance now into the very centre of the problem, and enquire how an emotion or a repressed emotional posture can be productive of a migraine. This is a special case of the eternal problem which Freud once designated "the mysterious leap from the mind to the body," and as such it is as dangerous as it is fascinating, for the discussion of mind:body relationships easily and insidiously decays into nonsense. We have acknowledged that our information is inadequate, and we will be forced, therefore, into a large measure of speculation; but we will stay close to clinical evidence at all times, and ensure that any suggestions made will be, in principle, fully verifiable or falsifiable.

This territory is best entered with the greatest of guides. Darwin's famous *Principles* of emotional expression, propounded in 1872, are the intellectual ancestors of everything that has since been written on the subject—the elaboration of the James-Lange theory of emotion, Freud's theory of conversion mechanisms, the experiments of Cannon and Selye, and the entire theoretical structure of current thinking in psychosomatic medicine—and these will form the nucleus of our own discussion. The third of Darwin's principles—that of "direct action of the nervous system"—is stated as follows:

> . . . certain actions which we may recognise as expressive of certain states of mind, are the direct result of the constitution of the nervous system, and have been from the first independent of the will, and, to a large extent, of habit.

Such direct actions may be of either motor or autonomic nature, although the latter tend to predominate. Darwin instances trembling as an example of such a motor expression, and glandular secretion, vasomotor action, visceral activity, etc., as examples of direct autonomic action. Direct action is seen "when the sensorium is strongly excited" (as in pain, rage, and terror), and under these conditions, Darwin postulates ". . . nerve-force is generated in excess, and is transmitted in certain directions, dependent on the connection of the nerve-cells . . ."

Such expressions of emotion, though dramatic in the extreme, are crude and stereotyped, and therefore inadequate to express finer shades of feeling. *These* are expressed, and freely modified, in accordance with Darwin's first principle—that of "Serviceable Associated Habits":

> Certain complex actions are of direct or indirect service under certain states of mind, in order to relieve or gratify certain sensations, desires, &c; and whenever the same state of mind is induced, there is a tendency through the force of habit and association for the same movements to be performed, though they may not then be of the least use.

This principle implies that the "complex action"—whether it is a movement or an autonomic reaction—*represents* the state of mind, and has become, through the force of habit and association (learning, conditioning, inheritance), a physical *symbol* of a particular state of mind.

Darwin was well aware that many forms of emotional expression utilised *both* of these principles. Weeping, for example, combined symbolic movements with involuntary secretions (". . . a man suffering from grief may command his features, but cannot always prevent the tears from coming into his eyes . . ."). Similarly the signs of rage, though due to direct action of the nervous system, ". . . differ from the purposeless writhings and struggles of one suffering from an agony of pain; for they represent more or less plainly the act of striking or fighting with an enemy" (Darwin, 1890, p. 74).

We must now consider how these principles may be applied to the expression of emotions which are both chronic and repressed, and, in particular, how we may interpret, in the irreducible terms which Darwin has provided, so complex a reaction as migraine. We will be compelled to introduce certain new terms, although these represent no more than an extension of the Darwinian concepts. Where Darwin speaks of "serviceable associated actions," we will now speak of "conversions," and where he speaks of "direct actions of the nervous system," we must speak of "vegetative neuroses." These psychopathological terms are narrower and more specific than the biological ones from which they are derived, and are used to denote physiological expressions of emotion which are chronic as opposed to acute, morbid as opposed to benign, and personal as opposed to universal; it is further implied that the emotional substrates of conversion-reactions and (vegetative) neuroses are repressed, or at least denied direct and adequate expression.

The use of these terms may be illustrated by a classical document of psycho-analysis (Freud, 1920, pp. 393–399):

> . . . The symptoms of an actual neurosis—headache, sensation of pain, an irritable condition of some organ, the weakening or inhibition of some func-

tion—have no "meaning," no signification in the mind . . . They are in themselves purely and simply physical processes; they arise without any of the
complicated mental mechanisms (i.e. conversion mechanisms) we have been
learning about . . . But then, how can they be expressions of the libido which
we have come to know as a force at work in the mind? . . . The answer to that
is very simple.

The "very simple answer" which Freud propounds is that these symptoms represent the direct somatic consequences of sexual disturbances,
an imbalance of some "sexual toxin." Thus, in the most general terms
(if we forget for the moment Freud's amazing and atypical postulate of
a "sexual toxin"), these neuroses are seen as the consequences of direct
nervous action, as stereotyped *concomitants* of chronic emotional tension.

A radically different mechanism is proposed with regard to the production of conversion (hysterical) symptoms. These are experienced in,
or manifested by, particular organs and parts of the body which have
become the representatives of an intense, displaced sexuality. In Freud's
words:

These organs thus behave as substitutes for the genital organs . . . Countless
sensations and innervations . . . in organs not apparently connected with sexuality, are thus discovered to be essentially fulfilments of perverse sexual
desires . . . the organs of nutrition and excretion, in particular.

This clear-cut distinction between (vegetative) neuroses and conversion
symptoms may, nevertheless, be blurred or difficult to make in certain
cases, for one may merge into the other, or be replaced by it, and Freud
is therefore compelled to make an additional reservation of great importance:

. . . The symptom of the actual neurosis is frequently the nucleus and incipient
stage of the psychoneurotic symptom . . . As an example, let us take an hysterical headache or backache. Analysis shows that by means of condensation
and displacement it has become a substitutive satisfaction for a whole series
of libidinal phantasies or memories; at one time, however, the pain was real,
a direct symptom of a sexual toxin, the bodily expression of a sexual excitation . . . All effects of the libidinal excitation upon the body are especially
adapted to serve the purposes of hysterical symptom-formation. They play
the part of the grain of sand which the oyster envelops in mother-of-pearl.

How may these concepts be applied to the understanding of migraine,
either isolated attacks which are generated by acute emotional disturbances, or recurrent attacks which occur in the context of chronic emo-

tional tensions? Are these vegetative neuroses, conversion-symptoms, or both? The literature on the subject is both confused and confusing, some authors (e.g. Alexander [1950], Furmanski *et al.* [1952]) conceiving migraine as a vegetative neurosis, and others (e.g. Deutsch [1948]) seeing it as a conversion-reaction. Deutsch represents an older school of thought which sees migraines, and indeed all psychosomatic symptoms, as the consequences of conversion-mechanisms:

> It must be assumed that a continuous conversion process, necessary for the maintenance of health and well-being, takes place in every normal individual. Let us think, for example, of blushing, of excessive perspiration, of spells of diarrhoea, of attacks of *migraine* . . . They all occur as discharges of pent-up libido . . . "Conversions" are necessary forms of a continual psychodynamic process which attempts to adjust the individual's instinctual drives to the demands of the culture in which he lives . . . One might say that human beings would be most unhappy or would take far more flight into a neurosis if they could not fall sick from time to time.

We must agree with Deutsch that functional illness is available to all of us as a perpetual alternative to intolerable feelings or the construction of neurotic defences, but we cannot endorse his view that all such ill-nesses are adequately described as conversion-symptoms; if this is done, no recognition is given to the far more universal principle of direct action of the nervous system, as Darwin describes this. Alexander, in particular, has taken strong exception to the indiscriminate or over-wide application of the notion of conversion to psychosomatic symptoms. He recognises, instead, two "fundamentally different" mechanisms at work, and dis-tinguishes these in the following terms (Alexander, 1948):

> I still uphold my original suggestion that we restrict hysterical conversion phenomena to symptoms of the voluntary neuromuscular and sensory per-ceptive systems, and differentiate them from psychogenic symptoms which occur in vegetative organ systems . . . Hysterical conversion symptoms are substitute expressions of emotional tensions which cannot find adequate out-let through full-fledged motor behaviour . . . the emotional tension is at least partially relieved by the symptom itself. We deal with a different psychody-namic and physiological situation in the field of vegetative neuroses . . . Here the somatic symptoms are not substitute expressions of repressed emotions, but they are normal physiological accompaniments of this symptom.

Alexander's distinction between conversion symptoms and vegetative neuroses is clear and concise: it makes extremely clear, for example, the fundamental differences between the mechanisms of a hysterical paraly-sis and an emotional hypertension, i.e. between an arbitrary symbolic expression and a physiological sign whose existence is unknown to the patient. It is less easily applied to certain vegetative symptoms, and here Alexander somewhat grudgingly concedes that both mechanisms may be involved. Migraine would seem to be an outstanding example of such a mixed device, and it is in these terms that we must consider it.

We stressed earlier (Chapters 1 and 5) the remarkable concomitance of mood and somatic symptom which may characterise every stage of a "typical" migraine, a synchronisation so striking and constant that we are almost compelled to defer to the terms of the James-Lange theory ("The emotion," James asserts, "is nothing but the feeling of a bodily state . . ."). Circumstantial migraines provoked by acute emotional excitement, for example, rage, may be considered, at least initially, as vegetative neuroses, whatever secondary and symbolic uses may subsequently be attached to them.

Thus a rage-migraine may be regarded as a complex but stereotyped reaction to rage, in patients who experience this. The earlier stages of such an attack (termed earlier the phase of "engorgement") are likely to be characterised, emotionally, by irritability and angry tension, and, physiologically, by vascular and visceral dilatation, fluid retention, oliguria, faecal retention, etc., the symptoms of a generalised sympathetic discharge. The patient is stuffed, impacted, and bloated with anger. The resolution of the attack may proceed by crisis (brief forceful vomiting, sudden passage of flatus and faeces, sneezing, etc.), or by lysis (diuresis, diaphoresis, epiphora, etc.). Thus the rage of such attacks is expressed in plethora, and discharged with a sudden visceral ejaculation (analogous to an oath or a blow), or a slow secretory catharsis (analogous to weeping). The expression of emotion proceeds by direct nervous action; it does not depend upon any intermediate conception, any conscious or unconscious symbolism uniting the affect and the physical manifestation. The symptoms of such a migraine, in Freud's terms, have no "meaning," no complex signification in the mind. Migraines of this type originate, as must all primitive reactions, in a region where emotional experience and its physiological counterparts are continuous and coextensive.

We cannot, however, construe situational migraines in terms as elementary as these, for these arise, not as expressions of acute emotional disturbance, but as expressions of chronic, and usually repressed, emotional needs. They are not simply reactions to emotion. They cannot be considered apart from their remote antecedents and effects. They have *functions*; they do *work*; they fill a dramatic role in the emotional economy of the individual; they perform, with greater or smaller success, a task of emotional equilibration, and as such are analogous to dreams, hysterical formations, and neurotic symptoms. If migraines are put to a special use, they must have a particular *meaning* for the patient; they must stand for something; they must allude to something; they must represent something. Thus it will be possible for us to approach a migraine not only as a physical event, but as a peculiar form of symbolic drama into which the patient has translated important thoughts and feelings; if we do this we will then be faced with the task of interpreting it as we would interpret a dream, i.e. discovering the hidden meaning of the manifest symptoms. Thus, the particular interest of situational migraines, and their special strategic value to the patient, is that *they represent biological reactions which can double as symptomatic acts or conversion symptoms.*[47]

We must allow the possibility that not only may the entire migraine have meaning for the patient, but that certain *individual* symptoms of the attack may also be invested with specific symbolic importance, and further, that they may be susceptible to modification in accordance with this importance. We have seen that nausea and vomiting are cardinal symptoms of migraine: these commonly signify disgust, often sexual disgust, and (in many cases of psychogenic vomiting) may be interpreted as efforts at symbolic expulsion of a disgusting (feared, hated) situation, person, etc.[48] The action of the bowels, initially determined by physiological needs and periodicities, may be further determined, often overwhelmingly so, by the (unconscious) symbolic values attached to faeces and defaecation. Constipation and diarrhoea, wreathed with a variety of symbolic meanings, are among the commonest of functional disorders and also, as we have seen, frequent and important parts of many migraines. Furmanski (1952), in an interesting character study of 100 migraine patients, has remarked on the frequency of "oral traits" and "anal traits" in this group, but has not attempted, regrettably, to determine

---

[47] Alexander has suggested that the term conversion should be restricted to motor and sensory symptoms, while excluding vegetative symptoms. But there is abundant evidence that many autonomic activities and symptoms, not generally considered to be under conscious or unconscious control, are in fact used as symbols, and modified accordingly. The clearest and most famous example of this is seen in the occurrence of hysterical stigmata.

Very important experimental evidence that vegetative processes can be *learned* has recently been obtained. Thus, it has been possible to train curare-paralysed dogs both to speed up and slow down their heart-rate, to relax and contract the intestinal muscles, to constrict blood-vessels in one ear while dilating vessels in the other ear, to control stomach contractions, urine formation, blood pressure and other responses.

[48] Vomiting is a primitive rejective reflex in many animals. Psychogenic vomiting may be regarded as a re-enactment of this reflex at a symbolic level. Nausea is *both* a sensation and an attitude, the affect and concept of "disgust" having been, apparently, derived from the rejective reflex, as pain (sensation, affect, concept) has been derived from nociceptive reflexes.

whether there existed any correlation between these traits and the *type* of migraine experienced. We would wonder, for example, whether a tendency to bilious attacks, or to migraines with conspicuous nausea and vomiting, is commoner in the "oral" group, as opposed to an increased incidence of bowel-disturbances in the "anal" group. Leaving aside the possibility of symbolic investment and interpretation of individual symptoms, we can readily conceive that the total migraine sequence may lend itself to valid interpretations. If, for example, the migraine has been generated in response to a painful or hateful situation, *this* (and its attendant feelings) may be symbolised (embodied) as a physical pain, a displaced form of suffering, and towards the end of the attack symbolically extruded by expulsive activities of viscera and glands. In such a case, which corresponds most closely to the apparent role of "encapsulative" migraines, the entire attack could be conceived in dramatic terms as a form of psychophysiological pantomime, or as an extended, unpleasant, visceral dream.

We have cited Freud's observation that the symptoms of a (physical) neurosis may act as the starting-point or nucleus of hysterical fabrications. We envisage that an analogous evolution may occur with the symptoms of a migraine, the initial physical symptoms becoming associated with specific emotional needs and phantasies, and thus assuming a second, symbolic, status. But a migraine is not in itself a hysterical artifice: its symptoms are real and rooted in physiological reactions. The language of hysteria is arbitrary and personal, and corresponds only to a moral, imaginative image of the body, and not to any physiological representation. In hysteria, the symbol is translated directly into a symptom: thus an arm which is, in phantasy, murderous, may be inhibited or punished by paralysis; but the hysterical paralysis does not correspond to any neurological deficit. In migraine, the symptoms are fixed and bounded by physiological connections; but its symptoms can constitute, as it were, a bodily alphabet or proto-language, which may secondarily and subsequently be used as a symbolic language.[49]

Thus, we must interpret situational migraines as if they were palimpsests, in which the needs and symbols of the individual are inscribed above, and yet in terms of, the subjacent physiological symptoms. Such

---

[49] The symbolism here considered has relation to various *symptoms* of migraine, not to any internal representations of the viscera, glands, etc. The inner body, unlike the surface of the body, is *not* represented topographically in consciousness. Hence the absurd images which most people entertain regarding the shapes and relations of their internal organs, and the hallucinatory projections of such images in the bizarre symptoms of hysteria and hypochondria: points which receive careful discussion in Dr. Jonathan Miller's book—*The Body in Question*. In migraine, symbolic significance is attached to actual symptoms: in hysteria, to imaginative or moral representations of the body.

an interpretation crosses the definitions of both conversion symptoms and vegetative neuroses, and in so doing makes the use of either term inadequate. And this, finally, need not surprise us, for the criteria which Alexander uses—symbolic expressiveness and physiological response—belong, as Starobinski and others have pointed out, to two different provinces of logical enquiry, either of which is capable of engrossing the entire problem of disease (Rieff, 1959, p. 10).

We must, therefore, return full circle to the Darwinian concepts with which we started. What starts as a direct action of the nervous system becomes, by degrees, a serviceable associated action: what starts as the physical aspect of an emotion becomes, insensibly, an allusion to, or token of, the entire affective situation. The reactions of the body contain the potential of a primitive bodily language—in migraine, a set of inner gestures, autonomic postures, analogous to involuntary facial expressions and motor gestures.[50] Much that Freud has said concerning the symbolism of dreams could be applied to the primitive physical symbolism of migraines. Freud sees the symbolism of dreams as archaic and universal, innate rather than individually acquired, and as representing the regressive use of "an ancient but obsolete mode of expression."[51] Similarly, and perhaps more plausibly, the symptoms of migraine and of many other psychosomatic syndromes, in their symbolic employment, may be seen as a reversion to an ancient and universal mode of expression—a primordial language of the body—implicit in the structure and functioning of the nervous system, and available for use when required.[52]

---

[50] The use of primitive neurological symptoms as personal symbolic expressions is readily exemplified in the area of motor mechanisms. Intermittent protrusion of the lips ("Schnauzkrampf") may be seen in diffuse cortical disease, frontal lobe lesions, schizophrenia, etc. Its occurrence, like that of snout and sucking reflexes, is dependent on diminished frontal lobe inhibition. It may, nevertheless, serve an additional symbolic purpose, especially in schizophrenia. In Bleuler's words: ". . . Schnauzkrampf is more readily understood as an expression of *contempt* than as a localised tonic contraction of the muscles which control protrusion of the lips . . . [it] is characterised by changes in intensity which, under psychic influences, may vary from zero to a maximum. The nature of these changes can only be understood if we consider at least their precipitations as a psychic process" (Bleuler, p. 448).

A much more familiar example is the use of yawning to express boredom.

[51] "The dreamer has at his command a symbolic mode of expression of which he knows nothing . . . These [symbolic] comparisons are not instituted afresh every time, but are ready at hand, perfect for all time . . . this we infer from their identity in different persons . . . We get the impression that here we have to do with an ancient but obsolete mode of expression . . . [which] goes back to phases in our intellectual development we have long outgrown. . . . It seems to me that symbolism, a mode of expression which has never been individually acquired, may claim to be a racial heritage." (Freud, 1920)

[52] An even more ancient mode of expression is the symbolic use of allergic reactions, reactions at cellular and tissue level which may be pressed into service in the emotional economy of the individual. We have seen how frequently emotionally-triggered allergic reactions may coexist with migraines, or serve as an alternative mode of bodily expression.

We have stressed, again and again, the countless variations, transitions and transformations of the migraine format, and the crucial fact that these may be employed, almost interchangeably, as "equivalents" of one another. Gowers laid great stress on this point, but offered no explanation, saying only: "... We can perceive the mysterious relationship, but we cannot explain it." We are no more certain concerning the factors which select or specify, from the many options available, the particular format of attack which a patient will actually adopt or "choose" at any given time. We consider it probable that there exist particular physiological idiosyncrasies, preferential pathways and mechanisms, which may predispose a patient towards one migraine-format rather than another, and we would suspect these to be particularly strong in certain rare and stereotyped forms of migraine, e.g. hemiplegic attacks and migrainous neuralgia. But in many other cases, these physiological factors appear to be weak, relative, or unstable, in that they allow profound changes of clinical pattern to occur. We must strongly suspect, therefore, that these physiological factors may be subordinated to psychogenic determinants, and that it is *these*, overruling or modifying all other factors, which may finally specify what form the protean migraine reaction will take. We must wonder whether the "mysterious relation" of which Gowers speaks is, in fact, a symbolic relation, the use of different types of attacks as *synonyms* for one another.

We have attempted to define, in the present chapter and its predecessor, some of the strategic functions of migraine. We have speculated that a hierarchy of determinants may be involved, from the most general reflex-reactivity of the organism, through a variety of physiological idiosyncrasies, to the most specific conversion-mechanisms of the individual patient. We have postulated that if the foundations of migraine are based on universal adaptive reactions, its superstructure may be constructed (and is certainly used and construed) differently by every patient, in accordance with his needs and symbols.

Thus we can now answer, in principle, the dilemma posed in Chapter 6, as to whether migraine is innate or acquired. It is *both*: in its fixed and generic attributes it is innate, and in its variable and specific attributes it is acquired. In an analogous manner, the universal "deep grammar" of all languages is innate (Chomsky), while every particular language is learned.

Walking, at its most elementary, is a spinal reflex, but is elaborated at higher and higher levels until, finally, we can recognise a man by the way he walks, by *his* walk. Migraine, similarly, gathers identity from stage to stage, for it starts as a reflex, but can become a creation.

CONCLUSIONS

We have portrayed the migraine *process* (or event) as a cycle of excitation
and inhibition of centrencephalic origin, subject to wide variations in
neural pattern and time-base. We have considered the part played by certain
local (vascular) and systemic (chemical) disturbances, but are persuaded
that these are variable in their occurrence, intermediary in role, and secondary to the primary neurophysiological disturbance of brainstem activity.

Feeling that a reaction so complex and versatile as migraine could
hardly have arisen *ab initio* in man, we have speculated on its possible
precursors and analogues in lower animals. We have envisaged that migraines were differentiated, *as reactions*, from a broad region of passive,
parasympathetically-toned, protective reflexes, such as many animals
employ in response to environmental or internal threats—cold, heat,
exhaustion, pain, illness, and enemies. All such reflexes, like migraine,
we have seen to be distinguished by regression and inertia, in contrast
to fight-flight responses.

Finally, we have considered migraines *as experienced and as used*, in
their relation to emotional life. Recurrent attacks, we have seen, constitute an available "flight into illness" for certain individuals, the motives
for such flight being as various as those underlying neurotic or hysterical
behaviour. We have further considered, more diffidently, that specific
symptoms of migraine may be linked to specific emotions or phantasies.

We have speculated that three forms of such psychosomatic linkage
may obtain in migraines: first, an inherent physiological connection between certain symptoms and affects; second, a fixed symbolic equiva
lence between certain physical symptoms and states of mind, analogous
to the use of facial expressions; third, an arbitrary, idiosyncratic symbolism uniting physical symptoms and phantasies, analogous to the construction of hysterical symptoms.

Whichever of these mechanisms is employed, migraine shows itself
both eloquent and effective in providing an oblique expression of feelings
which are denied direct or adequate expression in other ways. In this, it
is analogous to many other psychosomatic reactions, and no less analogous to the languages of gesture and of dreaming. In all of these we
employ an archaic language, one which evolved long before the language
of words. Why do we retain the language of autonomic symptoms, movements, and images, when we could use words? Such behaviour may be
regressive, but it will never be obsolete: in the words of Wittgenstein:

"What *can* be shown *cannot* be said."

"The human body is the best picture of the human soul."

PART IV

Therapeutic Approaches to Migraine

Introduction

It could be maintained that with the clarification of the nature of migraine, so far as we have been able to accomplish this, our task is finished, and that it would be a work of supererogation to provide a glossary of "treatments." Treatment, it might be said, is *implicit* in what has already been passed. One may write a treatise on "Aphasia" without the need to discuss speech-therapy. But our subject is not strictly comparable with this: migraine is common, inflicts widespread suffering or incapacity, tends to recurrence, is benign, and is peculiarly prone to misunderstanding or mistreatment, both by patients and physicians.

We have endeavoured, in the preceding portions of this essay, to present a coherent and logically consistent picture of the biology of migraine, and much of the therapeutic approach will be dictated by the considerations already implied. But medicine cannot be reduced to coherent and logically consistent terms—it is dependent on innumerable variables and intangibles, on "magic," and above all on the trusting relationship between physician and patient.

FOURTEEN

General Measures in the Management of Migraine

We have observed that roughly a tenth of the population suffer from common migraines, a fiftieth of the population from classical migraines, and a minute proportion from certain rare migraine variants (migrainous neuralgia, hemiplegic migraine, etc.). A further fraction of the population, not inconsiderable, experience migraine equivalents and isolated auras, but their numbers have not been estimated since their symptoms are generally the subject of misdiagnosis. Although headache is the commonest complaint presented to the practising physician, it is clear that only a small fraction of the migrainous population actually seek medical help. These are patients whose attacks are severe, frequent, or bizarre, and it is with them that we will be concerned in this chapter.

The physician must function first as diagnostician, then as healer or adviser. He has two diagnostic tasks: the identification of the complaint that is presented to him, and the elucidation of its causes and determinants. Let us assume that he has listened to the patient, perhaps observed an attack, undertaken all investigations he considers reasonable, and assured himself that the patient's problem is indeed one of recurrent migraines. The initial history will suffice, in some cases, to delineate the pattern of attacks and their chief causes; this is likely to obtain if the problem is one of periodic migraine (attacks regularly recurring, usually at intervals of 2 to 8 weeks, irrespective of the mode of life), or one of circumstantial migraine (in which the attacks have been clearly associated with specific provocative circumstances—excitement, exhaustion, alcohol, etc.). There will remain a large and severely-afflicted group of patients who suffer very frequent attacks without easily-defined antecedents, and such patients may have to be seen repeatedly, and studied carefully, before the determinants of their migraine are exposed. Two auxiliary measures may be of particular value in clarifying the patterns and determinants of repeated migraines: the keeping of two calendars (a migraine calendar and a general diary of daily events), which may reveal unsuspected circumstances as provocative of attacks, and (if deemed proper by the physician) the interviewing of close relatives who may provide invaluable information.

The physician becomes a therapeutic figure for the patient, whatever he says, whatever he does. He may see the patient once, a dozen times, or (if he is a psychiatrist) a thousand times. He may provide advice, support, or analysis, but whatever he elects to do, his relationship to the patient is pre-eminent. His authority, his sympathy, and the countless intangible and largely unconscious bonds which are forged in an effective doctor-patient relationship, are as important as the sense or otherwise of anything he says and does. This relationship, then, is central in the management of all patients with functional disease.

The question of *drugs* is likely to be raised at the outset, reluctantly, hopefully, or peremptorily. Innumerable drugs have been used in the treatment of migraine, many of which are successful, and a very few of which are specific (see Chapter 15), and attitudes to drugs, on the part of both patient and physician, may be extremely varied. My own attitude, in very general terms, is to prescribe some specific or symptomatic drug for the treatment of an acute attack, when seeing the patient for the first or second time, but to make clear to him, at the same time, my views on the place of drug-therapy in the management of migraine. It would be cruel and pointless to deny medication to an acutely-suffering patient, but it is another matter altogether to tout any form of drug-therapy as the sole treatment of severe, frequently-recurring migraines. I therefore present drugs as auxiliary and provisional measures, to be used while a fuller understanding of the patient's situation and his migraines is being achieved. There are some patients, of course, who insist on drug-treatment (or allergic or histamine "desensitisations," etc.) to the exclusion of any other therapeutic approach, and such patients must be treated in the only terms they allow.

The general therapeutic measures which have value for migraine patients are threefold: the avoidance of circumstances known to be provocative of attacks, the promotion of good general health, and, finally, social and psychotherapeutic measures. The first two of these may be considered together.

GENERAL MEASURES AND AVOIDANCE OF PROVOCATIVE CIRCUMSTANCES

One of the traditional roles of the physician is to tell the patient not to worry, take a holiday, get enough exercise, not stay up too late, etc., and this type of advice has been given to migraine patients, with varying success, since the time of Hippocrates. Thus Aretaeus, writing in the second century, made the following recommendations for epileptic and migrainous patients:

> Promenades long, straight, without tortuosities, in a well-ventilated place, under trees of myrtle and laurel . . . It is a good thing to take journeys . . . exercises should be sharper, so as to induce sweat and heat . . . cultivate a keen temper, without irascibility.

Peters (1853), writing seventeen centuries later, insists that the "hygienic" treatment of migraines is as important as the use of any drugs, and elaborates the advice of Aretaeus as follows:

> A general invigorating mode of life, diet and exercise are indispensable. Those who have brought them on by sedentary habits, much mental exertion and loss of sleep, must reform . . . avoid the excessive worry and perplexity of engrossing cares . . . abstain from the use of *black tea* . . . The shower-bath, and salt-water bathing, either at the sea side, or in the house, are often useful adjuncts . . . the bowels should be kept regular . . . The functions of the stomach and liver should be kept in as healthy a state as practicable . . . and those of the uterus by great care at the monthly periods . . . Those who will indulge in the dissipation of excessive pleasures, business, grief, or gormandising, will needs retain their headaches.

Liveing (1873), recognising that migraine is no respecter of social classes, provided memorable images of two groups of people driven to migraine by the circumstances of their lives. One group suffered from:

> the exhaustion which is produced by a poor and insufficient diet . . . and in women by too frequent suckling or child-bearing . . . excessive hours of labour, or occupations which entail a close confinement in the unwholesome and ill-ventilated workshops and dwellings of our crowded towns . . .

For these, the poor of London, Liveing would provide better living conditions, an adequate diet, and tonics—but alas! they are beyond his reach, for social reform must precede medicine. The second group of people prone to migraine were of a different class, students and professional men, engaged in

> the struggle for competence and professional position . . . the pressure and responsibilities of business, the competition and excitement of commercial speculation . . . or breaking down under the accumulating weight of family cares . . .

For *these* Liveing would recommend less ambition, less driving, more moral and emotional ease. Such advice is easily given, but is never taken. Alvarez, at the present time, has declared: "Better far perhaps is a healthy, happy rancher, than a headache-ridden professor!" but remains himself a headache-ridden professor.

Dutifully we exhort our patients, in words which have hardly changed from Aretaeus to Alvarez, and which must be construed, for the most part, as so much wasted breath. We are on firmer ground if we can counsel patients in the avoidance of specific circumstances provocative of migraine. There are countless such circumstances (many were listed in Chapter 8), and it is a test of the physician's acumen to pinpoint as many as possible.

Some such patients are sensitive to flickering light of certain frequencies, and need to have their television sets adjusted. Some patients cannot tolerate a missed meal, and others cannot tolerate a heavy meal. Some cannot take more than a single drink without risking a migraine. Some cannot tolerate loss of sleep, while others, conversely, will profit from rationing of sleep. In these and similar cases, the patient will learn that he faces a choice, to avoid the provocative circumstance or risk a migraine. But in the most important category of all, those patients in whom rage or other violent emotions may precipitate a migraine, the choice is not open. As John Hunter observed, with regard to his own attacks of angina which were precipitated by exertion or emotion: "A man may resolve never to move from his chair, but he cannot resolve never to be angry."

SUPPORTIVE AND PSYCHOTHERAPEUTIC MEASURES

Wolff (1963), in his excellent and full discussion of the psychotherapeutic approaches to migraine patients (a discussion whose scope is limited only by the fact that all Wolff's patients, like himself, exhibited the "migraine personality") makes three points which we must elaborate.

1. The precise method to be used in the management of migraine patients
   [Wolff writes] must ultimately depend on the physician's personal equipment and experience. A variety of approaches produces acceptable results.
   It is essential that the physician himself be aware of the advantages and
   shortcomings of the method he uses as a therapeutic agent.

We must add two comments in this connection relating to certain
dangers which may undermine the relationship of the migrainous patient
and his physician. The first is that the latter, his ambitions whetted by
psycho-analytic reading, but lacking analytic experience, will subject a
patient to impertinent, irrelevant, irresponsible, ill-timed, and frequently
incorrect "interpretations" of repressed feelings; the patient will usually
respond, and rightly so, by finding another physician. The second danger
is commoner and more serious, and lies in the failure of the physician
to appreciate the magnitude and severity of psychopathology in certain
patients who come to him with relentless unremitting migraines. We have
already indicated that some such patients are deeply disturbed (Chapter
12), and a very few ominously depressed or self-destructive. *These* patients, whose sufferings are out of proportion to their small numbers,
may be quite beyond the range of superficial psychiatric intervention,
and need to be referred for more specialised and intensive care.

The actual methods by which physicians may choose, or be forced,
to treat their patients is, of course, infinitely varied, as are the patients
themselves. Very few generalisations can be considered to have much
didactic value in this context. There is only one cardinal rule: one must
always *listen* to the patient. For if migraine patients have a common and
legitimate second complaint beside their migraines, it is that they have
not been listened to by physicians. Looked at, investigated, drugged,
charged: but not listened to.

The therapeutic interview, tied closely to consideration of the patient's
migraines in the first place, will gradually range further into other aspects
of the patient's life, and, particularly, with the stresses, fatigues, angers,
and frustrations which may be generated at work and at home. As the
physician listens, he clarifies: as he listens, he may drain off some of the
pent-up force of accumulated tensions; and, hopefully, he will be able
to point out to the patient how certain stresses may be sidestepped or
eased.

The power of direct advice and exhortation, in emotional spheres, is
extremely limited. Weiss and English (1957), in their textbook of psychosomatic medicine, provide 9 "simple rules" for the moral rearma-
ment of the migraine patient. These include such wholesome instructions

as: "Be satisfied with less . . . Stop being so critical . . . Approve of your-self . . . Stop feeling so guilty . . . ," etc. Such maxims may be framed and hung on a wall, but they cannot be emotionally assimilated through virtue of being uttered.

Wolff is particularly concerned with obsessive patients, driven by the harshness of their own standards and consciences, and imprisoned by reiterative conscious imperatives: I must do this, I must do that . . . He observes the tautness and anxious tension that characterise such patients, and his therapeutic concern, therefore, is with "repeated release of ten-sion through discussion . . ." and with "enabling the subject to become aware of his tension . . . fatigue . . . dissatisfaction . . . frustration, and the obsessiveness of his preoccupation with work or responsibilities."

But not all patients with habitual migraines are of this character type, a point which has already been demonstrated and discussed at length (Chapters 9 and 12). Many migraine patients, far from displaying over-activity and over-concern, show excessive compliance and passivity (combined with deeply-repressed rage and hostility, which is expressed in their migraines). Some show striking unconcern and denial of any problems and stresses (those with "dissociative migraines," analogous in their formation with hysterical symptoms). Another group of severely-afflicted patients are overtly depressed, masochistic, and alternate their frequent migraines with other self-punitive devices. It is particularly *these* patients which the physician will come to recognise, for they, unlike the majority of migraine patients, require sophisticated and intensive han-dling if any therapeutic success is to be achieved.

> 2. For the physician the preventive treatment of migraine patients is costly in energy. It is not a method that can be used by those who can give but a few minutes to an interview.

Here, again, Wolff's statement may be amplified. There are many migraine patients who come to a physician in the hope of receiving a correct diagnosis, a reassurance that their disorder is benign, a plain statement concerning its prognosis and management, and perhaps some medication for acute attacks. Included in this group will be all those patients who have relatively infrequent attacks, say 10 in a year. These patients need to be seen once or twice, to give them the "facts," and subsequently at widely-spaced intervals, once or twice a year, in order to check that the *status quo* is being maintained. More severely affected patients should be seen on a regular basis, at intervals—approximately, of 2 to 10 weeks—agreeable to both patient and physician. The early

interviews must be long and searching, in order to expose for both patient and physician the general situation and specific stresses which are
involved, while establishing the foundations of the physician's authority
and the patient-physician relationship; later consultations may be briefer
and more limited in scope, and will be chiefly concerned with the discussion of current problems as these are experienced by the patient and
expressed in his migraines. Cursory medical attention is disastrous, and
an important cause of allegedly "intractable" migraine.

> 3. One must appreciate that elimination of the headache may demand more
>   in personal adjustment than the patient is willing to give. It is the role of
>   the physician to bring clearly into focus the cost to the patient of his
>   manner of life. The subject must then decide whether he prefers to keep
>   his headache or attempt to get rid of it.

Wolff's statement stresses the limitations, as Groddeck questions the
propriety, of the physician who undertakes to treat psychosomatic illness. Both are concerned, implicitly, with the reality of the patient's
"choice"—to hold or relinquish his symptoms. Thus we come, finally,
to a definition of the aim of therapy.

This cannot be put in simplistic formulae of "cure" but must be conceived as a strategy individually plotted for each particular patient, an
attempt to find and secure the "best" *modus vivendi* for him. This is a
matter upon which there may exist a profound, if unconscious, disagree-
ment between the patient and his physician. We must speak of the extent
to which certain patients—a minority, but an important and often
deeply-incapacitated group of patients—may be *attached* to their symptoms, in *need* of them; the extent to which such patients may *prefer* the
migraine way of life, with all its torments, to any alternative which is
felt to be open to them. Wolff considers this possibility, but dismisses it
in a single phrase (". . . unwillingness to change may defeat all therapeutic effort"); we must, however, consider it at more length, particularly
in regard to that stubborn, tragic nucleus of patients whose migraines
have proved "incurable" despite a lifetime of seeking medical help.

We remarked, in the last chapter, that "conversion," or, in more general terms, the use of indirect physical means and illnesses to express
thwarted drives must be considered as a perpetual potential in all of us,
and we stressed Deutsch's wise comment: ". . . human beings would be
most unhappy or would take far more flight into a neurosis if they could
not fall sick from time to time." Patients with extremely severe, unremitting migraines fall into three groups: some face intolerable external

situations, some face potentially intolerable internal situations, and a very few (chiefly those who have had frequent classical migraines since earliest childhood, and often a strong family history of this) appear to have some idiopathic, physiological driving of their attacks analogous to that of epilepsy. It is only with the former two groups that we are here concerned. We have already implied that in such patients severe migraines may either coexist with severe neuroses, or occur in their place. The attempt to dislodge severe habitual migraines in a pathologically unconcerned or hysterical personality (Case 80, p. 168) may force the patient to face intense anxieties and emotional conflicts which are even less tolerable than the migraines. The physical symptoms, paradoxically, may be more merciful than the conflicts they simultaneously conceal and express. We may suspect this to be the case by observation of the personality and the symptoms, and we may verify that it is the case, on occasion, by the eruption of neurotic anxiety and conflict which may follow any therapeutic attempt to disturb the *status quo*. In such cases, migraines may fill the same paradoxical role, and be invested with the same unconscious ambivalence, as severe neurotic symptoms—they defend the personality, and offer certain advantages and securities, whilst preventing its expansion and freedom of action: the double role of city walls. Illness in such cases, to paraphrase the words of Groddeck, is both a friend and an enemy, and will only retreat if radically new choices can be offered to the patient.[53]

[53] Essentially the same point is made by Freud with regard to the management of neurotic symptoms and illness: ". . . Although it may be said . . . that he has taken 'flight into illness,' it must be admitted that in many cases the flight is fully justified, and the physician who has perceived this state will silently and considerately retire . . . Whenever . . . advantage through illness is at all pronounced, and no substitute for it can be found in reality, you need not look forward very hopefully to influencing the neurosis through your therapy" (Freud, 1920, p. 391).

FIFTEEN

Specific Measures During and Between Attacks

Many patients, and not a few physicians, perpetually await the appearance of a definitive *wonder-drug* for the specific treatment of migraine, and many new drugs introduced upon the market are greeted as such with rapture, and promoted at the expense of all existing remedies. Readers who have opened this book at this point may be assured that there have never been any such wonder-drugs, and never will be; readers who have reached this point by following the course of this book will appreciate the reasons for this. The specific treatment of migraine, like that of epilepsy or Parkinsonism, is a matter of trial and choice from among a considerable number of drugs which act on specific mechanisms in the nervous system, allied to symptomatic treatment, to the use of accessory drugs, and—not least—of important measures other than pharmacological ones.

The treatment of migraine attacks has always attracted an astonishing range of medical and surgical measures, not a few of which have been as radical as the stone-age measure of trepanning the skull. Medieval measures for the treatment of migraine included the use of every drug available at the time, and, if these failed, an appeal to blood-letting as a last resort.

Perhaps the first specifically useful drug discovered was *caffeine*. The drinking of much strong coffee was advocated by Willis, three centuries ago. Heberden, writing at the very start of the nineteenth century, recorded the use of ". . . valerian, the fetid gums, myrrh, musk, camphor, opium, extract of hemlock, sneezing powders . . ." as being fashionable in his day, but futile, and himself considered a draught of tartar emetic and tincture of opium as the most useful of prescriptions. Liveing, a century ago, advised the use of bromides and valerian as sedative measures, and of caffeine, belladonna and colchicine as specific measures to be used in the treatment of attacks. Gowers, assessing the treatments available towards the end of the last century, recommended the use of bromides as a staple measure, which might be combined with ergot. He considered that nitroglycerin could be exceptionally useful, especially in combination with tincture of gelsemium and nux vomica. The efficacy of such mixtures was increased by the addition of Indian hemp (see Appendix III).

Although ergot had been used intermittently and without great enthusiasm since the 1880s, it only came into vogue about 40 years ago with the advent of pure crystalline preparations, but since that time has held undisputed pride of place in the therapeutic armamentarium against migraine . An entirely different class of drug was introduced in the early 1960s as a consequence of chemical studies of the mechanisms of migraine; the best-known of these is methysergide, which is pre-eminent in the prophylaxis of migraine, as ergotamine is in the treatment of the acute attack.

This, very briefly, is the order in which pharmacologically-specific drugs for migraine were discovered. They are few in number, and their discovery has been a matter of difficulty, not because so few drugs may be of therapeutic use in migraine, but because any and every drug may work, given sufficient faith on the part of the patient. For every pharmacologically-specific drug which may be used in the treatment of migraine, a hundred others have been advocated: patent-medicines, home remedies, nostra, wonder-drugs, homeopathic drugs, placebos all of them, some merely charming or silly, others vicious or fraudulent. The mere listing of all the drugs which have been promoted for the treatment of migraine would compose a sizeable volume, and its contents would constitute one of the *curiosa* of Medicine.

DRUGS USEFUL IN THE TREATMENT
OF A MIGRAINE ATTACK

We must here consider three classes of drug: those which affect the actual mechanism of the migraine attack, in particular the dilatation of extra-cranial arteries which is responsible for headache; symptomatic drugs to diminish pain, nausea, and other concomitant symptoms; and accessory drugs, to promote relaxation or sleep.

ERGOTAMINE TARTRATE

Ergotamine tartrate is the best available drug for the treatment of *severe* migraine headaches; it is neither necessary nor advisable to use it in the case of milder attacks. The drug may be taken by mouth, by sublingual absorption, by suppository, by aerosol administration, or by injection, depending upon the desired rapidity of action, and upon individual tolerance or preference. Wolff favoured the use of ergotamine injection above other methods of administration, and there is no doubt that this may abort an attack when no other method of taking the drug has been useful. It can hardly, however, be advised as a routine or initial measure. If ergotamine is of value (as it will be in roughly 80 per cent of all migraine attacks), it must be administered as early as possible after the inauguration of migraine symptoms, for many attacks gather momentum very rapidly, and become increasingly less amenable to therapeutic intervention. An attack of migrainous neuralgia, for example, may achieve climactic intensity within a few minutes, and in such attacks oral ergotamine is absorbed too slowly to be of use (ergotamine tablets are absorbed within half an hour, if the stomach is empty; ergotamine suppositories and sublingual preparations within quarter of an hour; aerosol and parenteral administration may be effective within five to ten minutes). A classical migraine should be treated with ergotamine while the aura is in progress, and if the drug is taken at this stage, the headache and other ensuing symptoms of a full-blown attack may, with luck, be entirely averted. A common migraine should be treated as soon as the patient becomes aware of its inauguration.

Most therapeutic schedules advocate massive treatment with ergotamine within the first hour of the attack, during which a total dose of 4 to 8 mg may be taken orally or rectally, or a quarter of this amount if the drug is administered parenterally. Wolff advises that the maximum oral dose taken during the course of an attack should not exceed 11 mg. It is important to dissuade patients from taking repeated doses of ergotamine if the attack persists despite initial treatment. Although an injection of ergotamine may interrupt an attack which has been in existence for many hours, and is always worth trying *if* no ergotamine has been taken earlier, it may be stated, as a rough rule, that ergotamine affords an all-or-none treatment which will succeed, if it is going to succeed, within the first hour of the attack.

There are certain important contra-indications to the use of ergotamine. First and foremost, it must *never* be given during pregnancy; since, however, pregnancy itself procures some remission or even total exemption from migraine in a large proportion of patients (see Chapter 9), the withholding of ergotamine at this time may be no great hardship. It is also of importance to ascertain whether migrainous patients suffer from Raynaud's disease, Buerger's disease, or other problems compromising the peripheral circulation; the presence of any such conditions must also be regarded as an absolute contra-indication to the use of ergot. Coronary disease is a relative contra-indication, depending on its severity; patients with severe coronary disease should never take ergotamine.

Side-effects of ergotamine are prominent in some patients and negligible in others. The commonest of these are nausea and vomiting, and patients so affected may face a pretty choice between enduring a violent headache with relatively little malaise, or eliminating the headache at the expense of repeated nausea and vomiting. Other patients may experience a degree of faintness or drowsiness after taking ergotamine which is sufficient to prevent activity, but not to make the drug intolerable. The majority of patients, 9 out of 10, have no adverse effects from the drug.[54]

The therapeutic effects of ergotamine may be potentiated by combination with other drugs, particularly caffeine and belladonna, and there are many proprietary preparations on the market providing such combinations.

OTHER SPECIFIC DRUGS

Caffeine is a stimulant, a constrictor of cranial arteries and a diuretic. It is simple, non-toxic, and delightful to take, and should never be neglected in attacks of migraine which permit taking medication by mouth. Repeated cups of strong tea or coffee may always be recommended as worth taking in the earlier portions of an attack.

We have laid stress, in former chapters, on the strong parasympathetic predominance which characterises migraine symptoms, and we might therefore anticipate that parasympathetic blockers or sympathomimetic drugs would be of use. This supposition is borne out in practice. Such drugs are of particular use in cases where ergotamine is not tolerated, contra-indicated or ineffectual. I have prescribed tincture of *belladonna*, or related synthetic drugs, in a number of patients with relatively mild

---

[54]The clinical picture of ergotism, writes Wolff, is dramatic and terrifying. First there is vigorous vomiting, then the extremities, usually the feet, become pulseless, and swell with congestion and cyanosis. Ultimately gangrene develops. Although I have never seen ergotism of this degree, I have observed that a number of chronic ergotamine-takers (especially those who take in excess of 50 mg weekly) develop mildly ischaemic extremities, with pale, loose, mottled, cold-sensitive skin sometimes dotted with minute scars or micro-infarctions.

but very protracted migraines, with gratifying results. I cannot be sure whether these therapeutic results represent a specific pharmacological-effect or a placebo-effect; I know only that I have found the drug useful. Complementary to belladonna, and sometimes conveniently combined with it, is the use of *amphetamines*; I have prescribed these particularly for attacks of migraine or migrainous neuralgia which present themselves within a few minutes of waking in the morning.

Drugs of belladonna and amphetamine type carry obvious dangers of toxic effects, let-down reactions, and dependence; nevertheless, if used with discretion by suitable patients, they have every right to be included in the legitimate armoury of drugs specifically counteracting the mechanisms of migraine.

SYMPTOMATIC DRUGS

The outstanding symptom of common migraine is headache while nausea ranks next in frequency and severity. Analgesic drugs may suffice by themselves in the treatment of mild attacks of migraine, and many such attacks, without doubt, may be very adequately treated with aspirin. In the case of severe headache codeine or even morphine may be required. The use of narcotic pain-killers is conspicuous in a number of patients with severe and frequent migraines, and problems of dependence or addiction in such patients may constitute a problem additional to, and sometimes more malignant than, that of the migraine attacks themselves. Some of these patients may be weaned away from the stronger analgesics by the use of ergotamine, which they have never had occasion to take.

If nausea and vomiting are severe, it may be impossible to take any medication by mouth, and in such cases the best route (and the only alternative to injection) may be that of rectal absorption. Virtually every type of analgesic and anti-emetic drug is available in the form of suppositories.

ADJUNCTIVE DRUGS

The severest migraines are barely compatible with physical activity, and demand inactivity, and, above all, rest. All forms of sedative therefore have a place as adjuncts to specific and symptomatic treatment of migraine attacks. The most generally useful of these are barbiturates with a medium duration of action, and these are frequently combined with analgesics in various proprietary combinations. Tranquillisers also find a place in treatment of the acute attack, particularly if great irritability, anxiety or depression is present.

MISCELLANEOUS DRUGS

Innumerable other drugs have been used, and are still used, in the treatment of the acute migraine attack: nicotinic acid, anti-histamines, diuretics, etc. Only the last of these deserves serious consideration. A number of migraines, particularly menstrual migraines, may be preceded or accompanied by profound fluid-retention, and it has been found that *some* degree of fluid-retention accompanies at least a third of all common migraines (see Chapter 1). Wolff considered that this fluid-retention was not causally related to migraine headache, for the latter could not be influenced either by experimental diuresis or hydration.

At one time, I frequently prescribed the use of diuretics, particularly in the context of protracted menstrual migraines; I did this without serious anticipations of success, and I had no success with them. Physicians who *are* enthusiastic about the possibilities of diuretic therapy, and who communicate their optimism to their patients, frequently secure gratifying results by their use. These considerations suggest, without proving, that if diuretics are effective in the treatment of migraine, it is principally in view of their placebo-effects.

GENERAL MEASURES IN THE ACUTE ATTACK

A migraine of mild or moderate degree is entirely compatible with normal physical activity, and may be treated with medication (ergotamine and analgesics, etc.) while the patient is up and about. Severe attacks are barely compatible with normal activity, and may, in many cases, be exacerbated or protracted by continued activity. This, however, is by no means invariable, and a number of patients may find that they can work themselves out of an attack. Nevertheless, the *tendency* is for all migraines to be accompanied by some degree of lethargy, lowered muscular tone, and drowsiness (although these symptoms may be ignored in face of an overwhelmingly severe head-pain), and for the patient to *seek* rest. Ideally, therefore, the patient should be encouraged to secure the rest which the illness demands. In Wolff's words:

> Every administration of ergotamine should be followed by rest in bed for a period of not less than two hours. The desirability of this cannot be overstated, because the biologic purpose of the attack is defeated if the patient immedi-

ately resumes activity . . . If suitable relaxation and rest in bed is neglected after the abortion of an attack with ergotamine, headaches may actually occur with increased frequency.

Some patients may prefer to sit in a chair, finding that recumbency may aggravate their headaches. Local measures of use are pressure over the affected arteries, and the use of ice-packs over the forehead. There may be intense sensory and general irritability; the patient must therefore be shielded from light, noise, and intrusive attentions. He is likely to be very thirsty, and may become dehydrated from repeated vomiting, profuse perspiration, and, in some attacks, diarrhoea. Thin soups, with some added salt, may be recommended to maintain fluid and salt balance. There should not, however, be any attempts to give solid food; the patient will not suffer from a day's starvation, and his nausea will be minimised if the stomach is kept empty.

TREATMENT OF "STATUS MIGRAINOSUS"

The term "status" is reserved for the occurrence of confluent or continuous attacks of paroxysmal illness, whether this is epileptic, asthmatic, or migrainous in nature. True migraine status must be treated as a medical emergency. The patient is likely to have suffered excruciating headache for several days without pause, to be prostrated or collapsed from incessant vomiting, and seriously dehydrated. Status migrainosus can *feel* like a fatal illness, and the patient may be intensely apprehensive or depressed to near-suicidal degree.

The first acts of the physician must be reassurance and protective seclusion, for the intensity of the patient's anxiety, and the agitated movement of relatives milling around in a well-intentioned but intensely irritating manner, are likely to be important factors in perpetuating the state. Intensive domiciliary care must be provided, or, in the severest cases, admission to hospital. The patient will be in need of massive medication: parenteral barbiturates, codeine or morphine, anti-emetic drugs, and frequently strong tranquillisers such as chlorpromazine. All supportive measures must be taken, among which intravenous feeding of fluids is of crucial importance. Ergotamine is *not* indicated in this situation, and is prone to aggravate rather than ameliorate the symptoms.

The use of *steroids* must be considered in every case of true migraine status, provided their use is not contra-indicated on other grounds.

When the status is finally over, and the patient has returned to his normal health, he must be encouraged to place himself under continuing medical care. Attacks of migraine, in their nature, tend to be of limited duration, but attacks of migraine status are nearly always associated with intense if hidden emotional stresses, the desperate quality of the symptoms reflecting the intensity of the underlying emotional substrate.

PREVENTION OF MIGRAINE ATTACKS

Drugs employed in the prophylactic treatment of migraine fall into two classes: the first group is constituted by drugs considered to modify the migraine-mechanisms and specific migraine-reactivity, and the second group, of no less importance, aims to diminish emotional reactivity where this is considered to be a major determinant of frequent migraines.

It is evident that only a limited proportion of migraine patients are actually in need of any prophylactic therapy. Patients with isolated attacks coming at relatively infrequent intervals are obviously not candidates for preventive therapy. The group of patients we are here concerned with are those with frequent, severe, unremitting attacks: the most severely-affected patients may, for example, suffer as many as five attacks of migraine weekly, and be seriously incapacitated on a chronic basis. Another group of patients to whom prophylactic treatment is a necessity are those with cluster headache, overwhelmingly painful attacks of migrainous neuralgia, as many as 10 a day, throughout the 2- to 8-week duration of the cluster. A third group of patients who are in need of preventive therapy are those with severe, protracted menstrual migraines.

The most potent drugs with specific prophylactic power against migraine attacks are ergometrine and methysergide (Sansert in USA, Deseril in UK). Belladonna compounds are of some prophylactic use; anti-histamines, though widely used for this purpose, are of unproven efficacy. The use of steroids, already mentioned in connection with the treatment of status migrainosus, has a further use—if methysergide has failed—in the treatment of cluster headache.

Methysergide (lysergic acid butanolamide) was introduced for the prophylaxis of migraine almost a decade ago, following the studies of Sicuteri, and his demonstration of the remarkable anti-serotonin effects of methysergide. Indeed, the drug was introduced *as* an anti-serotonin agent; it has, however, anti-inflammatory, anti-histaminic and many other pharmacological properties, and it is far from certain that its therapeutic effectiveness is due to its anti-serotonin effect. Its initial effectiveness, in the early sixties, appeared astounding, and it was claimed that upwards of 90 per cent of all cases of severe migraine could hope for dramatic improvement while taking it. It was widely held that the wonder-drug for migraine had at last arrived; the expectation of its healing powers doubtless contributed to those powers. However its efficacy and its reputation have both declined over the years; in unison, it may now be said that methysergide benefits no more than a third of all patients with severe, frequent migraines. Nevertheless, methysergide is still the most powerful prophylactic agent available, and should be tried in all cases of "intractable" migraine provided that it is not contra-indicated on medical grounds, and provided that adequate vigilance is exercised, both by physician and patient, in the avoidance of side-effects or toxic effects.

Methysergide is available in 2 mg tablets, and at one time patients were given daily doses as high as 20 mg daily. The reasonable maximum daily dose is now considered to be 8 mg daily, for while there is no added benefit beyond this dosage, there *is* a sharp increase in toxic effects. Common initial side-effects are those of nausea, drowsiness, or abnormal wakefulness; these are likely to be tolerable and transient, and are mimimized if the full therapeutic dosage of methysergide is achieved gradually, e.g. over a period of a week or 10 days. This length of time is commonly required before its full therapeutic power is manifest, and this also must be made clear to patients. The other and more serious side-effects of methysergide fall into several categories: disorders of high cerebral function, vasomotor problems, vascular insufficiency, and fibrotic problems.

Possible disorders of neurological function are many and bizarre; most physicians with appreciable experience of the drug have come across a number of these in patients taking methysergide, but I am not aware that they have ever been systematically surveyed. Persistent insomnia or persistent drowsiness may occur; a number of patients may become significantly depressed while on the drug (methysergide has been employed, in preliminary studies, for the treatment of mania); a few patients may experience bizarre disorders of voluntary movement— states of catalepsy, fascination, and statuesque immobility, or states of psychomotor excitement and compulsive movement: symptoms more familiar in certain forms of Parkinsonism, catatonia, and some intoxications (phenothiazides, bulbocapnine, LSD, L-dopa, etc.); a very few patients may experience unusually vivid dreaming, or waking dreamy-states with odd perceptual changes or hallucinations (methysergide is an exceedingly close chemical relative of LSD, lysergic acid diethylamide).

The vasomotor and vasoconstrictive effects of methysergide may be responsible for elevations of blood-pressure (especially in previously hypertensive patients) and, more seriously, compromise of the blood-supply in the extremities or internal organs. Compromised circulation in the arms or legs may be experienced as numbness, coldness, or tingling in the fingers and toes; rarely, there may be ischaemia of the entire limb, with disastrous consequences if untreated. All major internal arteries may be affected, in particular coronary and mesenteric arteries.

The third category of toxic problems occurs only in relation to long-continued use of the drug, and consists of fibrotic indurations in the pleural or pericardiac spaces, rarely, and retroperitoneal fibrosis, of which nearly a hundred cases associated with methysergide administration have been reported. The former may present as breathlessness or pleuritic pain, and the latter as back-pain, loin-pain, haematuria, etc. It is of particular note that methysergide-induced retroperitoneal fibrosis may be clinically silent, proceeding in the absence of symptoms to severe unilateral hydronephrosis.

This formidable list of potential side-effects does not imply that the drug should not be used; *what it does imply is the necessity of painstaking periodic examination of the patient, allied to the use of certain routine tests.* Patients on methysergide should be seen at intervals of a month, or at most 6 weeks; they must be closely questioned regarding any untoward symptoms (chest-pain, shortness of breath, coldness and numbness of fingers, etc.), while the clinical examination will include auscultation of the chest, recording of blood-pressure, and careful examination of all peripheral pulses. Maintaining the blood-pressure cuff above the systolic pressure may induce tingling in the fingers within a few seconds if there is significant but as yet asymptomatic compromise of the peripheral circulation; an ischaemic cuff can normally be tolerated for at least 60 seconds without the production of any paraesthesiae. The most important laboratory investigations to be performed are three-monthly blood-counts, chest X-rays, and electrocardiograms. An abbreviated intravenous pyelogram should be performed at the inauguration of long-standing methysergide administration (e.g. after one month of treatment, if the latter is so successful as to indicate the patient's continuance on the drug), followed by further pyelograms at intervals of 6 months (Elkind et al. 1968).

We have devoted considerable space to the discussion of side-effects and their avoidance, for the outstanding danger in the use of methysergide is *negligence* on the part of patient or physician. The drug is never one to be used casually. Having said this, one must emphasise that methysergide, when properly used, is outstandingly effective in the prophylaxis of migraine in many patients who have proven refractory to all other specific therapeutic measures, and its use should always be considered in such patients. I have kept upwards of 200 patients on methysergide for as much as 2 years, without encountering any untoward effects, and some of the patients I have seen have taken it for 8 years, with highly satisfactory results.

It is advisable to take long-term patients off the drug for one month every 6 months, for this apparently reduces the likelihood of any side-effects. The dose should be reduced gradually at such times, for abrupt cessation of the drug may cause a violent rebound phenomenon, a status migrainosus, analogous to the status epilepticus which may occur if patients are suddenly taken off anticonvulsant drugs.

The prophylactic use of ergot drugs was practised long before the appearance of methysergide, but has somewhat fallen into disuse with the rise of the newer drug. I have had a number of patients who have taken ergot drugs prophylactically for many years with very satisfactory effects, but I have never had occasion to make an adequate comparison of the relative efficacy of ergot drugs and methysergide. Such a comparison has very recently been performed by Barrie *et al.* (1968). These workers have compared the effectiveness of ergotamine tartrate (0.5 to 1 mg daily), ergometrine maleate (1 to 2 mg daily) and methysergide (3 to 6 mg daily). Remarkably little therapeutic difference was found in this trial; the ergot drugs showed themselves almost as effective as methysergide, and their use was associated with fewer side-effects, and less defaulting from the trial. In all cases, the higher dosages were more effective than the lower ones.

The contra-indications regarding the use of methysergide are essentially those which have been mentioned with regard to ergotamine; it is worth reiterating that the drug should *never* be used if a patient has Raynaud's disease or Raynaud's phenomenon.[55] A number of workers consider that methysergide is contra-indicated by coexistent collagen dis-

---

[55] A number of previously asymptomatic patients may develop their first *overt* symptoms of vascular sensitivity when placed on methysergide; these idiosyncratic reactions are especially common, and to be guarded against, in those who have a family history of Raynaud's disease. Some physicians attempt to "titrate" such patients with small doses of ergot or methysergide. This procedure is to be avoided, for it may lead to progressive ischaemic damage of the extremities.

ease; it is certain that *if* retroperitoneal or other fibroses develop while on methysergide (these are potentially reversible unless advanced), the drug should not be given again.

There is a large group of patients who experience several relatively mild migraine attacks each month, and are in need of some prophylactic medication, but not of methysergide or ergotamine in high doses. My experience has been that belladonna may provide a specific prophylactic medication of adequate power in many such patients, and is perhaps best combined with small amounts of ergotamine and phenobarbital: many such proprietary preparations are available.

It is illegitimate to use steroids on a long-term basis for the prevention of migraine, save in the special case of cluster headache. This is the least bearable of all forms of migraine during the duration of a severe cluster, for the patient may be driven to desperation by experiencing as many as a dozen individual attacks daily, each of excruciating severity.

The individual attacks may be treated with a quickly-absorbed form of ergotamine with variable success, but prophylactic treatment must supplement this. It is always worth using methysergide in such cases, but this will only disrupt the cluster in a proportion of cases. If the cluster continues with undiminished intensity after two weeks of methysergide administration, it is worth supplementing it with one of fluorinated steroids in high dosage; and to both of these a tranquilliser may be added with advantage.

NON-SPECIFIC DRUG-TREATMENT IN THE PROPHYLAXIS OF MIGRAINE

Clinical observation of migraine patterns indicates that a majority of patients with extremely frequent, severe, intractable migraines are caught in a situation of severe emotional stress or conflict (of which they may or may not be aware) and that this drives the migraine as a psychosomatic expression of their underlying emotional problems. We have indicated that there exist a small proportion of patients who have experienced incessant migraines since earliest childhood (usually of the classical variety), who appear to suffer from a truly idiopathic form of the illness; this latter group is also likely to be emotionally disturbed, although the disturbance in their case may be secondary to intractable migraine, rather than its cause. Both groups may stand in need of prophylactic medication *additional to* methysergide, ergotamine, etc. The choice of such medication is, of course, dependent on the severity and type of emotional distress which may be exhibited, the patient's actual reactions to trial of one medication or another, the presence of any medical contra-indications, and the physician's individual preferences.

Some patients may be "held" by mild medications such as phenobarbital (1/4–1/2 gr. t.d.) or meprobamate; others will need compounds of the chlordiazepoxide type (Librium, Valium, etc.), and the most severely disturbed will require phenothiazine tranquillisers, or anti-depressants (Tofranil, etc.). In the case of more severely disturbed patients, some form of psychotherapy may be indicated or demanded, from simple supportive therapy and regular attention from a physician to intensive psychotherapy.

MISCELLANEOUS DRUGS IN THE TREATMENT OF MIGRAINE

It has been indicated that a limitless variety of drugs have been promoted at one time or another in the treatment of migraine, and that many of these have been dramatically successful, despite the improbability of any chemical rationale for their action, or indeed in the absence of any chemical activity whatever. Migraine is notoriously (and fortunately) sensitive to therapeutic suggestion, and the assessment of true pharmacological activity is made extremely difficult by the existence of outstanding placebo-response in many patients. A few such drugs may be alluded to very briefly.

HISTAMINE "DESENSITISATION"

Horton introduced the technique of histamine "desensitisation" for migrainous neuralgia on the supposition (subsequently refuted) that such attacks represented an abnormal response to endogenously-produced histamine. The treatment was outstandingly successful in the charismatic hands of its originator, but generally of indifferent success in the hands of others. The mystique (and perhaps also the masochistic gratification) of repeated histamine injections, coupled with the attention of an enthusiastic physician, is no doubt the secret of success when histamine desensitisation is of value. It may be recommended as an innocuous placebo-procedure, especially for patients who have heard of the technique and clamour for injections.

ALLERGIC "DESENSITISATION"

This too, like histamine desensitisation, has been promoted on the basis of an erroneous theory, but is frequently of use in certain patients. The most suitable patients, as might be predicted, are those who deny the possibility of any emotional distress or driving of their migraines, and believe implicitly in the allergic origin of their attacks. Such patients may do extraordinarily well in the hands of an attentive allergist who shares their beliefs, and who will combine injections with the therapeutic emotional contact of which the patient stands in need.

HORMONE TREATMENTS

The general subject of hormones in relation to migraines has already been considered at length (Chapter 8), and at this point we need only recall the conclusions there reached: that the majority of such studies have been conducted without adequate controls, and that their results, accordingly, admit of many interpretations. We have noted, also, that certain hormone preparations may *aggravate* migraine, in addition to exposing the patient to a number of unwanted and incalculable side-effects.

For these reasons, hormones cannot be considered as harmless placebos, comparable to nicotinic acid, glucose tablets, or histamine injections. The entire matter is urgently in need of experimental clarification, and must be considered *sub judice* at the present time. These considerations predispose me against any attempted use of hormone-preparations other than in the context of a controlled experiment, and I have both avoided, and advised against, the use of hormone-preparations in my own practice.

SURGICAL PROCEDURES

Credulous and desperate sufferers from migraine have presented a perennial target for well-meaning surgical procedures, which at best may be worthless or procure transient remission, and at worst may be grossly fraudulent or mutilating.

A number of *local* procedures have been advocated, and are still advocated, such as ligation or denervation of one temporal artery in cases of severe, persistently unilateral migraine. These and other procedures have been discussed in great detail by Wolff (1963), and we can do no more than restate his assessment of such procedures, namely that they only procure transient benefit.

A different and altogether more horrifying problem is that of *general* surgical procedures which may be performed for the treatment of migraine, procedures which may vary from simple removal of all the teeth, or the tonsils, to near-evisceration of the patient: gall-bladder, uterus, and ovaries are the usual sacrifices to the surgeon's knife. A particularly common victim is the migrainous woman of middle age, who has been submitted to hysterectomy in the hope of eliminating frequent migraines. Characteristically many such operations are followed by a period of remission from migraine, but the attacks are subsequently likely to re-establish themselves in the same or another pattern. *If* permanent exemption from migraine is secured, we must envisage the surgery as filling the role of a particularly monstrous placebo or satisfying some intense masochistic need. Although some patients will continue to clamour for operations, and some surgeons will respond to their requests, it cannot be stated too strongly that surgical procedures have no place in the treatment of migraine.

We may wonder whether there is not an implicit *moral* basis (masochistic or punitive) underlying the performance of mutilating surgical operations in this context, and we may remind ourselves of certain Victorian treatments of epilepsy, in which the existence of such a basis is more openly admitted:

> Castration has been proposed as a remedial measure . . . circumcision, if effectually performed, is usually successful, and should be adopted in all cases in which there is a reason to associate the disease [epilepsy] with masturbation. (Gowers, 1881)

CONCLUSIONS

There is only one cardinal rule: one must always listen to the patient; and, by the same token, the cardinal sin is not listening, ignoring. Prior to any and all specific approaches, there must be this general approach, the establishment of a relation, a communication with the patient, so that patient and physician understand each other. A relationship, moreover, in which the patient is not entirely passive and compliant, believing and doing what he is told, and taking what is "ordered"; a relationship which is, essentially, collaborative.

The history of "treatments" for migraine is largely a story of medical "overkill" and patient exploitation, and the first thing to be understood by the patient, if and when the time comes for him to seek medical advice, is to insist on a full and careful *discussion* between himself and his physician, a discussion which defers to the special knowledge and skill of the latter, but is none the less a discussion between one adult and another. The wise physician will *wish* to be conservative, knowing as he does the wisdom of the body, and the natural tendency toward resolution seen in migraine—and similar disorders. He will be *against* massive "intervention" and "fussing-around," knowing (as Hippocrates did) that this is not only inane but counterproductive and may complicate the situation and *delay* its resolution.

The vast majority of migraine attacks, by virtue of the fact that they move toward resolution, after running their course of so many hours, require nothing more than the simplest measures to make these hours bearable: namely, strong tea (or coffee), rest, darkness and silence. The simplest of analgesics—aspirin, or something comparable—will take the edge off the pain in a majority of attacks; and with the diminution of the pain, there is likely to follow a diminution of nausea and other symptoms, if present (apparently by "sympathy" within the body, so that a return to health or "valescence" of one affected organ will lead the way to a "convalescence" of them all).

By the same token, any measure, taken for any one symptom, can help dissipate them all. If nausea is intense, an anti-emetic will help; and help *not only* the nausea, but the headache as well. A very mild sedative—a little phenobarbital, librium or valium (the equivalent of Gowers's bromides) will tend to alleviate *all* the pathological excitements—the pounding head, the irritability, the restlessness, the anxiety—and allow the fastest possible resolution of attacks.

In the original edition of this book I spoke much of ergotamine and other drugs that can *abort* an attack, just as there are physiological measures (exercise, sleep, etc.) which may also achieve this. I am now less certain of the wisdom of aborting attacks, and instead of advising such drugs straightaway, I would have the patient consider the pros and cons of letting the attack develop naturally. The following case history will illustrate this:

Case 75   A middle-aged professor, of fiery temperament, who tends to get classical migraines on Friday afternoons, following his inspired and stormy

teaching sessions. He has scarcely time to rush home from these before scotomata and other symptoms make their appearance, followed within minutes
by violent hemicrania, nausea, and vomiting. If these symptoms are *endured*,
they run their course and resolve in three hours, leaving a wonderful sense of
refreshment, and almost of rebirth. If, on the other hand, they are *aborted*
(as they may be by ergotamine, exercise, or sleep), there is a persistent malaise
throughout the entire weekend. Thus this patient is presented with a *choice*:
to be violently ill for three hours, and then perfectly well; or to be vaguely ill
and wretched for two to three *days*. Since realising his situation, he has given
up the use of all abortive measures, finding a severe but brief migraine altogether preferable to a mild but greatly extended one.

There are different moods of medicine in different times—and different places. We fuss about the migraineur now, with injections and interventions, in a way which would have horrified Liveing, or the Victorians,
and it is precisely this sort of fussing which makes migraine worse so
that, paradoxically, the very intensity and incessancy of "treatment,"
these days, may serve to aggravate, not alleviate, the malady it seeks to
help. The best migraine clinic I have seen was one where the sufferer was
led, without an unnecessary movement or words, to a darkened cubicle,
where he could lie down and rest, and receive a pot of tea and a couple
of aspirin.

The results of this simple, natural regiment, even with classical attacks
of great severity, were far more impressive than anything I had seen in
other clinics; and brought home to me with an overwhelming conviction
that, for the vast majority of patients and attacks, the answer does not
lie in ever-more-powerful drugs, and medicamental aggressiveness, but
a sensitive feeling for suffering, and nature; a deep sense of the healing
power of nature itself (*vis medicatrix naturae*), and the humility which
seeks to woo nature, but never to bully it.

For though a migraine is a physiological event, it is not *just* a physiological event, but one that tends to be strongly related to, and determined by, the affected *individual*—his character, his "needs," his circumstances, and his mode of life. Thus it is insufficient to look for purely
physiological remedies, when what one may have to remedy, if it can be
remedied, is a whole way of life, a whole life.

This was always the central motto and message of Hippocrates, the
Father of Medicine: that one must not treat the disease, but the afflicted
individual; that though the doctor must be knowledgeable and expert
about diseases, drugs, physiology, and pharmacology, his ultimate concern must be for the individual himself.

The physician must not dominate or be dogmatic to the patient, must not play the expert, insist "I know best"; he must listen to the patient, listen beneath words; listen to his special, unspoken needs; address his dispositions, the patterns of his life; listen to what his illness, the migraine, is "saying." Only then will the path of healing become clear.

SIXTEEN

Recent Advances in the Treatment of Migraine

That attacks of migraine may be provoked by sudden emotions, or related to the patterns and stresses of a life, or to the personality of the individual, has often given rise to the notion that migraine is "functional" or "psychosomatic"—but this represents a failure to appreciate that the phenomena of migraine are extraordinarily specific, and must have an equally specific mechanism and basis. We have had, since antiquity, a notion of the *general* circumstances which may provoke migraines, and of the *general* measures by which one may alter these. But it is only relatively recently—and most especially in the past twenty years—that we have started to come to grips with some of the *specific* mechanisms involved, and the equally specific measures which may be used to alter these.

This change in atmosphere, in our thinking about migraine, can be traced with precision to the year 1960, when the drug methysergide was first used. Neil Raskin (1990) writes:

> I was still in training when methysergide was introduced in 1960. It was quite astonishing how this drug changed physicians' thinking about the nature of migraine. Prior to that time . . . migraine was thought to be predominantly psychosomatic . . . Suddenly, patients could take a few tablets of methysergide and within a week they were headache-free. No change in their internal milieu. Cured . . . [56]

[56] Similar changes in thinking occurred at this time with regard to other neurological conditions. Thus in 1960 it was also found that the drug haloperidol could drastically reduce the bizarre phenomena of Tourette's syndrome. Before this, Tourette's had been seen as purely psychogenic, as "Freudian," and patients tended to be subjected to lengthy,

Drugs used prior to this time (the ergotamines were introduced in the 1920s) suppressed specific symptoms of migraine; there had been no drug able to "reset" the basic mechanism, because we had no idea, until the 1950s, what the basic mechanism might be. In the 1950s it was found that migraine attacks might be associated with abnormalities of the neurotransmitter serotonin, and methysergide was devised as a serotonin antagonist. At that time there were thoughts of a single, simple "serotonin system" in the brain, whose abnormalities might give rise to migraine on the one hand, but also to anxiety, depression and sleep disorders on the other.

The simple picture of this time has disappeared. We now know that there are upwards of forty neurotransmitters in the brain, and that all neurotransmitter systems are complex in the extreme: thus there are three main families of serotonin receptors, with many subtypes in each family. But it was only in the 1980s that it became possible to dissect this complicated system, and to develop very selective drugs to act on particular parts of it.

But these developments relate only to one aspect, the chemical aspect, of migraine: what of the other aspects, the vascular and electrical aspects, which had seemed, even to Liveing, to be equally important? What of the physiology of the migraine aura—and of the headache and head pain? Lashley, measuring the advancing margin of his own migraine aura, inferred that this must reflect a wave of excited-then-depressed activity in the cerebral cortex, advancing across it at the rate of 2 to 3 mm per minute. No such process had ever been observed in man, but a perhaps similar process, called "spreading depression," had been observed by Leão in the exposed cortex of experimental animals (see p. 190). Early in the 1970s, Olesen in Denmark, using a new technique of measuring cerebral blood flow with radioactive tracers, found a slowly spreading wave of reduced blood flow in the cerebral cortex, moving forward across the visual cortex at precisely the same rate. This was strongly suggestive that such a process did occur in the human brain, though still left open was the question of whether the spreading depression was the cause or the effect of this spreading change in microcircu-

---

well-meaning but wholly ineffective, psychoanalyses. With the discovery of haloperidol's effectiveness, there was a sudden (and perhaps excessive) switch, and Tourette's was now seen as purely "chemical," as due to genetically unstable dopamine systems in the brain. Now, in turn, there is something of a reaction to this reaction, for a syndrome impinging on character and emotions, on daily experience, like Tourette's, has to have psychodynamic and environmental determinants no less than chemical ones—and this must be true, if to a lesser extent, of migraine as well.

lation. Just in the past year or two, it has become possible to measure the brain's neuromagnetic fields through the skull, and this has shown that a magnetic wave, with excited spikes at its advancing rim and depressed slow waves in their wake, moves across the visual cortex at 2 to 3 mm per minute during visual migraine auras—confirmation at last that "spreading depression" does indeed occur in man, and is the immediate cause of the singular cortical phenomena of the aura.[57]

But, as seemed clear even to Liveing and Gowers, though the aura might be cortical, the origin of migraine was not; but seemed, rather, to arise from some abnormal neural activity or reactivity deep in the brainstem. This too was my own feeling, on general clinical and biological grounds—that there must be massive, slow potentials emanating from the brainstem, and projected from this both "upstream" and "downstream" in the nervous system. The bizarre, huge, long-duration action potentials recorded by magnetoencephalography give the first direct evidence for this, the first direct evidence that, whatever vascular or other changes may occur, migraine is first of all a neural phenomenon, generated by the abnormal activity of neurons deep in the brain. Are such neurons demonstrable in the brain? Can their involvement in the origination of migraines actually be documented? Answers to these questions have been provided by many researchers, pre-eminently Neil Raskin at the University of California, San Francisco, and by James Lance at the University of New South Wales in Sydney, Australia.

Both the San Francisco and the Australian workers have been interested in pain, and its "gating," especially by a newly-defined pain-modu-

---

[57] Most of the triggers of migraine were recognised long ago, but one new one—not described in the medical literature, at least, until 1972—is so-called "footballer's" migraine: the prompt elicitation of phosphenes, scintillating scotomata, extinction of colour perception, and even cortical blindness, followed by unilateral headache, vomiting, etc. a few minutes after "heading" a football. This could occur in any player, even in someone who had never had a migraine. It seems probable that blows to the head may cause a prompt "spreading depression" in the visual cortex, which then leads into a migraine directly, bypassing the usual "idiopathic" mechanisms.
There is evidence, both clinical and electrophysiological, that the visual cortex may be unusually sensitive to excitation and disturbance in sufferers from classical migraine, even between attacks. Purely visual stimuli can provoke a migraine aura: Liveing describes a patient whose attacks were set off by the sight of falling snow, and I have seen many patients whose auras were set off by disturbances in the visual field (the rippling of water or foliage, most commonly; and, in one patient (Case 90, p. 151), by asymmetries—the sight of an asymmetrically-buttoned jacket, for example), which would initiate a spreading perceptual disturbance, a distortion in the visual field, spreading out from it in all directions. Flickering light can provoke a migraine in some people, and even when it does not actually do this, tends to cause an excessive "driving" of the EEG in the visual parts of the brain. The study of visual evoked potentials shows potentiation of these in migrainous patients, both in the primary visual cortex and in the visual association areas, even between attacks. These observations strongly support the notion that migraine is primarily a neural event, a neural reaction, based on innate and specific neuronal sensitivities.

lating system descending from the brainstem to the spinal cord. Neurosurgeons had found that they could sometimes greatly reduce lower-back or limb pain (though not pain from the head or neck) by implanting electrodes in the brainstem, and stimulating neurons in the grey matter around the cerebral aqueduct. Many of these patients, when the electrodes were activated, started to develop typical migraines, with severe, pulsating, unilateral headaches (usually on the same side as the implants), vomiting and visual disturbances. That these were indeed typical migraines was shown by their sensitivity to intravenous dihydroergotamine. *But these were patients who had never had migraines before.* This constituted the first clearly-demonstrated example of an *acquired* or experimental migraine—a migraine acquired in consequence of the artificial electrification of so-called raphe neurons in the brainstem by an implanted electrode. The exciting electrode caused these neurons to fire, but their firing produced a typical migraine. Did spontaneous or normally occurring migraines, it was immediately wondered, have a similar genesis in an increased firing of these raphe neurons?

Additional studies by Lance, in monkeys and cats, show that direct electrical or chemical stimulation of these nuclei can produce the vascular changes typical of migraine. These brainstem nuclei, Lance has further shown, as well as projecting upward to the cerebral cortex, also project downward to a "pain-gating" system descending from the brainstem to the spinal cord, the upper three segments of which can form a "pain centre" for the head. Patients often have a period of emotional excitement—anxiety, sometimes elation—a prodrome, for several hours *before* the aura, and this suggests that higher-order mechanisms, in the hypothalamus or diencephalon, may play some part in initiating the overall sequence.

How then do all these different mechanisms fit together to produce the entire sequence of a classical migraine? The most general hypothesis is that of Lance (see Lance, 1982, pp. 169–171), who envisages the initiation of attacks in the hypothalamus, whether on the basis of a built-in periodicity, or in response to sensory stimuli from the cerebral cortex. Once initiated, impulses descend from the hypothalamus to the periaqueductal grey matter, thence to the raphe nuclei, and here, as we have seen, they can affect the cortical microcirculation, constricting it, initiating "spreading depression" in the cortex (and thus producing the aura phase of the attack), and at the same time reducing pain perception by closing the (enkephalinergic) "gate" in the spinal cord.

This phase, which depends on hyperactivity of both noradrenergic and serotonergic brainstem systems, is succeeded by one of reduced monoamine transmission, and with this the "pain gate" in the cord opens, flooding the head with previously-inhibited pain, and simultaneously the afferent gate to the special senses is opened, producing the characteristic and intolerable heightening of sights, sounds and smells.

Various vicious circles also come into operation. The convergence in the spinal cord of afferent fibres from the upper three cervical nerves with the descending tract of the trigeminal nerve means that pain can be referred from the neck to the temples, and back again. The trigeminal impulses, additionally, by a neurovascular reflex, still further increase extracranial blood flow. This leads to more pain, and still more vasodilatation, so that the migraine can get trapped in a steadily worsening vicious circle, that self-perpetuation which is so characteristic of attacks (see pp. 160–161). Thus to stop or reduce the pain of a migraine is not merely to alleviate suffering, but to prevent its self-perpetuation *by* pain, through this trigeminovascular reflex.

With this work, we see the identification, in principle, of all the major elements involved in the genesis of a migraine—and we see how they could work, in unison, to produce one. We see too how it might be possible, by interfering with a critical link—that is, with the primary pathogenic process in the brainstem—to prevent a migraine, or to greatly modify its course.

Let us return, now, to the role of neurotransmitters. There are at least half a dozen neurotransmitters involved in the production of a migraine —noradrenaline, acetylcholine, dopamine, histamine, GABA, enkephalins—and 5-hydroxytryptamine, or serotonin. There is evidence that all of these can be influenced by different drugs, and this is why, until very recently, it was often necessary to use three or four drugs simultaneously—to use, for severely affected patients, what Lance calls a "frantic polypharmacy."

The range and safety of this polypharmacy has been much increased since the original publication of *Migraine*, when, basically, there was ergotamine for acute attacks, and methysergide, which, because of its side-effects, one hesitated to use freely.

If patients have one attack a month or less, individual attacks may be treated as they come, but medication to prevent attacks should only be taken by those patients who have two attacks a month or more. Sometimes more than one agent may be used in combination. All of them must be used only with medical supervision.

The best-known and most important new drug is *propanolol*, which was introduced in the 1970s. Propanolol belongs to the newly-developed category of beta-adrenergic agents, which block beta-2 receptors in arterial walls and elsewhere (as well as being a serotonin antagonist). Propanolol is as effective as methysergide for long-term use in the prevention of migraines—and notably safer. Besides its effects in preventing the incontinent dilatation of the extracranial arteries which occurs in migraine, it has a number of general autonomic effects (on blood pressure, cardiac rate and rhythm, etc.). These, indeed, may be therapeutic, and propanolol is especially useful for the hypertensive migraineur, although it should be avoided if there is any tendency to hypotension, or bronchospasm.

Alpha-adrenergic agents, like *clonidine*, were also introduced in the 1970s—clonidine is now widely used as an antimigraine drug in Britain, but has not been well-received in the United States. An occasional patient, however, may do very well on it.

Safer than propanolol, but (by the same token) milder and less effective, is *pizotifen*, which certainly reduces the severity and frequency of migraines in most patients, though not as powerfully as either propanolol or methysergide. Pizotifen blocks the vasodilator action of histamine, and has somewhat complex action on the vascular effects of serotonin.

Among other new agents, with definite effectiveness in reducing the frequency of migraine attacks, as well as the severity of individual attacks, is the class of non-steroidal anti-inflammatory drugs (NSAIDs): *naproxen, tolfenamic acid* and *mefenemic acid* are probably the most effective of these. It should perhaps be mentioned here that *aspirin* has been finding a new use as a preventive agent against migraine; it reduces platelet aggregation and prostaglandin synthesis (both of which may be subsidiary mechanisms in the pathogenesis of migraines). The NSAIDs and aspirin, if they are tolerated (they may have troublesome gastric and other effects) have a distinct place in the prophylaxis of migraine.

The herb *feverfew* has become a cult remedy for the prevention of migraine—it is not clear, as yet, whether it has better than placebo effects (but see Johnson et al., 1985).

Another wholly new category of drug is the calcium channel blocker, which can have a variety of important autonomic effects. These drugs can prevent migraine (as well as peripheral vasospasm and angina); *verapamil* is usually considered one of the most effective of these.

An unexpected resource in the last twenty years has been the use of various antidepressants, although the antimigraine effect of these is apparently quite independent of their antidepressant effects. Among the tricyclic antidepressants, *amitryptaline* is the most potent—it appears to block the reuptake of serotonin at central synapses. Amitryptaline has the same physiological effects as all the tricyclics, and should be used cautiously, if at all, if there is any history of seizures, of cardiovascular symptoms, of narrow-angle glaucoma, or of urinary retention.

Another and very potent category of antidepressants—the mono-amine oxidase (MAO) inhibitors—may be highly effective for migraine prevention in otherwise resistant patients; *phenelzine* is especially used here. But there are major hazards associated with the use of MAO inhibitors, and the strictest precautions must be observed, in view of the reactions between these agents and various foodstuffs (and drugs) which may cause dangerous (even fatal) hypertensive crises. Patients must meticulously avoid cheese, meat extracts, red wines, broad beans, pickled herrings, chicken livers, etc. (as well as opiates, amphetamines, tranquillisers, sedatives, nasal decongestants, bronchodilators, etc.). The MAO inhibitors should not be taken concurrently with any of the tricyclic antidepressants. Given these precautions, however, MAO inhibitors can be taken safely for years.

In general, of course, one would begin with the mildest (and safest) of these medications, and only if these are not effective proceed to those which are most potent (but, by the same token, requiring more precautions). Lance, for example, may start patients on pizotifen, and if there is no improvement after a month, move to propanolol; if this fails, to methysergide; if all of these fail, to phenelzine; and if this too fails, as a last measure, he may try intravenous procaine or lignocaine. Another physician might do things very differently, and have a preference for calcium blockers, clonidine, or amitryptaline. A third may have yet another favourite regime. There are many paths here, and no single one is best; each individual doctor, each individual patient, will discover what is best for them.

This list could be greatly extended. What remains remarkable is the unpredictability of response, as was observed by Gowers a century ago (". . . the measures that do good in one case will fail in another, apparently quite similar"). This means that one cannot treat patients by rote; that there is no scheme or formula which fits every patient; that there must be, for those who have several attacks a month, a patient and painstaking trial of every drug and every drug combination available, in the hope of finding something which suits that individual.

Might there, however, at least in principle, be something beyond this —a pharmacological way of altering the first, critical link? Might there be an "ideal" migraine drug? If so, what sort of drug might it be?

Attention has been drawn, since the 1950s, to the role of the brain's serotonergic systems in migraine. The data were at first very confusing—migraine seemed to reflect a serotonin *deficiency*, and yet to be helped by methysergide, a serotonin *antagonist*. This paradox was solved by the discovery of different families of serotonergic receptors (known in the trade as 5-HT_1, 5-HT_2 and 5-HT_3 receptors), which themselves had antagonistic but reciprocally-linked roles. Methysergide, and indeed all drugs hitherto used for migraine, are "dirty"—dirty in the sense that their actions are not specific, that they affect several systems. Methysergide, it was found in the 1980s, is a powerful blocker of 5-HT_2 receptors, which are antagonistic in function to the 5-HT_1 receptors. Was there then some way of stimulating these 5-HT_1 receptors, of finding a "pure" serotonin antagonist which would activate *just* these? This quest—very different from the sort of empirical, "shotgun" drug trials of earlier times—finally led, in the late 1980s, to the synthesis of an agent called sumatriptan. The first, highly-successful trials of this new drug were reported in late 1988.

5-HT_1 receptors are especially distributed in the carotid circulation, but the action of sumatriptan appears very specific, constricting only the microcirculation, and the peculiar arteriovenous channels which are so plentiful and important in the carotid circulation. (It was precisely the opening of such channels, Heyck hypothesised in 1969, that led to the shunting of blood away from the cerebral cortex in a migraine.) But Lance has shown that sumatriptan not only affects the microcirculation in this way, but also has a direct effect on the raphe nuclei. Thus if it is dropped directly on to the cells of the nucleus raphe magnus, it strongly inhibits the firing of these cells—it turns them, and their pathological reactivity, off.

There is always a temptation, and always a danger, in the beguiling notion of "wonder" drugs. I speak of this at the start of the last chapter of this book (and it is a central theme in another book, *Awakenings*, 1973). In this chapter, originally drafted in early 1967, I wrote:

> Readers who have opened the book at this point . . . may be assured that there have never been any wonder-drugs for migraine, and never will be . . . The specific treatment of migraine, like that of epilepsy or Parkinsonism, is a matter of trial and choice from among a considerable number of drugs which act on specific mechanisms in the nervous system, allied to symptomatic treatment, to the use of accessory drugs.

The month after I wrote this, a new drug, L-DOPA, was announced for the treatment of Parkinsonism—an agent so dramatic and fundamental in its effects as to transform, from this time on, the life of Parkinsonian patients. I had to eat my words, in relation to Parkinsonism; will I have to eat them, too, for migraine?

I was confident, when I first wrote *Migraine*, that no such drug could be found:

> There may be as many ways of concocting a migraine as of cooking an omelette. If one particular intermediate link, one mechanism, is eliminated, the whole system can be reorganised . . . Excise one temporal artery, one end-organ, and another one will be pressed into use; endeavour to block attacks with, say, a serotonin-inhibitor, and attacks are likely to recur utilising a different intermediate mechanism.

I think now that I made an error in seeing migraines as having a complex "plastic" structure analogous to that of motor tasks or actions (as suggested on pp. 218–219). Whatever the strategic use of migraines—and I continue to think that, on occasion, this may be of great importance in some patients—we can scarcely speak of a migraine having a *tactic*; a migraine has a mechanism, but a mechanism which can be understood, and, in principle, greatly modified.

We have, in the last twenty years, been closing in on the final common pathway of migraine, an abnormal firing of neurons in brainstem nuclei on the basis of some intrinsic (but probably chemical) excess of sensitivity. If this is indeed the final common pathway (if migraine *has* a final common pathway)—despite the immense range and variety of its phenomena and triggers—we may finally be in sight of drugs sufficiently specific for us to renounce the "frantic polypharmacy" which has characterised its treatment for decades, and to offer our patients a potent and harmless specific agent.

I wonder, in my conclusions to the original edition, whether I was not "unduly pessimistic" with regard to the treatment of migraine. The advances of the last twenty years have made me less pessimistic, but a certain cautious scepticism remains: I will not believe in a breakthrough, a wonder drug, a specific, until I see its effect with my own eyes.

The highly "chemical" orientation of the 1960s was succeeded, in the following decades, by a swing to other forms of medicine—to holistic notions of stress reduction, relaxation, meditation, yoga; and to notions of self-help using the will or the mind, aided by the newly-developed techniques of biofeedback. "One cannot will," writes Nietzsche, "one can only will *something*." The essence of biofeedback was to make some normally-invisible "something," some normally-invisible physiological parameter, strongly visible and present to consciousness, so that the will could apprehend, and hopefully change it. A very early use of biofeedback was with regard to the visualisation of brain waves for epileptic patients—which was, and is, highly successful for many. Can one apply similar techniques to migraineurs? What parameters in them can be brought under voluntary control?

The most obvious correlate of migraine headache is the pulsation of the frontal branches of superficial temporal arteries, and such pulsations are easily measured and shown on a monitor. Vascular headache is usually accompanied by some degree of tension headache, and it is easy to monitor the tension of scalp and neck muscles using electromyography. It is easy too to measure skin temperatures in migraine—either of the face and temples or of the hands (the notion of monitoring the temperature of the hands, which seems strange, arose from the self-observation of many migraine patients that their hands became cool in an attack, but warm again as it subsided).

Using such feedback devices (pulsometers, thermometers, electromyography, etc.) the patient concentrates on what is being presented to him, and tries to change it, by force of will. Thus one may learn to diminish the pulsations of one's own temporal arteries—this can have a dramatic effect in reducing a migraine headache, and, with its reduction, many other migrainous symptoms which are dependent on the intensity of the pain. One can learn to raise the skin temperature of one's hands voluntarily, and by this achieve, through a reflex, a restoration of tone to the dilated migrainous arteries.

That one may learn to intervene, in this way, and modify one's own erring or aberrant responses, is now well established. Whether such methods will constitute a widely useful, major and revolutionary mode of therapy—as its proponents sometimes claim—is still unclear.

In some instances, biofeedback may be crucially effective. One patient wrote to me that she was wholly refractory to all medications—like Willis's patient (p. 304), "deaf to the charms of every Medicine." This woman, tormented by constant common migraines, often wondered if life could be borne, until, dubiously, she tried biofeedback, and has since found herself virtually free of her migraines. But equally, I know of some patients who have had little or no success with biofeedback, and other patients—a majority—who have had a limited success. Here then, as with drugs, there is great individual variation: it is difficult to predict, but it is always worth trying, and most migraine clinics are now equipped with biofeedback equipment.

The question arises, with some of these undoubtedly effective feed-back techniques, as to what exactly is going on—whether one is wholly focused on a specific parameter like skin temperature or pulse volume, or whether one is achieving, assisted by a feedback device, some general relaxation, with a reduction of all excessive somatic and psychic excitations.

Stress and psychosomatic disorders have become more common in our lives, and the need for reducing stress, for relaxation, becomes continually more pressing. Certainly this is so in the self-management of migraine, both with regard to going through an acute attack and, not less, in the prevention of attacks. Two techniques which became popular in the 1970s were yoga and transcendental meditation (which is little more than the repetition of a self-hypnotising mantra). Such regimens and meditations are not to everyone's taste, but there is little doubt that they can be helpful with some patients.[58]

Acupuncture has played a traditional role in Chinese medicine for more than 2,000 years, but has only been introduced into Western practice—half-seriously, half-faddishly—in the last twenty years. Some patients improve with this—one uncontrolled study claimed benefit in a third of the migraine patients treated—but it is not clear whether this improvement represents a specific effect of acupuncture, or, like the seeming success of so many other treatments, a placebo effect related to therapeutic attention. We need strictly controlled, double-blind studies; but this is not easy when what is to be tested is a needling and not a drug. There is evidence that acupuncture can have physiological effects, in regard, particularly, to the endogenous opiate systems of the body—and perhaps it may play some useful role in migraine. Lance's experience has been that while patients may improve while undergoing treatment, they relapse shortly thereafter; this, of course, could go equally with a specific or a placebo effect.

Finally, we return to the afflicted individual, the *person* who has migraine. There is indeed a mechanism, perhaps several migraine mechanisms, but the mechanisms are embodied in a life, in a person. Migraines are clearly physiological events, but they become (how can they not?) historical events too, part of the intricate texture of a lived life, of that

---

[58] I once had occasion to observe the immediate and total termination of a Tourettic "fit"—with violent tics, barking, cries, and jerks—by self-induced hypnosis (in the form of TM). I would not have thought such an effect physiologically possible, and have had more respect, since, for the powers of such techniques.

lifelong pattern (as Dr. Gooddy puts it) of "ever-changing features and factors which the patient with migraine both suffers and creates." We may abstract particular attacks, particular mechanisms, but they are parts of this migrainous space-time continuum.

The first problem, the purely medical problem, is clarifying the phenomena, making a diagnosis, understanding what is happening—understanding, for example, that a migraine aura is *not* a stroke (a thought which occurs to many people experiencing one for the first time), and, equally, that it is not a "somatization" or a hysteria (the burden of so much accusation and self-accusing), but a real and morally neutral event, which is organic, indeed, but essentially benign. A simplistic medical approach, having clarified this—and this may, in itself, be an enormous reassurance to the patient—will go on from here to prescribe medication.

But a migraine patient is not just complaining of a recurrent dysfunction—he is telling us, if we will listen, the story of his life, of patterns of living, and patterns of reacting, and (perhaps) deep patterns of which he has no conscious awareness, any or all of which may be relevant to his migraines. We cannot know in advance, on first meeting him, what is relevant or irrelevant. It is crucial to enquire minutely into all the circumstances of attacks—when they are most common, when they are rarest, what are their patterns and provocative triggers. But at a deeper level, one needs to know the "economy" of a life, the psychological and physiological "needs" of an individual. And this is not something which can be ascertained in a quick or casual way—it requires a relation between patient and doctor, and an insight, on the sufferer's part, not to be achieved in a moment, as to the connections between his patterns of life and his migraines. It requires, to some extent, making the unconscious conscious or, in Freud's words, replacing an "It" with an "I."

Thus, with patient 18 (p. 42)—one of the first patients I saw, and a patient I saw at a time when I thought purely in physiological terms—there was a singular "replacement" of migraines by asthma. At this point we had a strange conversation: "Do you think," said the patient, "that I *need* to be ill on Sundays, that I *need* to have migraines, asthma, whatever?" I found this a startling question—I had not thought in such terms, although I had observed, as had he, that when his migraines were treated, he became "bored" on Sundays, and felt he had "nothing to do." At this point, then, the "treatment," and the dialogue and the relationship between us, became somewhat different—questions of economy and of need became central, in place of the earlier accent on the purely physiological. With further and searching discussion of the question he had raised—the putative "need" for illness in his life, the putative role his Sunday migraines might be playing—his migraines (and asthma) entirely disappeared, and this without any further use of drugs. He became able to *enjoy* Sundays, and lost the need to be ill.

"Economic" considerations were also forced on my attention by another patient, the migrainous mathematician (patient 68, p. 29), who was also among the first I saw. With this patient, to continue the history, it was easy to find effective antimigraine drugs. Ergot worked, and worked very well; but when I cured him of his migraines, I cured him of his mathematics too—he seemed, however paradoxically, to need one for the other. At this point, he said, "I'll keep my migraines—I think we better keep everything as it is." This experience also served to reduce my own impatient need to "treat," and disposed me to listen more carefully to patients, to that whole pattern of "ever-changing features and factors which the migraine patient both suffers and creates."

Such considerations do not arise, or arise less, when migraine is occasional—when attacks come, for example, once a month or less. But if migraine is severe, if it intrudes more into life, then complex interactions are bound to occur, and treatment should not be "purely physiological." One would not, of course, deny physiological treatment—one would seek out whatever drugs, or other measures, to help the patient. But, at the same time, one should search more deeply, both patient and physician should search more deeply; for migraine, when frequent, is not just a disease, but a whole way of being, which forces the organism into special adaptations and identities.

One sees this frequently in patients with lifelong epilepsy, who suddenly find themselves, through development of new medication, "bereft" of seizures. Having been "an epileptic" for so many years, they cannot instantly lose the special adaptations they have made; they may still retain, despite the absence of seizures, an "epileptic identity."[59] It was precisely this—or something akin to this—a "migraine identity"—which my "Sunday migraine" patient had to become conscious of, to work through, and renounce.

It is, paradoxically, not so easy to be well—it is easier in some ways to have a limited life, to be ill. With frequent migraines, with all-intrusive

---

[59] In "Witty Ticcy Ray" (*The Man Who Mistook His Wife for a Hat*, 1985), I relate my attempts to treat a young man who had had Tourette's syndrome since early childhood. It was necessary for him to relinquish his lifelong "Tourettic identity," to face the challenge of being Tourette-free and well, *before* he could react properly to specific medications.

symptoms, one adapts, one learns, in a paradoxical way, to be ill. As new drugs and other new measures are developed, as the physiological affliction begins to retreat, one needs to convalesce, to have an interim period to recover—one has, now, to *learn* to be well. Only with this, and gradually, with insight and care, is the shadow of the once all-pervasive illness finally left behind, and the possibilities of full recovery open before one.

PART V

Migraine as a Universal

SEVENTEEN

Migraine Aura and Hallucinatory Constants

with Ralph M. Siegel, Ph.D. [*]

What *are* these Geometrical Spectra? and how, and in what
department of the bodily or mental economy do they
originate?

—Herschel, *On Sensorial Vision* (1858)

INTRODUCTION

The visual disturbances of migraine are common—they affect at least
10 per cent of the population—and often startling, and as such they have
attracted attention and curiosity since antiquity. Thus Aretaeus, in the
second century, observed that attacks might be accompanied or preceded
by "flashes of purple or black colours before the sight, or all mixed
together, so as to exhibit the appearance of a rainbow expanded in the
heavens."

Detailed descriptions—and, above all, self-descriptions—appeared
by the score in the late eighteenth and nineteenth centuries, provided
both by scientists (George Airy, the Herschels, Arago, Brewster, Wheat-
stone, etc.) and physicians (Hubert Airy, Wollaston, Parry, Fothergill,
etc.). One sometimes feels that every scientist and physician of note, at
this time, actually had migraine, and that all of them vied in trying to
describe and explain it.

Of particular interest are the beautiful descriptions and illustrations
provided by Hubert Airy in 1870, depicting that most characteristic phenomenon, the expanding, scintillating, zigzag arc, which Aretaeus had
compared to a rainbow:

> When it was at its height it seemed like a fortified town with bastions all
> around it, these bastions being coloured most gorgeously. . . . All the interior

[*]Center for Molecular and Behavioral Neuroscience, Rutgers University, Newark,
New Jersey

of the fortification, so to speak, was boiling and rolling around in a most wonderful manner as if it was some thick liquid all alive.

The appearance of these brilliant, luminous "fortifications" as an invariant perception or hallucination in every attack disposed Airy to feel that they constituted a "photograph" of some equally invariant structure in the brain. The younger Herschel, while clearly experiencing the same phenomena ("a pattern in straight-lined angular forms, very much in general aspect like . . . a fortification, with salient and re-entering angles, bastions, and ravelins") was moved, however, to a more complex sort of explanation. The movement of the fortification, he felt, was incompatible with any "possible regularity of structure in the retina or optic nerve." Clearly the fortifications arose at a higher level—in the brain or in the mind. Yet they were quite different from imagination or imagery as normally conceived, ". . . the exercise of calling up representations . . . of persons or scenes," or imagining "faces in casual blots, or . . . pictures in the fire." For representations are personal, whereas Geometrical Spectra (as he liked to call them) are abstract; and imagination (as ordinarily conceived) depends on associations, on memory, whereas Geometrical Spectra seem to arise *de novo*. Do such spectra, such patterns, come from "the mind"? If they do, Herschel argues, they must come from an impersonal and unconscious part of the mind—an elemental, "geometrizing" part of the brain or mind, "working within our own organization [but] distinct from that of our own personality." Perhaps, Herschel concludes, taking the most natural optical model as an analogy, perhaps "there is a kaleidoscopic power in the sensorium to form regular patterns by the symmetrical combination of casual elements." And with the notion of such a permuting, synthesising power his discussion ends.

Thus, where Airy thinks of a fixed *structure*, Herschel thinks in terms of an *activity*, an organising, geometrising mechanism or Intelligence. Migraine hallucinations, for Airy, allowed one to see, quite directly or literally, straight into the structure of the brain, and for Herschel, to see the workings of the mind. Both thought that the phenomena illuminated something fundamental.

TYPES OR LEVELS OF HALLUCINATION

Gowers was fascinated by "Subjective Visual Sensations" (as his 1895 paper was titled), and wrote of them repeatedly throughout his long life. Constrasting the sensory auras of migraine and epilepsy, he stressed that the former consisted, almost exclusively, of "elementary" hallucinations—luminous blobs, stars, fortifications, as well as more complex, variable, geometrical forms; whereas, in epilepsy, there was less tendency to geometrical forms, but a much greater disposition to dramatic hallucinations of complex events and scenes. Most commonly, Gowers felt, the epileptic discharge tended to "ascend," from the lower sensorial centers of the brain to the highest, "ideational" ones, with sensory hallucinations, if they occurred, being rather brief and simple—over in seconds, and a mere prelude to the more complex forms of aura. Thus in one epileptic patient

> first the beating of the heart was felt . . . [then] it seemed to become audible as sound . . . then two lights appeared before the eyes . . . [then] the figure of an old woman in a red cloak, who offered something that had the smell of Tonquin beans; [then consciousness was lost].

Whereas in migraine, the discharge did not tend to ascend in the same way, but tended rather to "lodge" in the lower centers—the primary visual and tactile regions of the sensory cortex. This difference, Gowers thought, might have something to do with the time-course of the discharges—the nimble epileptic aura lasted only a few seconds, whereas the slow excitations of a migraine aura might continue for half an hour, stirring up a much more complex, albeit "elementary," disturbance confined to the lower centers.

Complex, "personal" hallucinations *do* occur, very occasionally, in migraine, either concomitantly with the elementary sensations, or, with the passage of time, reverting to these, as in a case described by Kinnier Wilson:

> . . . a personal friend used at first to see a large room with three tall arched windows and a figure clad in white (its back towards him) seated or standing at a long bare table; for years this was the unvarying aura, but it was gradually replaced by a cruder form (circles and spirals), which, later still, developed once in a while without subsequent headache.

But it is the "cruder" forms of aura that we need to attend to, and which we need now to categorise further for analysis. One may distinguish, usefully, three "levels" of geometrical hallucinosis.

The first is, colloquially, "seeing stars" (phosphenes); the second is the classical expanding spectrum or scotoma, with its edge of fortifications; the third—less described, but no less common—consists of rapidly-changing, intricate geometrical patterns. There is a certain tendency for these three levels to occur in this order, the sequence being launched with phosphenes:

The simplest hallucination takes the form of a dance of brilliant stars, sparks, flashes or simple geometric forms across the visual field. Phosphenes of this type are usually white, but may have brilliant spectral colors. They may number many hundreds, and swarm rapidly across the visual field.

Sometimes there is no more than such a dance of phosphenes, although with some patients this may be more than an aura, may indeed last (along with other signs of extreme visual excitability) throughout the course of the entire attack. Sometimes there may be elaborations of phosphenes, as in a case recorded by Gowers, when the patient would see "a luminous disc, which would ascend, break into a four-leaved object, and then disappear."

Some patients (not all) may proceed from these phosphenes to the second stage—fortifications, or scintillating scotomata, (other patients experience this at once, without any preceding phosphenes). This, as shown in Airy's descriptions and illustrations, starts as a sort of explosion, a blinding light near the fixation point, and then moves outward across the visual field, in the form of a giant crescent or horseshoe. The excitation is very intense—the advancing margin or a scotoma is as bright as a white surface in the noonday sun. Its transit across the visual field takes about twenty minutes, and its rate of scintillation is about ten per second.

Most descriptions of migraine aura confine themselves to these two— the phosphene and the scotoma—but there are other, more complex phenomena that are equally characteristic:

> . . . a form of visual tumult or delirium, in which latticed, faceted and tessellated motifs predominate—images reminiscent of mosaics, honeycombs, Turkish carpets [and so on] . . . or moire patterns. . . . These figments and elementary images tend to be [brilliantly luminous, coloured] . . . highly unstable, and prone to sudden kaleidoscopic transformations.

Polygonal shapes—squares, rhomboids, trapezoids, triangles, hexagons, or more complex shapes, sometimes containing tiny replicas of themselves—may dominate the picture in this third stage. These later elaborations were not at first observed by Herschel, but they became more apparent over the years, as he indicates in a letter to Airy:

> Since I wrote to you I have been very frequently visited with the phenomenon . . . and it has assumed some new features, viz. patches of a kind of coloured chequer work in some of the corners of the fortification forms . . .
> Here is what I find recorded in a memorandum of June 22 ult.—"The fortification pattern twice in my eyes today . . . Also a sort of chequer work

filling in, in rectangular patches, and a carpet-work pattern over the rest of the visual area." (Letter of November 17, 1869, cited in Airy, 1870)

Here lattice and carpet patterns are described in the context of migraine auras, especially as arising, at times, near the active angles of the fortifications.[60] But Herschel is not content with this: he gives us fascinating descriptions of complex geometrical patterns seen by him under "the blessed influence" of chloroform (he had to have some minor surgery), namely, "a kind of dazzle in the eyes, immediately followed by the appearance of a very beautiful and perfectly regular and symmetrical 'Turks-cap' pattern, formed by the mutual intersection of a great number of circles outside of, and tangent to, a central one"; and detailed descriptions of several "spontaneous" attacks, the etiology of which is not made clear:

> In the great majority of instances the pattern presented is that of a lattice work; the larger axes of the rhombs being vertical. Sometimes, however, the larger axes are horizontal. Occasionally at their intersections appears a small, close, and apparently complex piece of pattern work . . . [sometimes] the lattice pattern is replaced by a rectangular one, and within the rectangles occur in some cases a filling in of a smaller lattice pattern, or a sort of lozenge of fillagree work. . . . Occasionally too, but much more rarely, complex and coloured patterns like those of a carpet appear, but not of any carpet remembered or lately seen, and in the two or three instances when this has been the case, the pattern has not remained constant, but has kept changing from instant to instant, hardly giving time to apprehend its symmetry and regularity before being replaced by another; the other, however, not being a sudden transition to something totally different, but rather a variation of the former.

A contemporary description is provided by Klee (1968):

> Case 10 reported that she saw red and green triangles which seemed to move towards her, while at the same time they became larger. There was often a shining circle inside the triangles. She might also see hexagonal figures with a shining ring inside, and she also experienced a shimmering of red and yellow which looked like a waving, checked blanket.

[60] Fortifications, Lashley notes, are extremely brilliant—comparable to a white surface reflecting the noonday sun. Chequer-works, lattice-works, filigrees, etc. are much fainter, so may fail to be noticed even if they are present. But with some patients it may be as Herschel describes—that attacks first consist only of phosphenes and fortifications, and only later develop chequer-works and subtler forms. The stereotyped format of medical questioning may also serve to conceal the frequency of the more complex geometric forms. Thus, very recently (March 1992), I elicited startling descriptions of mosaic vision from two people met by chance: both of them, I found, had sought medical help, and had been asked whether they experienced "classical" scotomas, but neither had been asked about the much stranger attacks of mosaic vision they were also subject to. This important symptom, which seemed to them both beautiful and terrifying, had failed to be "elicited" by simplistic medical questioning.

More commonly the polygons come together to form the "meshes" of what patients variously compare to spiderwebs, honeycombs, mosaics, networks, lattices. Such lattices, again, are characteristically mobile —the meshes are apt to change shape (from almost circular to rhomboidal to trapezoidal, whatever) and change scale, in seconds, or fractions of seconds, in a way which seems spontaneous and autonomous, and unaffected by thinking or will.

If the polygonal latticeworks are not too intense, they appear superimposed on whatever the subject is seeing, like a faint, delicate, everchanging web or grid (this is beautifully illustrated in Plates 7A and 7B). If the gridding is very intense, it will actually break up the image into irregular, crystalline, sharp-edged fragments, a bizarre phenomenon sometimes termed "mosaic vision" (Plate 6). When the fragmentation is gross, patients may compare the effect to that of Cubist paintings, and if the fragmentation is very fine, to pointillist paintings. Typically there is movement—a continual changing of scales—and often, simultaneously, an admixture of several scales.

Again, patients may perceive during an aura complex rounded forms of all sorts, like Kinnier Wilson's patient who saw circles and spirals. These too tend to be changeable and unstable, and tend to show rapid modulations of form and size and motion: circles may spin, rotate into spirals, a spiral may deepen into a vortex, a large vortex may break up into little scrolls or eddies. The whole visual field—or half of it—may be taken over by a violent, complex turbulence, sweeping the perceived forms of objects into a sort of topological turmoil; straight edges of objects may be swept into curves, bits of a scene magnified or distorted as if stretched on a rubber sheet. Klee speaks of *metamorphopsia* here— the contours of objects being altered and modulated. "In one patient," he writes, "linear parts of the machine at which she worked apparently bent in waves." (See Plates 5A and 5B.)

Finally, the perceptual world, in such states, seems to run completely amok, everything moving and alive, in a state of gross distortion and perturbation. There may be a sense of winds and waves and eddies and swirls, of space itself—normally neutral, grainless, immobile and invisible—becoming a violent, intrusive, distortive field.[61] Yet, fascinatingly,

---

[61] Thus Airy, in the journal he kept as a schoolboy of fifteen, spoke of the interior of the fortification "boiling and rolling around in a most wonderful manner, as if it was some thick liquid all alive," and in his 1870 paper he adds other images of almost meteorological turbulence he experienced in several attacks. He repeatedly speaks of a slow "rolling,"

such gross, torrential disturbances may be completely confined to one-half of the visual field, the other half remaining calm and imperturbable (Plate 2A and 2B), or confined to a small area, or areas, within the half-field. The luminous arc of a scintillating scotoma, by contrast, though it may be imposed upon, or obscure, part of what one is looking at, or edge an object with iridescent needles, does not distort space, distort the perceptual field, in this sort of way (see Plates 1A and 1B). Distortions only occur with this third level of disturbance.

The instability of these third-level disorders is very remarkable; there are not only rapid modulations, but swift (and seemingly instantaneous) fluctuations: a rotation will suddenly reverse itself, seemingly without any slowing, or "in-between"; one pattern of whorls or lozenges will abruptly, kaleidoscopically, be replaced by another. And yet, after a period, despite the intense and continuing sensory excitation, the turmoil of the aura tends to change to a calmer, more organized, more geometrical whole. Regular scrolls may spread across the field. Complex lattices appear and reappear; sometimes these may be multiple and superimposed, giving rise to complex interference and moire patterns. Higher-order geometrical forms may now appear too. These seem to be elaborations of polygonal networks, and may be compared to cone-shells or sea urchins, or to the complex, "Fullerenic" forms of radiolaria.

Sometimes these networks have an acicular or crystalline appearance, and may grow visibly, sometimes with sudden jerks, "like frost on a windowpane," or "primitive plants." Sometimes there are radially symmetrical forms like flowers or pinecones, continually unfolding in a constant revelation of themselves. Or "maps," "landscapes," pseudogeographies of great complexity, which constantly create themselves before the inward eye, enlarging endlessly in a self-similarity. These "geographic" patterns are never of actual or specific places, but are synthetic or imaginary geographies, so to speak, created by the excited brain. These too fade in time, and everything resumes its normal appearance. The aura is

---

"heaving," or "swaying" of parts of the visual field—quite separate from the rapid "tremor" of the fortifications, and in one almost poetic description he tells us that

> the outskirts of the visual area seem to be boiling over with tumultuous light, that may be seen at times to collect itself in a rallying point here and there [a century later, we might speak, perhaps, of an "attractor" here] and presently to stream away again along the shore of the seething sea, splendid with large gleams of blue and red and green.

over, there may or may not be a headache. But there will have occurred, perhaps, in the space of twenty minutes, such a revelation of bewildering (and perhaps beautiful) complexity as the mind may never be able to forget.

The observing mind usually remains clear in a migraine, even in the stormiest migraine aura. The mind remains able to attend and observe, to describe, to analyze, to depict, to remember. Thus, despite all expectations, we have remarkable paintings of what some of these deep aura states are like, paintings which if they are not exact "photographs" or reproductions, may at least be counted as painstaking reconstructions.[62] And, as will be apparent in the next section, we have not only descriptions, but detailed analyses of analogous phenomena in a variety of other neural states.

HALLUCINATORY CONSTANTS

Geometrical forms very similar to what may be seen in migraine may also occur with various intoxications. This has been very carefully documented in relation to mescal by Kluver (1928) and in relation to cannabis by Ronald K. Siegel (1975, 1977). The closeness of these experiences to those of migraine can be brought out by some of the cases cited by Kluver:

> Immediately before my eyes [stated one subject, after an injection of 0.2 gm. mescaline sulphate] are a vast number of rings, apparently made of extremely fine steel wire, all constantly rotating in the direction of the hands of a clock; these circles are concentrically arranged, the innermost being infinitely small, almost pointlike, the outermost being about a meter and a half in diameter. . . . As I watch, the center seems to recede into the depths of the room, leaving the periphery stationary, till the whole assumes the form of a deep funnel of wire rings. The wires are now flattening into bands or ribbons, with a suggestion of transverse striation. . . . These bands move rhythmically, in a wavy upward direction, suggesting a slow endless process of small mosaics, ascending the wall in single file. The whole picture has suddenly receded, the center much more than the sides, and now in a moment, high above me, is a dome of the most beautiful mosaics. . . . The dome has no discernable pattern. But circles are now developing upon it; the circles are becoming sharp and elongated . . . now they are rhomboids, now oblongs; and now all sorts of curious angles are forming; and mathematical figures are chasing one another wildly across the roof.

[62] The Boehringer-Ingleheim archive contains examples of migraine art, with hundreds of paintings by patients of their own auras. Ninety of these were recently exhibited at the Exploratorium in San Francisco, in an exhibit entitled "Mosaic Art."

Now one of Kluver's personal experiences:

Half an hour after a second dose of mescal buttons. . . . Tail of a pheasant (in center of field) turns into bright yellow star; star into sparks. Moving scintillating screw; "hundreds" of screws. . . . Sparks having the appearance of exploding shells turn into strange flowers . . . Forms in different colors. Gold rain falling vertically . . . rotating jewels revolving around a center. Then, with a certain jerk, absence of all motion. Regular and irregular forms in iridescent colors reminding me of radiolaria, sea urchins and shells, etc. . . . Slow, majestic movements along differently shaped curves simultaneously with "mad" movements. Feeling there is motion *per se* . . .

Proceeding from his own experience, and accounts of mescal intoxication which are singularly similar, despite very different cultural origins and contexts, Kluver extracts certain *universals* of hallucinatory experience, or, as he calls them, "form constants." "One of these form-constants," he writes, "is always referred to by such terms as *grating, lattice, fretwork, filigree, honeycomb* or *chessboard* design. . . . Closely related to [this] is the *cobweb* figure." A second form constant, he continues, "is designated by such terms as *tunnel, funnel, alley, cone*, or *vessel*. A third form constant is the *spiral*." With this, as with other form constants, the hallucination may be experienced by touch as well as by sight, as in the following account cited by Kluver:

. . . a luminous spiral forms itself through the active movement of stripe. This quickly rotating spiral is moving back and forth in the visual field. At the same time . . . one of my legs assumes spiral form. . . . The luminous spiral and the haptic spiral blend psychologically . . . one has the impression of somatic and optic unity.

Similar fusions have been described with lattice hallucinations, which may not only be seen, and not only projected upon the body surface, but may cut it up, or replace it—so that the body itself is felt as a mosaic or lattice. Again Kluver cites a description:

The subject states that he saw fretwork before his eyes, that his arms, hands, and fingers turned into fretwork and that he became identical with the fretwork.

Such simultaneous occurrences of complex hallucinations in both visual and haptic spheres is not uncommon in migraine aura—there were several paintings, in the recent exhibit called "Mosaic Vision" (at San Francisco's Exploratorium), of such lattices becoming somatic as well as visual, being felt as "nets" or "cobwebs" on the body. This shows us, importantly, that these are not just visual phenomena, but *sensory* form constants; or, put most generally, forms of organisation, presumably physiological, which can become apparent to any spatially-extended sense.

Some years after completing *Mescal*, Kluver returned to what he clearly felt was a subject of great importance and wrote a wide-ranging essay on "Mechanisms of Hallucination" in 1942. In this he explores the "geometrisation" expressed in these form constants, a tendency which does not stop with the production of the major patterns (lattice, spiral, etc.) but goes on to a multiplication or reiteration of these, sometimes on a smaller and smaller, even "microscopic" scale:

> The tendency towards geometrization as expressed in these form-constants is also apparent in the following two ways: a) the forms are frequently repeated, combined, or elaborated into ornamental designs and mosaics of various kinds; b) the elements constituting the forms have boundaries consisting of geometric forms.

This "geometrical ornamental structure," as Kluver calls it, may enlarge, in the course of an intoxication or an aura, through many degrees of magnitude, but in doing so endlessly reproduces itself (since it is composed of self-similar structures differing chiefly in scale).

It is this endless geometrisation—this geometrisation to infinity— which Herschel speaks of, with regard to his own Geometrical Spectra; and which Louis Wain, the psychotic artist, illustrates in his "mosaic" cat (Figure 5 C). (And it is this endless geometrisation, and self-similarity, of course, which distinguishes fractal patterns as they are generated.) Such an endlessly geometrised kaleidoscopic form pattern (induced by cannabis) is beautifully illustrated in Siegel and West's 1975 book *Hallucinations* (Figure 10).

Kluver draws attention to the fact that similar hallucinations, similar form constants, may appear in a variety of other conditions: in certain hypnagogic hallucinations, in entoptic phenomena,[63] in insulin hypoglycemia, in fever deliria, in cerebral ischemia, in some epilepsies, and with exposure to rotating or flickering visual stimuli. Nor does he omit mi-

---

[63] Simple geometrical patterns can be elicited by pressure on the eyeballs, and apparently arise within the eye. Such patterns were illustrated by Purkinje almost two centuries ago. It is possible that the retina itself is capable of generating such patterns, and of a limited degree of "self-organisation." But in migraine, as was evident even to Herschel, the patterns originate in the brain, for they have characteristically hemianopic distributions, and other evidences of a "higher" origin. Such patterns may also be seen—and this is also true of the elementary hallucinations induced by cannabis and mescal—in total darkness, or by blind subjects in whom the eyes are enucleated.

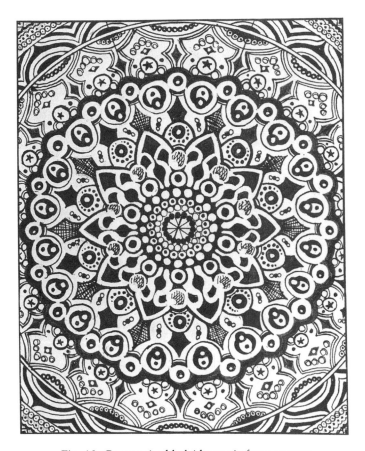

Fig. 10. Geometrised kaleidoscopic form pattern.
(Courtesy Dr. Ronald K. Siegel)

graine. (Kluver's list could be greatly extended: an important "negative" inducement to hallucinations, studied in detail by Hebb, is sensory deprivation, where, characteristically, the deprived brain starts by generating simple hallucinations—"dots, lines, or simple geometric patterns"; goes on to "something like wallpaper patterns"; then to "isolated objects, without background"; and finally to "integrated scenes usually containing dreamlike distortions."[64]

So many etiologies, so many causes, producing the same phenomena;

[64] The generation of such patterns, as well as higher-level images, with sensory deprivation is of particular interest, for it suggests that there is a continual autonomous cortical activity, even at rest, and that this may become exaggerated and pathological, not only with overstimulation of the cortex, but with removal of the normal perceptual constraints.

there must be, Kluver infers, some common path, some "fundamental mechanism" at work, in the sensory cortex. The form constants, despite the most varied origins, must be constants of cortical structure or organisation, must tell us something deep about the functioning of the sensory cortex, and the nature of sensory perception and processing.

Kluver's work, in the twenties, was one of report and review, collecting and analyzing narratives of drug action. The use of mescaline was rare and esoteric in the twenties, whereas the use of cannabis, and the psychedelics, became epidemic in the sixties. It was time for another, and more exacting, analysis—and this was provided, in the early seventies, by Ronald Siegel of UCLA. Siegel's approach was experimental and quantitative, where Kluver's had been more anecdotal and qualitative. Realising almost from the start that his subjects taking cannabis (and dimethyl tryptamine) experienced essentially similar hallucinations to those described by Kluver, Siegel spread his net wider than Kluver, and not only analysed "constants" of form (here using nine categories where Kluver had used four), but constants of movement as well (concentric, rotational, pulsating, etc.). Thus there emerged a clearer picture of the *flow* of hallucinations and perceptual changes in the experience, its dynamic and complex organisation in space and time.

It is important to stress the instability, the fluctuations, made explicit in Siegel's analysis—Kluver's use of the term "form constants," with its purely spatial connotations, gives a misleading impression of stability and invariance in time. This is not a stable, equilibrium state, but a highly unstable, far-from-equilibrium state, which is continually reorganising itself. There is incessant movement at this stage of hallucinosis, not only concentric, rotational, and pulsating—some form of oscillation is almost invariable—but with sudden fluctuations as well, sudden replacements of one pattern or one image by another, which Herschel, a century earlier, had called "kaleidoscopic." These kaleidoscopic changes, Siegel estimates, may occur at the rate of ten per second. Siegel, moreover, extends his analysis to higher levels than Kluver, and concerns himself not only with elementary time-space patterns of hallucinosis, which are abstract, independent of experience, and context-free, but with the formation of *images* in his subjects.

It had been hinted by Kluver—and is hinted too in those rather rare migraine experiences where seeing geometrical patterns goes on to hallucination of scenes and images—that the geometrical patterns might form a "screen" or "matrix" upon which, or within which, true images could arise—often tiny images of people and places *within* the interstices or links of the lattice.[65] This was amply confirmed by Siegel in his studies, and his publications (1975, 1977) contain beautiful illustrations of this happening. Such images, like all images, always have a personal quality, exhibit the particularity of imagination and memory of the individual, and must be constructed at levels higher than primary sensory cortex.

But the higher cannot occur without the lower. One knows that the primary visual cortex, though it cannot generate complex imagery by itself, is none the less a prerequisite for its generation—patients with extensive damage to primary visual areas, or ablation of these, are not only blind, but unable to evoke inner visual images. The course of hallucinations, in intoxications, as in migraine, hinted at the sort of activity, of "preprocessing," which might need to occur in the sensory cortex in order to ready it for more complex imagery. Cortical activity clearly assumed a grossly pathological form in these conditions—it became visible, hallucinatory, unconstrained, autonomous—yet it might cast light on normal mechanisms too: this indeed, is the use of pathology.

MECHANISMS OF HALLUCINATION

The simplest migraine hallucinations, as we have said, are phosphenes— simple, almost structureless, moving lights in the visual field. Phosphenes virtually identical to these are readily elicited by direct electrical stimulation of the visual cortex, either in the primary area (Brodmann area 17) or the surrounding visual association cortex. Such stimulation evoked, in Penfield's studies

> . . . flickering lights, dancing lights, colors, bright lights, stars, wheels, blue, green and red colored discs, fawn and blue lights, colored balls whirling [etc.] . . .

It seems probable, then, that migraines begin with a similar, internally-generated excitation of the visual cortex (and there is direct physiological evidence of this, from electroencephalography and measuring visual evoked potentials of such a stimulation occuring in migraines). But nothing *other* than simple flashes and phosphenes can be elicited by direct stimulation of the primary visual cortex. One never observes more

[65] See Appendix II: Cardan's Visions.

complex forms, or forms evolving over a considerable time. Penfield and Rasmussen themselves remark that "the detailed zigzag outlines of migraine images have not been described to us." And to this Kluver adds that the form constants seen in mescaline intoxication are also not elicitable by occipital-lobe stimulation. Both of these, it is clear, demand another explanation, make us visualize a more complex, longer-lasting, cortical disturbance.

What then is the nature of this peculiar, long-lasting, irradiating cortical process? Gowers wrote, almost a century ago:

> The process is very mysterious. . . . There is a peculiar form of activity which seems to spread, like the ripples in a pond into which a stone is thrown . . . [and] in the regions through which the active ripple waves have passed, a state is left like molecular disturbance of the structures.

Forty years later, Lashley made a minute study of his own migraine scotomata, plotting their contours and enlargement as they traversed the visual field. He observed that the scotoma always remained constant in *form* as it expanded, as if there were some even, uniform, centrifugal process underlying it. The neurological atmosphere at this time was characterised by a passion to localise, to see the brain as a mosaic of innumerable, tiny centers. Lashley, against this, had long thought that there must be other, more global processes at work, capable of integrating large (and perhaps widely separated) areas of the brain. He had speculated at length about this, in an earlier (1931) paper, when he envisaged a wavelike "diffusion" or spread of nerve impulses through a homogenous cellular network, a spread with analogies to that of physical wave motion or chemical diffusion, and, like these, producing characteristic interference patterns of a complex type.

The spread of his own migraine scotomata seemed to Lashley to be an example of such a wavelike excitation propagating across a sheet of cortical matter—a propagation which, in this instance, had a slow and uniform course. By plotting the rate of enlargement of his scotomata, and comparing it with the known dimensions of the striate cortex, Lashley could now calculate that the wave of excitation, from its first appearance near the macula, must then spread out across the cortex at about 3 millimeters per minute.

When Gowers had written, in 1904, about "ripple-waves" in the cerebral pond, this had been no more than a metaphor. And when Lashley had speculated about wave motions in his 1931 paper, he was careful to say that such notions as "mass action" and wave action in the cortex could not but appear "highly metaphoric," but, he added, "Yet the facts demand something of the sort." Now, in 1941, from his own self-observations, he could be more confident that such wave motions did in fact exist—Gowers's "ripple-waves" had become more than a metaphor, they had become a quantitative, measurable fact.

But what of the organization of this wave, its patterns of activation—how were the fortifications to be understood? Lashley observed that when there were fortifications, these maintained their characteristic pattern in each area, being typically finer and less complicated in the upper quadrants, and coarser and more complex in the lower quadrants of the visual field. They did not, he observed, increase in size with increasing size of the scotoma—additional ones were instead added as the activated area grew. The scintillations, he added, "seem to sweep across the figure towards the advancing margin and are constantly renewed at the inner margin, like the illusion of movement of a revolving screw." Their rate of scintillation (about 10 per second), and patterns (of lines and angles) seemed to be the same for everybody who experienced them.

Lashley observed that such repetitive patterns of activity also occurred in other pathological conditions—he cited Kluver's studies of mescal—and seemed, therefore, to represent not just a specific migraine process, but a universal of cortical reaction and activity. Such repetitive patterns, he concluded, "should have been predicted from the free spread of excitation through a uniform neural field (having the structural arrangement of reverberatory circuits described by Lorente de Nó) . . . the patterning represents the type of organisation into which the cortical activity falls as a result of inherent properties of the architectonic structure."

Lashley was heavily criticised, and often dismissed, by his contemporaries, who could not understand his dissatisfaction with the accepted notions of localisation, or his fantastical (as they saw it) invocation of "mass action" and "waves." But the sweep and prescience of his thought is remarkable—we are in a better position to see this than his contemporaries—and it is sad that he did not live to see some of the empirical confirmations and applications of his thought. For, shortly after Lashley's 1941 paper, Leão was able to demonstrate that, following cortical injuries in animals, there might occur a slowly-diffusing "spreading depression" in the cortex with exactly the properties and rate of propagation that Lashley had calculated from his scotomata. And very recently, using new techniques of magneto-encephalography, it has been confirmed that precisely such a slow wave of excitation and inhibition, slowly spreading across the striate cortex, may actually be visualised during the course of migraine auras (Welch, 1990).

Nothing could be said about the architectonic structures which might be organising this excitation until the 1960s, when Hubel and Wiesel were able to demonstrate the existence of a variety of "feature detectors" within the visual cortex—detectors which were, characteristically, organised into small "columns." This allowed a new approach to the problem of the fortifications of migraine, and in 1971, such an approach was made by Richards, using—as had Lashley, Herschel, and Airy before him—his own scotomata as a field for observation.

What is so striking about the fortifications—and this is brought out by every description from Herschel to Lashley—is the *orientation* of their constituent parts ("straight-lined angular forms . . . with salient and re-entering angles, bastions, and ravelins"), and this suggests that the neurons of the cortex being activated either have such orientations themselves (if there is a literal correspondence between cortical patterns and hallucinatory patterns), or are sensitive to different orientations. The latter, of course, is precisely what Hubel and Wiesel were able to demonstrate in 1963. But the dimensions of the columns of Hubel and Wiesel's orientation detectors are 0.2 millimeters, whereas the size of the serrations, Richards calculated, each correspond to about 1 millimeter of cortical distance. Therefore, Richards argues, the advancing wave activates not individual columns, but groups or pools of them responding to the same orientation. Thus (as Lance puts it) a wave of excitation, advancing over the cortex, could throw one group after another into activity, and by causing a direct electrical stimulation of these cause the patient to "see" bars of light at different angles, shimmering as column after column is stimulated. "In this way," writes Richards, "the migraine fortification is an excellent natural experiment: the advancing waves of disturbance draw continuous traces across the cortex and in less than half an hour reveal part of the secret of its neuronal organization."

Writing at the time, in 1970, I felt that the Lashley-Richards theory of the scotoma and fortifications, while (perhaps) needing correction on details, might be adequate in principle to explain these. But no such scheme—of cytoarchitectonic patterns being activated by an excitatory wave—seemed to me applicable to the third, "Kluveresque" level of hallucinosis in migraine: the appearance of tesselations and lattices, continually modulating in scale and form; of curved organising forms, like spirals and cones; and of higher-order geometrical forms, like Turkish carpets and radiolaria, with their proneness to sudden, kaleidoscopic transformations. "It is evident," I wrote in the first edition of *Migraine*, in 1970, "that we must here postulate some form of functional schematisation *above* anatomically fixed cytoarchitectonic patterns." I put forward several theories, including one of perceptual units ("gnostic units") able to vary in size (p. 198), but felt dissatisfied with them all. And indeed, one could not go farther in 1970, could not move beyond the intuition that a radically new principle or theory was required, because the needed empirical and conceptual advances still lay in the future. We stood in need of a deeper understanding of the functional anatomy and physiology of the visual cortex; the development of a mathematical theory for the propagation of complex waves in an excitable medium; and, not least, a way of simulating or modelling larger numbers of interconnected neurons. Perhaps too we needed a radically new way of looking at complex systems and their self-organisation in time—the as-yet scarcely-born science of nonlinear dynamical systems, or (in short) chaos theory.

SELF-ORGANIZING SYSTEMS

The problem one faced was one of *morphogenesis*, the origin and growth of biological forms, albeit forms of a rather simple geometric type. Such a concern, both at this simple level and at much more complex levels, goes back to Aristotle, and was a particular passion of that strange blend of classicist, mathematician and biologist, D'Arcy Thompson, whose *Growth and Form* is one long meditation on the subject. A migraineur, or anyone with personal experience of Kluver's constants, cannot open *Growth and Form*, cannot see its pictures of radiolaria and heliozoa, of starfish and sea urchins, of pinecones and sunflowers, or spirals, lattices, tunnels, and radial symmetries, without a startled cry of recognition.

This was very much in my mind when I originally drafted a Part 5 of Migraine, in 1968, but the purely topological approach used by D'Arcy Thompson, it seemed to me, though it might explain the slow transitions of forms or patterns into one another—for example, of a plane lattice into a curved one (see Plate 7)—could not explain the sudden, global changes, the fluctuations, the kaleidoscopic switches, so characteristic of migraine aura. For this reason I abandoned this Part 5.

A different sort of approach was needed to explain these—and this was not available to D'Arcy Thompson at the time he wrote (nor to me, when I wrote *Migraine*). It was first intimated, perhaps, albeit in a wholly theoretical form, by the mathematician Alan Turing, when, in one of his late papers, he examined the problems of morphogenesis, and how these might be modelled, or initiated, by a wave, such as the waves or patterns of chemical concentrations which he showed might be generated at a critical point in a complex chemical system in a diffusing medium (Turing, 1952).

Such a system was to be discovered a few years later by Belousov, and independently by Zhabotinski, examining complex mixtures of cerium sulphate, malonic acid, and potassium bromate dissolved in sulphuric acid. If these reagents are arranged in a thin layer and unstirred, various geometrical wave forms spontaneously appear and grow—circular waves expanding concentrically from a fixed center, spirals that twist outward, clockwise or anticlockwise, and so on. If the reagents are kept moving and stirred, we see not spatial patterns, but equally remarkable temporal patterns, sudden switches or oscillations, the entire mixture turning blue for a minute, then red, then blue again, with such regularity as to constitute (in Prigogine's words) a chemical clock.

Many other such chemical systems have now been discovered, or devised, capable of generating the most complex geometries in space and time, but all of these with certain basic forms akin to Kluver's hallucinatory constants, or, for that matter, to the elements combined in Herschel's sensorial kaleidoscope. Thus Muller *et al.* (1989) note:

> As complex as the observed chemical patterns may be . . . it is obvious that a certain number of basic structure types can be extracted from them. . . . These are singular points, branching points with frequently triangular geometry, sharp bands, diffuse stripes, circles, patches with a varying degree of regularity, spirals and helices. Dislocations, polygons or targets are already compositions of such elements. . . . Frequently, these are implemented on different spatial scales.

These spontaneous organisations of matter into complex patterns might have seemed, did seem, mere oddities, freaks of nature, until Ilya Prigogine realized the literally cosmic (or cosmogenetic) importance of such systems, and in a single stroke resolved a scientific and philosophical dilemma which had stimulated thinkers since the time of the Greeks.

Aristotle saw the production of organic forms as a consequence of a Purpose, a Design; Democritus as a result of chance juxtaposition of atoms. Idealism and materialism have vied for 2,000 years and more, yet neither, it is clear, can explain Nature (or indeed anything). Herschel, indeed, vacillated between such explanations for his Geometrical Spectra, seeing them either as expression of "a Thought, an Intelligence" or as the result of a purely mechanical Device, the then very popular kaleidoscope of Victorian drawing rooms. Clearly he is satisfied with neither of these teleological explanations—and, indeed, neither will work.[66] An entirely different principle has to be invoked, a principle of emergence or evolution, a principle which does not imply any preexisting pattern or design, but rather a spontaneous emergence of order and form.

This new principle Prigogine called "self-organisation," and he sees it as a universal creative power in nature, creating order, creating complexity, creating "the arrow of time," a spontaneous self-organisation emerging in nature at every level, from the cosmic to the physico-chemical, to the biological, to the cultural. It becomes an entirely new view of nature—or God.

The principle of self-organisation, spontaneously emerging complexity, opens up to us a new and entrancing view of nature—a creative or evolutionary perspective in place of (or to supplement) the "clockwork" and "heat-death" ones. Self-organising systems are indeed the rule in nature, yet paradoxically, these were only "discovered" thirty years ago, and only given a full mathematical analysis with the development of chaos theory years after this. We now see, as Prigogine reminds us, that nature "thinks" in nonintegrable differential equations, "thinks" in terms of chaos and self-organisation, "thinks" in terms of nonlinear dynamical systems. ("The universe," Prigogine says, "is like a giant brain.") Such systems tend to hover far from equilibrium, and it is this far-from-equilibrium position which gives them their sensitivity, their criticality, their capacity to change radically and unpredictably, to generate, to evolve, new structures and forms. Such systems, with their "universal behaviours," as chaologists call them, though so widespread, are hidden for the most part, not seen, not suspected, in the course of our daily lives.

Paul Davies, the cosmologist, writes:

For three centuries science has been dominated by the Newtonian and thermodynamic paradigms, which present the universe either as a sterile machine, or as a state of degeneration and decay. Now there is the new paradigm of

---

[66] As Prigogine says, "The idea of an immanent organising intelligence is thus often opposed to by an organisational model borrowed from the technology of the time (mechanical, heat, cybernetic machines), which immediately elicits the retort: 'Who' built the machine, the automaton that obeys external purpose?"

the creative universe, which recognizes the progressive, innovative character of physical processes. (1988)

If we ask why this new view did not emerge in science before (it has always, in a sense, been obvious to intuition), we will find a partial answer in the *ideal* quality of science, with its use of ideal, simplified models which rarely correspond to the complexity of reality. Classical dynamics is founded on such simplifications—we analyse the movement of a pendulum (while ignoring friction), or the movement of two celestial bodies (while ignoring all others). These simplified or ideal systems lie in eternal equilibrium; there are no perturbations, there is no "arrow of time."

But natural systems, in general, are not closed, but open to the environment—part of the world, with all its vicissitudes. This openness to the environment causes unpredictable fluctuations, and these force the system farther and farther away from equilibrium. Soon there comes a critical point—these are the singular points to which Clerk Maxwell refers (p. 139)—and at this point an abrupt change, a so-called bifurcation occurs, at which the now enormously amplified fluctuation drives the system into a new phase, which may in turn move to a new point of bifurcation. Thus a rapid divergence occurs, with the opening of innumerable alternate pathways. In classical, closed systems fluctuations are rapidly damped and suppressed. In open systems, real systems, the reverse tends to be true, and fluctuation becomes the "go," the "engine," of the whole process. Prigogine calls this phenomenon "order through fluctuations," and he sees it as a fundamental organising principle in nature.

It has not, of course, been Prigogine alone at the helm of these new discoveries, this new wave of thinking. There has, indeed, been an independent occurrence, and yet concurrence, of discoveries in a dozen unrelated fields, and only now do we see how, at the deepest level, these are all related. Thus one complex open system which has always frustrated long-term prediction is the weather. It was imagined, until the early 1960s, that if only one had sufficient information and computing power, one would be able to make accurate long-term predictions. Edward Lorenz showed that this was not the case, because the systems involved behave in a nonlinear fashion, and the partial differential equations representing them do not converge to a single solution, but instead diverge and bifurcate into innumerable alternatives.

This realm has burgeoned into an entire new field—that of chaos theory, or nonlinear dynamics. And chaos theory, we are finding increasingly, provides a fundamental key to understanding complexities and irreversibilities throughout the whole of nature.[67]

Another approach has been that of Benoit Mandelbrot, and his discovery of fractional ("fractal") periodicities and dimensions. In his book, *The Fractal Geometry of Nature*, Mandelbrot provides computer patterns with an uncanny resemblance to clouds, trees, snowflakes, mountain ranges, and so on, an entire world of "natural" landscapes, varying in scale from the geologic to the microscopic. It is characteristic of natural forms that they exist simultaneously on many scales and preserve their forms, and are isomorphic, whatever the scale. Thus the famous "Mandelbrot set," when it is magnified or analysed on a computer, yields an endless succession of self-similar patterns, all of which, so to speak, were in it from the start. It is similar with the "geometrical-ornamental structures" of which Kluver speaks, which have a potentially infinite succession of self-similarities on finer and finer scales. Such phenomena are unintelligible given the conventional view of a "normal" Euclidian world, but appear perfectly natural, indeed inevitable, given the idea of fractional dimensions or fractals.

Thus a new revolution has been afoot in the last twenty years, bringing together the concepts and discoveries of many fields and disciplines, until now, in Feigenbaum's phrase, we start to see "universal behaviours" at work, at every level from the cosmic to the neural (Feigenbaum, 1980). The enormous complexity of these universal behaviours is a rebuttal to those who feel that reality must be "simple"—and these universal behaviours have required, for their formal illustration or solution, the development not only of new branches of mathematics, but supercomputers of enormous power.

A NEW MODEL OF MIGRAINE AURA

These exciting developments have led us to re-examine the previously intractable problem of the complex, evolving forms of the aura, and of hallucinatory form constants in general, in a way which was not possible

[67] Mitchell Feigenbaum and others have been leading theorists here, Feigenbaum being especially pre-eminent for his discovery of so-called "period-doubling" bifurcations. This refers to the changing of frequencies of the system by exact multiples of two, as some parameter is altered. What is critical is that the bifurcations occur in a precise geometrical sequence (the "Feigenbaum sequence"), which cannot be predicted from the basic description of the system. Such period doublings are seen in a surprisingly large number of natural systems, from dripping faucets to cardiac rhythms to the chaotic motions of Pluto's orbit.

when this book was first written. Equally important has been the new power of simulation—namely, designing model networks of neurons, endowed with at least some of the properties of real cortex, and visualising with a supercomputer their behaviour when stimulated, to see whether, if driven to critical, far-from-equilibrium conditions, they actually generate spatial and temporal patterns similar to those of the aura. This we are currently attempting to do.

It is in the nature of models to simplify; we cannot give our model what the cortex itself has—a hundred million cells, twenty cell types, six layers, an infinity of connections both intrinsic and extrinsic. But we can simulate some realities, above all, that of time (Siegel, 1991). The neurons of the cortex have action potentials which result from the movement of ions in and out of the cell in a complicated, time-dependent manner. Indeed, these action potentials are the very basis of neural function—they are the sole means of communication between neurons. Action potentials do not propagate instantly through a network, but take time to propagate through the axon and across the synapse. This time factor cannot be ignored: migraine auras occur in time, evolve in time, develop in time; they do not consist of time-independent spatial patterns. Thus our model, though it consists of only 400 "neurons" (disposed in a 20 by 20 square array), and only a single (excitatory) "cell type," is nevertheless endowed with these time-related properties which physiology shows to be crucial: action potentials, propagation delays (i.e., the time needed for an action potential to go from one neuron to the next), and synapses, which make for a "functional anatomy," a connectivity, resembling that of actual cortex. All of these parameters can be separately varied, as well, of course, as the stimulus itself.

When this network is analysed on a small supercomputer, we may see three quite different sorts of behaviour, depending on the parameters used. A single focussed stimulus can cause waves to propagate away from the stimulus point, until (with the all-or-none quality of action potentials) they suddenly collapse, cease to exist. Such waves, in their initiation, we may regard as analogous to phosphenes, and in their subsequent spread outward across the nerve net as analogous to the symmetrically spreading cortical waves which underlie the uniform enlargement of scotomata. It should be emphasised that such waves, in our model, are created by the excitation and propagation of action potentials; they are not purely physical diffusions or radiations.

With different parameters, the primary wave of activity may provoke the production of secondary and tertiary waves—each excited neuron, potentially, can be a source for such subsidiary waves—and these secondary and tertiary waves can then collide in constructive and destructive interference, apparently in a random fashion, to produce a seething mass of excitation. This may be regarded as analogous to the violent disorder and turmoil we may see in the earlier, turbulent phases of the third stage, prior to its self-organisation into lattices and other forms.

With yet different parameters, an entirely new and remarkable phenomenon occurs: the emergence and evolution, quite spontaneously, of complex geometrical patterns in space and time. Some of these geometric patterns are relatively simple, corresponding to the lattices, radial forms, and spirals seen in migraines; others are more complex, and hint at the more elaborate "ornamental" forms described by Kluver.

The three distinct and distinctive behaviours our net shows can be elicited by varying a single parameter—for instance, the strength of synaptic connectivity. But the patterns are not only dependent on synaptic strength; they can, equally, be found with variations in the propagation delay. It seems as if the system itself has only a certain range of behaviours, and that these behaviours are "universals" of the system, the result of a spontaneous "self-organisation" in the network. It is as if a field, a whole field of neurons, is being excited here, which organises itself and behaves as a coherent whole; as if such a field, once excited, embarks on a free course of its own, a course determined only by its global properties and connectivity. It is our hypothesis that the neurons of the primary visual cortex too form just such a "field"—a "field" in Lashley's sense—in which complex neuronal events and integrations are determined less by local considerations of microanatomy and nuclei and columns and centers than by global considerations of wave actions and interactions in an alive, spontaneously active, enormously complex neuronal medium.

Such global, field paradigms have been exceedingly useful in understanding cardiac rhythms, the electrical "complexion" of the heart, and its geometries in space and time and, most especially, the pathology of such activations, when the normal patterns of self-organisation and chaos can become hugely amplified and destructive. One would certainly expect them to be no less useful in understanding cerebral activity, the more so as so many of the "classical" mechanisms show themselves limited, and indeed bankrupt, when we try to come to grips with complex, evolving, or rapidly changing patterns of activity. This limitation is very evident at "higher" levels; but it is evident also at the level of primary visual cortex, where the elementary Geometrical Spectres of migraine, and other conditions, are generated and evolve.

Similar thoughts were inspired in Ermentrout and Cowan, who were already working on the visual system, when they became acquainted with Kluver's work on hallucinatory form constants—indeed, they dedicate their 1979 work to him. Ermentrout and Cowan also wondered whether an analysis of wave propagation in the primary visual cortex could explain the form constants seen in migraine and other conditions. The model they used was not too realistic—wave propagation was instantaneous, there was no consideration of time—and yet, when they came to analyse their equations with the mathematics of group- and bifurcation theory, they too found solutions of these in doubly periodic stationary states, as spatial "rolls" and "grids" which, if projected on the retina, would be perceived as the form constants which Kluver describes.[68] There is thus a convergence between their results and ours, between the results of a formal mathematical analysis and an actual computer simulation.

It is possible, of course, that this is a mere coincidence—that we are generating geometrical patterns of a "cortical" type in a way which has nothing to do with the actual functioning of the cortex, imitating the brain but not truly modelling it. But that the brain should fail to avail itself of so simple and natural a mechanism—a mechanism, indeed, of a sort universal throughout nature—and employ instead some other necessarily more complicated and cumbersome mechanism (for producing the same result) seems improbable.

And so we come full circle, almost a century and a half after Herschel,

[68] It had been proposed earlier, by Cowan and others, that there was a "conformal" projection of the visual field onto the cortex, that is, a formal mapping of its circular structure onto the rectilinear structure of the cortex. The conformal mapping is, in essence, a stretching and bending of the visual world. Such a projection meant that straight wavefronts in the cortex could be perceived, or hallucinated, as curved structures in the visual field.

Conformal projection showed that the four form constants of Kluver corresponded with simple bands of excitation on the cortex. Given this, Kluver's circular, spiral, and radial form constants become simple rectangles, or "rolls," while the lattice and web constants become rectangular "grids" in the cortex. Ermentrout and Cowan's analysis generated such grids and rolls, and we have seen similar grids and rolls in our own simulations. But we have also seen lattices, spirals, tunnel-like forms as such (see Plate 8). One must hope that advances in brain imaging—perhaps especially in PET scanning and SQUID (magneto-encephalography), conducted during migraine auras—will be able to demonstrate the presence of such forms as electromagnetic patterns at the same moment as patients see them internally. Such imaging would provide an objective "photograph" of migraine processes, where hallucinations can only provide a subjective one.

brooding on his Geometrical Spectra, wondered whether there was not "a kaleidoscopic power in the sensorium." Now, at the close of the twentieth century, we can mimic the sensorial kaleidoscope by letting a self-organising neural network create its own patterns; we can picture a spontaneous and dynamic "kaleidoscopy" in the brain. Our model net—and the brain itself—creates these geometries out of energy and time. Sherrington spoke of the brain as "an enchanted loom," weaving ever-changing, dissolving, but always meaningful patterns. But he was speaking of thoughts and images, whereas we are concerned here with something at once more elementary and elemental—the creation, the play, or pure patterns, pure forms.

It must not be imagined that such self-organising activity, the complex patterns of order and chaos, occur only in pathological conditions. There is increasing evidence to show that chaotic and self-organising processes occur normally in the cortex, and that they are, indeed, a prerequisite for sensory processing and perception, as well as being constrained by these too. One of the clearest signs of this is their emergence in grossly exaggerated form if there is no sensory input to constrain them (see p. 283). But the processes of chaos and self-organisation in the cortex are normally local, microscopic, and, as such, invisible—it is only in pathological conditions that they cohere, synchronise, become global, become visible, take over, and thrust themselves as patterned hallucinations into awareness. Our own model was designed to show normal activity, the normal processes of self-organisation, and it was only when we altered certain parameters that these became pathological—that, so to speak, our model had a migraine.

Our view of Nature has changed in the last twenty years—we have come to recognize nonlinear dynamical processes, chaotic and self-organising processes, in a vast range of natural systems, and to realize that these play an essential part in the evolution of the universe. But we do not need to go far afield for examples—to the aggregation of slime-fungi or the motions of Pluto—we have a natural laboratory, a microcosm, in our own heads. It is in this sense, finally, that migraine is enthralling; for it shows us, in the form of a hallucinatory display, not only an elemental activity of the cerebral cortex, but an entire self-organising system, a universal behaviour, at work. It shows us not only the secrets of neuronal organisation, but the creative heart of Nature itself.

The Visions of Hildegard

The religious literature of all ages is replete with descriptions of "visions," in which sublime and ineffable feelings have been accompanied by the experience of radiant luminosity (William James speaks of "photism" in this context). It is impossible to ascertain, in the vast majority of cases, whether the experience represents a hysterical or psychotic ecstasy, the effects of intoxication, or an epileptic or migrainous manifestation. A unique exception is provided in the case of Hildegard of Bingen (1098 to 1180), a nun and mystic of exceptional intellectual and literary powers, who experienced countless "visions" from earliest childhood to the close of her life, and has left exquisite accounts and figures of these in the two manuscript codices which have come down to us—*Scivias* and *Liber divinorum operum simplicis hominis.*

A careful consideration of these accounts and figures leaves no room for doubt concerning their nature: they were indisputably migrainous, and they illustrate, indeed, many of the varieties of visual aura earlier discussed. Singer (1958), in the course of an extensive essay on Hildegard's visions, selects the following phenomena as most characteristic of them:

> In all a prominent feature is a point or a group of points of light, which shimmer and move, usually in a wave-like manner, and are most often interpreted as stars of flaming eyes [Figure 11B]. In quite a number of cases one light, larger than the rest, exhibits a series of concentric circular figures of wavering form [Figure 11A]; and often definite fortification figures are described, radiating in some cases from a coloured area [Figures 11C and 11D]. Often the lights gave that impression of *working*, boiling or fermenting, described by so many visionaries . . .

Hildegard writes:

> The visions which I saw I beheld neither in sleep, nor in dreams, nor in madness, nor with my carnal eyes, nor with the ears of the flesh, nor in hidden places; but wakeful, alert, and with the eyes of the spirit and the inward ears, I perceived them in open view and according to the will of God.

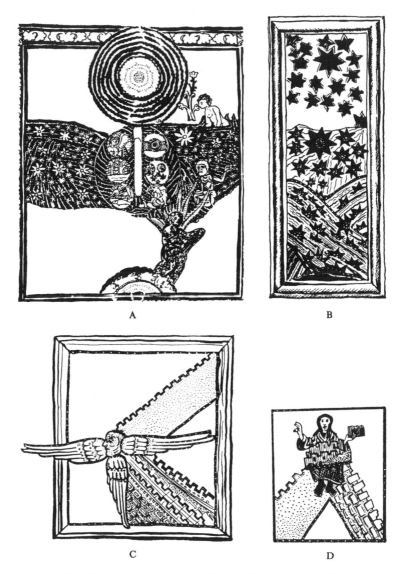

A

B

C

D

Fig. 11.   Varieties of migraine hallucination represented in the
visions of Hildegard

Representations of migrainous visions, from a MS. of Hildegard's *Scivias*, written at Bingen about 1180. In Figure 11A, the background is formed of shimmering stars set upon wavering concentric lines. In Figure 11B a shower of brilliant stars (phosphenes) is extinguished after its passage—the succession of positive and negative scotoma: in Figures 11C and 11D, Hildegard depicts typically migrainous fortification figures radiating from a central point, which, in the original, is brilliantly luminous and coloured (see text).

One such vision, illustrated by a figure of stars falling and being quenched in the ocean (Figure 11B), signifies for her "The Fall of the Angels":

> I saw a great star most splendid and beautiful, and with it an exceeding multitude of falling stars which with the star followed southwards . . . And suddenly they were all annihilated, being turned into black coals . . . and cast into the abyss so that I could see them no more.

Such is Hildegard's allegorical interpretation. Our literal interpretation would be that she experienced a shower of phosphenes in transit across the visual field, their passage being succeeded by a negative scotoma. Visions with fortification-figures are represented in her *Zelus Dei* (Figure 11C) and *Sedens Lucidus* (Figure 11D), the fortifications radiating from a brilliantly luminous and (in the original) shimmering and coloured point. These two visions are combined in a composite vision (Frontispiece), and in this she interprets the fortifications as the *aedificium* of the city of God.

Great rapturous intensity invests the experience of these auras, especially on the rare occasions when a second scotoma follows in the wake of the original scintillation:

> The light which I see is not located, but yet is more brilliant than the sun, nor can I examine its height, length or breadth, and I name it "the cloud of the living light." And as sun, moon, and stars are reflected in water, so the writings, sayings, virtues and works of men shine in it before me . . .
>
> Sometimes I behold within this light another light which I name "the Living Light itself" . . . And when I look upon it every sadness and pain vanishes from my memory, so that I am again as a simple maid and not as an old woman.

Invested with this sense of ecstasy, burning with profound theophorous and philosophical significance, Hildegard's visions were instrumental in directing her towards a life of holiness and mysticism. They provide a unique example of the manner in which a physiological event, banal, hateful, or meaningless to the vast majority of people, can become, in a privileged consciousness, the substrate of a supreme ecstatic inspiration. One must go to Dostoievski, who experienced on occasion ecstatic epileptic auras to which he attached momentous significance, to find an adequate historical parallel.[69]

[69] "There are moments [Dostoievski writes of such auras], and it is only a matter of five or six seconds, when you feel the presence of the eternal harmony . . . a terrible thing is the frightful clearness with which it manifests itself and the rapture with which it fills you. If this state were to last more than five seconds, the soul could not endure it and would have to disappear. During these five seconds I live a whole human existence, and for that I would give my whole life and not think that I was paying too dearly . . ."

Cardan's Visions (1570)

Among the earliest "clinical" autobiographies we have is the fascinating *Book of My Life*, written at the age of 70 by the Italian physician Jeronimo Cardan (Cardano). In Chapter 37 ("On Certain Natural Eccentricities; and Marvels, Among which, Dreams"), Cardan describes the strange visionary attacks which he experienced between the ages of three and six. In these he would see innumerable tiny creatures and scenes, moving in a semicircle, the tiny images set in, or projected upon, a latticework of tiny rings. These visions would be followed by a persistent coldness from the knees down. Though no headache is described, and no clearcut scotoma, they could nonetheless well have been migrainous (see p. 100):

> I used to vision, as it were, divers images of airy nothingness of body. They seemed to consist of very small rings such as compose vests of chain mail— although up to that time I had not yet seen a linked cuirass. These images arose from the lower right-hand corner of the bed, and, moving upward in a semicircle, gently descended on the left and straightaway disappeared. They were images of castles, of houses, of animals, of horses with rider, of plants and trees, of musical instruments, and of theaters; there were images of men of divers costumes and varied dress; images of flute-players, even, with their pipes as it were, ready to play, but no voice or sound was heard. Besides these visions, I beheld soldiers, swarming peoples, fields, and shapes like unto bodies which even to this day I recall with aversion. There were groves, forests, and other phantoms which I no longer remember; at times I could see a veritable chaos of innumerable objects rushing dizzily along *en masse*, without confusion among themselves, yet with terrific speed. These images were, moreover, transparent, but not to such a degree that it was as if they were not, nor yet so dense as to be impenetrable to the eye; rather the tiny rings were opaque and the spaces transparent.

I was not a little delighted with my vision, and gazed so raptly upon these marvels, that my aunt on one occasion questioned me whether I saw aught. And I, though I was still a boy, took counsel with myself: "If I tell, she will be displeased at whatever causes the passage of this proud array, and she will do away with my phantom festival." Even flowers of many a variety, and four-footed creatures, and divers birds appeared in my vision; but in all this exquisitely fashioned pageant there was no color, for the creations were of air. Accordingly I, who neither in youth nor yet in my old age have been given to falsehood, stood still for a long time before I replied.

Thereupon she asked, "What makes you stare so intently?" I no more remember what I replied to her; I think I said, "Nothing."[70]

. . . Following this period of visions, I scarcely ever, until nearly daybreak, had any warmth from my knees down.

---

[70]Complex migrainous hallucinations or "visions" may be particularly terrifying for children—such children may fear (like Cardan) to mention their experiences to anyone, lest they be thought fantastical, or liars, or mad, or worse. Dr. J. C. Steele and his colleagues, working with migrainous children in Toronto, not only established the frequency of such "visions" but were able, in many instances, to persuade these children to paint their aura-visions, or to collaborate with a medical artist in reproducing them (some of these paintings are included in Hachinski et al., 1973). Dr. Steele indicated to me the immense relief which was shown by these "visionary" children when they were able to admit their strange experiences, and especially to depict them, and to encounter a friendly, sympathetic understanding—instead of the tellings-off, the scoldings, that they had previously met.

Remedies Advised by Willis (1672), Heberden (1801) and Gowers (1892)

It is of more than historical interest to observe the remedies of former ages. Below are cited, in part, accounts of treating migraine given in three famous texts: those of Willis (1672), Heberden (1802) and Gowers (1892).

REMEDIES OF EVERY KIND FOR THE CURING THIS HEADACH, TRY'D IN VAIN

For the obtaining a Cure, or rather for a tryal very many Remedies were administered, thorow the whole progress of the Disease, by the most skilful Physicians, both of our own Nation, and the prescriptions of others beyond the Seas, without any success or ease; also great Remedies of every kind and form she tryed, but still in vain. Some years before, she had endured from an ointment of Quicksilver, a long and troublesome salivation, so that she ran the hazard of her life. After twice a Cure was attempted (though in vain) by a Flux at the Mouth, from a Mercurial Powder, which the noted Emperick Charles Hues ordinarily gave: with the like success with the rest she tryed the Baths, and the Spaw-waters almost of every kind and nature: she admitted of frequent blood-letting, and also once the opening of an Artery; she had also made about her several Issues, sometimes in the hinder part of her head, and sometimes in the forepart, and in other parts. She also took the Air of several Counties besides her own native Air, she went into Ireland and into France; there was no kind of Medicines both Cephalicks, Antiscorbuticks, Hysterical, all famous Specificks, which she took not, both from the Learned and the unlearned, from Quacks and old women: and yet notwithstanding she professed, that she had received from no Remedy, or method of Curing, any thing of Cure or Ease, but that the contumacious and rebellious Disease refused to be tamed, being deaf to the charms of every Medicine.

Willis, *De anima brutorum*

In the attempts to cure this malady, evacuations have proved not only useless, but hurtful; and bleeding in particular has been very detrimental. Cataplasms have not been very well borne, and have rather added to the misery of the patients. The Peruvian bark has very often been tried in vain, and so have the root of valerian, the fetid gums, myrrh, musk, camphor, opium, extract of hemlock, sneezing powders, blisters, deep caustics, electrifying, fomentations made of a decoction of hemlock, warm pediluvia, epithems of aether, anodyne balsam, sp. vini, linimentum saponaceum, and oil of amber, opening the temporal artery, and drawing some of the teeth; nor has a supervening fit of the gout made any alteration in this obstinate ailment. But still the bark has now and then succeeded, and not so seldom but that it is advisable to recommend it in the first place: an ounce of it, or not much less, should be given every day for a week. Blisters behind the ears have appeared to abate the violence of the fits; and instances have not been wanting of the good effect of as much extract, cirutae, given daily as could be borne without giddiness. In some cases, where everything else had failed, a draught with one quarter of a grain of tartar emetic and forty drops of tincture of opium, taken at bed-time for six nights, has made a lasting cure.

Heberden, *Capitis Dolores Intermittentes*

The special treatment consists, first, in the continuous administration of drugs during the intervals, with the object of rendering the attacks less frequent and less severe; and secondly, the amelioration of the attacks themselves. As a rule, the measures that do good when employed during the intervals have no influence on the attacks . . . As already mentioned, *the measures that do good in one case will fail in another, apparently quite similar* . . .

. . . The influence of *bromide* in epilepsy naturally leads us to turn first to this as likely to be of service in a malady that has so many features in common with that disease . . . It is most likely to be efficacious in the cases in which there is no change in the colour of the face, or in which the face is flushed throughout the attack. *Ergot* may often, then, be usefully combined with it. In the majority of cases, however, and especially in those in which there is conspicuous pallor in the early stage, the drug that has most influence is *nitroglycerine*. Given regularly during the intervals, just as bromide is given for epilepsy, it has a striking effect in many patients . . . A very useful combination is with tincture of nux vomica, tincture of gelsemium, and dilute phosphoric acid, or with citrate of lithia and the acid syrup of lemons. Sometimes more benefit is derived from the combination of this with bromide . . . I have found such combinations of the liquid preparation of nitroglycerine with other drugs far more useful than the administration of nitroglycerine in tablets. It is not well to continue it during an attack; at the very onset a dose may be taken, but if this is not effective the medicine should be omitted till the attack is over; it seldom gives relief to the symptoms, and occasionally makes them worse . . .

During the attack absolute rest is essential . . . All strong sensory impressions should be avoided . . . Relief is afforded to the pain by a full dose of bromide, and its effect is increased by the addition of five to ten minims of tincture of *Indian Hemp*; this may be repeated every two or three hours . . . Drugs that cause contraction of the arteries are almost powerless; all that a full dose of ergotin does is to lessen the throbbing intensification of the pain complained of by some patients. Strong tea and coffee are popular remedies, and occasionally give some distinct relief, which may also be obtained from a few grains of *caffeine* . . .

Repeated galvanisation of the sympathetic has been recommended as a remedial measure . . . The value of the treatment is, to say the least, seldom perceptible.

Gowers, *A Manual of Diseases of the Nervous System*

Glossary of Case-Histories

		Attacks only at full moon. Lunar migraines sometimes alternate with "lunacy."

39   58   Classical migraines with severe precordial ("pseudo-anginal") pain accompanying headache. Precordial migraines also occurring without a headache component.

39, 167   76   Common migraines and stuporous migraine equivalents in response to conventual restrictions.

39, 46, 47   49   Polymorphous syndrome: post-prandial torpors: common migraine and continuous "latent" vascular headache; paroxysmal nocturnal salivation or diaphoresis; orthostatic hypotension; paroxysmal bowel-colics; narcolepsy and cataplexy.

41   32   Sudden transition from menstrual cramping to severe premenstrual migraine headaches.

47, 66, 86,   75   Migraine auras of many different forms: nightmares and
253   "daymares" (delirious auras) with specific sensory hallucinations, aphasia and sleep-paralysis on occasion: ecstatic aura with Jacksonian paraesthesiae: also many migraine equivalents.

47, 48   64   Polymorphous syndrome: paroxysmal asthma, recurrent peptic ulceration, rheumatoid arthritis, angioneurotic oedema, and common migraines.

48, 171   62   Polymorphous syndrome: common migraine, ulcerative colitis, psoriasis, associated with environmental "trapping" and secondary guilt reactions.

48, 49   61   Polymorphous syndrome in patient and family: common migraine, psoriasis, hayfever, asthma, urticaria, Menière's syndrome, peptic ulcer, ulcerative colitis, Crohn's disease.

48, 49   21   Polymorphous syndrome: classical migraines, nightmares, pre-menstrual syndromes, paroxysmal abdominal syndromes, syncopal attacks, urticaria.

63, 66   67   Classical migraines and isolated auras, with marked analepsis preceding scotomata.

83   72   Classical migraine with delirious aura.

83   19   Classical migraines and isolated auras of unusual complexity with scintillating scotomata, auditory misperceptions, epigastric aura, syncopes, hallucinations and deliria on occasion.

84   11   Classical migraine (aura only in pregnancy). Scintillating scotomata precipitated by flickering light. Feelings of "angor animi" in some auras.

84   16   Classical migraines and isolated auras, latter often accompanied by "forced" thinking and reminiscence, and pleasant affect.

84   65   Severe, infrequent classical migraines, with conspicuous aphasia, and hilarity during aura.

85	69	Classical migraines and isolated auras. Elated prodrome and aura. Higher-order visual misperceptions with scintillating scotomata.
85	70	Classical migraine and isolated auras. Some of the latter characterised by "mosaic vision."
85	14	Classical migraines in adolescence, isolated auras thereafter. Latter may take many different forms; scotomatous, paraesthetic, affective or syncopal.
91	98	Complex "migralepsies" associated with temporal lobe angioma.
94, 151	90	Physician with server negative *scotomata* presenting as gaps or holes in reality.
95	91	Patient with transient "extinction" of left half of visual field, left half of body field,and leftness generally, due to a discharging parieto-occipital lesion.
96	92	Patient with permanent "extinction" of all perception and idea of leftness, due to a sensory "stroke" affecting the right cerebral hemisphere.
101	1	Cluster headache, with attacks of both migrainous neuralgia and common migraine in each cluster.
101	2	Migrainous neuralgia and cluster headache.
101	3	Migrainous neuralgia. Attacks preceded by lacrimation, and "defused" by histamine.
102	5	Classical migraine and cluster headache.
102	6	Common migraine and migrainous neuralgia.
102	7	Cluster headache with prominent prodrome. Permanent partial Horner's syndrome.
102	8	Annual clusters of migrainous neuralgia except during a period of psycho-analysis.
102	9	Migrainous neuralgia: one attack seen to be greatly modulated by state of mind.
104	23	Classical migraines with occasional hemiplegic attacks.
104	25	Classical migraines with protracted facioplegia.
105	24	Infrequent common migraines, with three attacks of ophthalmoplegic migraine at widely-separated intervals, each preceded by a barrage of common migraines
105	73	Classical migraines in childhood, with a single attack of ophthalmoplegic migraine.
105	99	Ophthalmoplegic migraine recurring for 25 years, with persisting deficits.
106	26	"pseudo-migraine," i.e. misdiagnosed attacks termed "classical migraine" in fact resulting from occipital lobe angioma.
107	48	Temporal arteritis misdiagnosed as "migraine."
107	50	"Pseudomigraine" due to occipital-lobe infarction.
128	15	Classical migraine in childhood and old age, with 52-year remission in between.

128	38	Severe common migraines presenting in late middle-age, following administration of hormone preparation.
135	52	Annual "clusters" of common migraine.
138	74	Menstrual migraines continuing to appear at strictly monthly intervals after menopause.
145	54	Common migraines attributable to severe functional hypoglycaemia.
147	43	"Migraine status" and other depressive and parasympathetic symptoms following withdrawal from "Ritalin" addiction.
155	4	Migrainous neuralgia consistently preceded by constipation, and controllable by laxatives.
158	31	Severe menstrual migraines ceasing on administration of contraceptive hormone-preparation.
167	78	Migraines coupled with anxiety concerning husband's health.
167	79	Migraines associated with repressed hostility to overprotected, over-demanding children.
168	80	Very severe ("habitual") migraine associated with hysterical denial of environmental stress.
168	81	Classical migraines "driven" by severe depression, guilt and self-reproach. Exemption from migraines after "accidents" (to which patient was prone), and during periods of melancholia and institutionalisation.
169	56	Remission of habitual migraine during pregnancy, mourning, and illness.
170	82	Repeated severe migraines associated with sado-masochistic relationship between patient and spouse.
170	84	Symptomatic migraines and belching associated with impotent resentment at intolerable working conditions.
170	55	Migraines following sexual intercourse.
171	83	Sunday (Sabbatical) migraines in an obsessive "migraine-personality."

Note: The above case-histories are quoted *in extenso* in the text. Other case-histories are alluded to more briefly, and reference to these must be sought in the Index.

Glossary of Terms

ACETYLCHOLINE   Naturally occurring "neurotransmitter," tending to serve parasympathetic and inhibitory systems, and thus antagonistic to those served by adrenalin and dopamine.

ADRENALIN AND NOR-ADRENALIN   Naturally occurring "neurotransmitters" in the nervous system, especially serving sympathetic and excitatory activity.

AGNOSIA   Inability to perceive through inability of the brain-mind to relate, or integrate, the components of perception. This is neither a paralysis nor a hysterical disorder, but a specific disturbance of higher brain functions.

AMUSIA   An alteration or deprivation in the perception of music—either in the perception of melody, or of tonality (see *Aphasia*).

ANALEPTIC   Exciting the nervous system (*cataleptic*, strictly, would be depressing the nervous system. Tranquilizers and mood-changers are sometimes called *neuroleptics*).

ANESTHESIA   A complete deprivation of sensation and feeling: see also *Paresthesia* which are distortions of sensation and feeling.

ANEURYSM, ANGIOMA   Rare abnormalities of blood vessels, which may, very rarely, cause migrainelike symptoms. An *aneurysm* is a thinned-out, balloonlike swelling. An *angioma* is a tumorlike cluster of abnormal blood vessels. Properly speaking an angioma is a malformation—not a tumor.

ANGIONEUROTIC EDEMA   Swelling of the face and scalp tissues, occasionally the tongue: sometimes allergic, sometimes "nervous," sometimes seen in a migraine.

ANGOR ANIMI   Fear for the soul, sense of imminent dissolution, overwhelming dread and conviction of death. A peculiar and terrible form of fear, perhaps only seen with organic disturbances (migraine, angina, etc.)

APHASIA   Inability, or diminished ability, to understand or use language (the former being a "receptive," the latter an "expressive" aphasia, either of which

311

may occur independently of the other). The "three As"—apraxia-agnosia-aphasia—are not uncommon in migraine aura, at least to a mild degree (see chapter 3).

APRAXIA   Inability to act through inability of the brain-mind to place in relationship, or synthesize, the components of the act. This is neither a paralysis nor a hysterical disorder, but a specific disturbance of higher brain functions.

ATONIA, HYPOTONIA, HYPERTONIA, AND SO ON   Absent, diminished, or increased muscle tone. (Muscle tone is usually increased in the early, tense phases of migraine, and reduced or collapsed in the exhausted, late phases.)

AURA   This term is now used for the many weird and wonderful symptoms which commonly precede the headache of migraine—and frequently replace it altogether. The word *aura* was first used by Pelops, the master of Galen, who was struck by the phenomenon with which many attacks begin. The sensation having been described to him by patients as "a cold vapor," he suggested that it might really be such, passing up the vessels then believed to contain air. Hence he named it "spirituous vapor" in Greek.

AUTOMATISM   A trancelike state in which a person may perform simple habitual actions, or behave repetitively and automatically, without any consciousness or recollection afterward.

AUTONOMIC (VEGETATIVE)   That part of the nervous system, centered in the brain, but spreading into nerves and nerve plexuses all over the body, which regulates the tone and activity of blood vessels, glands, involuntary muscles, and so forth, and which is wholly automatic and unconscious in its functions. It is sometimes called the vegetative nervous system. One may say that it is disturbances of autonomic or vegetative function, above all, which dominate the picture of common migraine. Common migraine is essentially a vegetative disorder (see also *Sympathetic/parasympathetic*).

BORBORYGMI   An onomatopoeic word, referring to noises and spasms in the distended, flatulent gut.

BRADYCARDIA   See *Tachycardia*.

CATAPLEXY   A sudden loss of muscular tone, sometimes brought on by sudden emotion, or migraine: sometimes associated with narcolepsy, sleep paralysis, and the like.

CATARRH   Excessive secretion from the nose (or, indeed, anywhere else: thus older physicians might speak of a bladder catarrh, etc.).

CEPHALALGIA (USUALLY SHORTENED TO CEPHALGIA)   Head pain—nothing more.

 Similar words in the older literature—gastralgia (stomach pain), pectoralgia (chest pain). The only "algia" commonly spoken of now is *neuralgia*.

CHEMOSIS   An inflammation and exudation at the surface of the eye, making it moist and shiny. Chemosis is very frequent in migraine attacks (see page 19).

CHOLECYSTITIS   Inflammation of the gallbladder.

CHOREA (LITERALLY, "DANCE")   An odd, dancing, twitching movement, moving desultorily from one part of the body to another. Most commonly seen in certain diseases (Huntington's chorea, etc.), or in Parkinsonians treated with L-Dopa, it may sometimes occur for a few minutes in a migraine (chapter 3. Complex choreic movements have some resemblance to *tics*.

CONSTITUTION, (PRE)DISPOSITION, DIATHESIS   Archaic but powerful general terms indicating a radical (and perhaps ineradicable) psychophysiological character or *nature*, which makes one peculiarly susceptible to migraine, or whatever else is in question. It is often implied that this character or nature is *innate*, as opposed to something learned or acquired.

CROHN'S DISEASE   Regional inflammation of the small bowel or *ileum*.

"DAYMARE"   A nightmarelike experience occurring while awake, side by side, so to speak, with normal, waking consciousness.

DEPERSONALIZATION, DEREALIZATION, EGO DISSOLUTION   Loss of the sense of one's self, and of one's world, or "reality" (see page 93). Common in schizophrenia, but also acute migraine, and other organic disorders.

DETUMESCENCE   A subsidence, after an engorgement: as with a genital reaction, a rage, a creative furor—or a migraine.

DIAPHORESIS (DIAPHORA)   Sweating, especially excessive sweating.

DIATHESIS   See *Constitution*.

DIURESIS   Excessive production of urine.

DOPAMINE   Allied to adrenalin—a neurotransmitter—especially concerned with "tuning up" levels of neural activity.

DYSRHYTHMIA (SEE *ELECTROENCEPHALOGRAPHY, EEG*)   A special vocabulary has grown up to describe the appearance of the brain waves, as these may be recorded by EEG. Normal brain waves are remarkably rhythmical, and regular, in appearance: a lack of proper rhythm is called a *dysrhythmia*. Excessive excitement—as in an epilepsy, or some migraine auras—may make the waves high, sharp and steep, culminating in the formulation of *spikes*. There are also characteristic changes during sleep, lethargy, inattention, and sometimes migraine.

ECCHYMOSIS   Spontaneous bruising, or suffusion of blood.

EDEMA   Swelling of tissues, an organ, or a limb, and so forth due to abnormal accumulation of body fluids.

EGO-DISSOLUTION   See *Depersonalization*.

ELECTROENCEPHALOGRAPHY (EEG)   Recording cerebral activity (brain waves) through electrodes on the scalp.

ENCEPHALIZATION   The ascent of neural functions to higher and higher levels of the brain.

ENOPHTHALMOS, EXOPHTHALMOS   Sunken-eyedness, or pop-eyedness, respectively. Both may be seen during migraine attacks, and reflect alteration in the tone or tuning of eye nerves.

EPIGASTRIC   Just above the stomach.

ERYTHEMA (OR RUBOR)   Redness.

EXUDATION   See *Transudation*.

FIELD   The way in which the brain maps and organizes sensations conveyed to it from the senses. Most commonly we speak of the *visual* fields. A gap, defect or hiatus in a field is a *scotoma* (see *Scotoma*). Special forms of field defect have other special names, for example, see *Hemianopia*.

FIGMENTS   Half-formed, fragmentary sounds, and sights, below the level of recognizable images. Very characteristic of migraine aura, delirium and other cerebral excitements.

FORCED THINKING   Trains of thought, reminiscence, ideas, feelings, and other occurrences which appear to be forced on one, and which one is compelled to pursue. Common in schizophrenia, but equally common in organic disturbances like migraine, epilepsy, fever, delirium.

FORMICATION   A crawling feeling, as of ants on the skin.

GENETIC, GENES, AND SO ON.   Inheritance (of mental and physical traits, inheritance of constitution, and of particular diatheses, etc.) is considered to be based on one's genetic character; the constellations of hereditary particles, or *genes*, in one's make-up. Such genes, or gene groups, are described as dominant, recessive, of such-and-such penetrance, and so forth depending on their power to determine or predetermine traits.

HEBETUDE   A *dullness* of sensation, emotion, and other feelings, often seen in the late, exhausted phases of migraine.

HEMIANOPIA   A peculiar sort of blindness, arising from disorder in the brain, in which there is loss of *half* the visual field. The lost part does not look *dark* (as in ordinary blindness), but nonexistent. Thus a person may not be aware of hemianopia (or scotoma)—not only losing the sight of one half, but also losing the *idea* of this half (see chapter 3).

HEMIPLEGIA   Paralysis of one side, seen in strokes, tumors, and (very rarely) migraines. A hemiplegia follows upon depression or destruction of the motor areas in one half (hemisphere) of the brain. A *hemianopia*—much commoner in migraine—upon involvement of the visual areas. *Hemisensory* deficits, or *hemianesthesia* may result from involvement of the general sensory or tactile areas.

HIGHER INTEGRATIVE (OR CORTICAL) *FUNCTIONS*   The neuropsychological (brain-mind) functions required for the putting together of speech, complex actions, perceptions, and the like. When disturbed, we find such disorders as *agnosia, aphasia, apraxia, amusia*.

HISTAMINE   An amine found in the nervous system and other tissues, which can serve as a transmitter of nerve impulses (see Histamine headache, chapter 4).

HOMEOSTASIS   The maintenance of physiological constancy and stability. This (according to Claude Bernard, who introduced the concept) is the "purpose" of all physiological controls, and is "the condition of a free life." In disease, and in migraine, homeostasis is disturbed, and with this diminution in stability comes a corresponding reduction in freedom of activity.

HORNER'S SYNDROME   An inhibition or paralysis of the sympathetic nerves to the eye, so the eye droops, produces tears, has a small pupil, and so on. May occur transiently in migraine, most especially migrainous neuralgia (see chapter 4).

HYPERTENSION, HYPOTENSION   Respectively, an unusually high or low "tension" or level of blood pressure.

HYPOGLYCEMIA   Abnormally low blood-sugar—an occasional cause or concomitant of migraine.

ICTUS   A seizure, or attack of any kind. Prior to a seizure there may be *pre-ictal* excitement, and, succeeding it, *post-ictal* exhaustion (and immunity).

IDIOPATHY   A feeling or malady arising *on its own*, and not obviously in response to some other cause. Thus idiopathic migraines come out of the blue, while symptomatic ones may follow a Chinese meal or a rage (see chapter 7).

INDURATION   Inflammatory thickening.

LACRIMATION   Tearing: specifically, a physiological, involuntary, nonemotional production of tears.

LARYNGISMUS   A spasm of the larynx (compare, vaginismus, tenesmus, and similar formations).

LATENT, DORMANT, AND SO ON.   Latent means "hidden," dormant "asleep." It is commonly held that one does not *acquire* migraine out of the blue, but that one may have some "latent" or "dormant" tendency to it, which is made actual, or *manifest*, under provocative conditions.

MEISOSIS, MYDRIASIS   Contraction and dilatation of pupils respectively.

METAMORPHOSES   Transformations. Specifically, here, the transformations of migraine into (or from) other disorders—transformations which involve *equivalence* in some sense(s) (see chapter 2).

MIGRAINE   Derived from *hemicrania* (half head), indicating that its headache is commonly confined to either side (or sometimes, alternating sides) of the head. Despite the word, headache is *never* the sole feature of a migraine (see page 11).

MIGRAINEUR/MIGRAINEUSE   A male/female sufferer from migraine.

MIGRALEPSY   Hybrid word for a hybrid attack which combines features of both migraine and epilepsy.

MOSAIC VISION, CINEMATIC VISION   In mosaic vision the sense of *spatial* articulation and continuity is lost, and one sees a flat mosaic, without spaciousness or meaning. In cinematic vision the sense of *time* is fractured, the sense of continuity, articulation, and development in time; and one sees the world as a sequence of motionless stills.

MYOCLONIC JERKS   Violent jerks involving large portions of the body's musculature. Such jerks happen to everybody, on occasion, while falling asleep. They tend, however, to be especially common before and during some migraines.

NARCOLEPSY   A brief, sudden, usually dream-charged sleep, which may be of compelling power and gives little warning. Narcolepsy is often related to nightmares, sleepwalking, sleep paralysis (when one is awake, but unable to move), and other phenomena. All such sleep disorders are related to migraine.

NEURALGIA   The pain of an irritated, inflamed or injured nerve. Such pains tend to be excruciatingly, wincingly violent—though often very short-lived ("lightning pains"). They are seen especially in migrainous neuralgia (chapter 4). The quality of pain is very characteristic, and quite different from that of *vascular pain* (the pain of swollen, throbbing blood vessels) and of *muscular* pain (the ache of muscles tensed, or in spasm), which are much commoner in migraine.

NEUROGENIC   Produced by the nervous system. Thus one may experience fever in a migraine, not due to any inflammation or infection, but purely "neurogenic."

NEUROPSYCHOLOGICAL   The relation (or correlation) of altering conditions of the nervous system with altering states of perception, feeling, and of mind; the grounding of psychology in neurology and physiology. All the phenomena of migraine allow neuropsychological study, but the most wonderful such correlations are to be found in the migraine *aura* (see chapter 3).

NOR-ADRENALIN See *Adrenalin.*

OLIGURIA Scanty urine production.

ONEIRIC Of, or belonging to, dreams.

OPHTHALMOPLEGIA Partial or complete paralysis of eye movement—which may occur very rarely (and transiently) in migraine—due to disorder of the eyes' controls in the brain (chapter 4).

ORTHOSTATIC HYPOTENSION Inability to maintain normal blood pressure when standing; so, liability to feel dizzy, or faint, on sudden standing.

PANCREATITIS Inflammation of the pancreas.

PARESTHESIA Tingling feelings, in any part of the body produced by disorder of the nervous system. *Un*pleasant tingling may be called *dysethesia.* Other disturbances of feeling (e.g., the sensation of a tight band, of a plaster cast, of subjective heat or cold)—all disturbances of normal feeling may be called paresthesia. If the disturbances are very complex, and assume the form of images, we speak of *phantoms.* The most complex paresthesia and phantoms are only seen in migraine *aura* (see chapter 3).

PATHOGNOMONIC Symptoms and signs considered wholly characteristic—or *diagnostic*—of a particular disorder.

PHOSPHENES Tiny, subjective radiances or sparks, very common in the early stages of a migraine—even commoner than full-fledged scotomata.

PHOTOPHOBIA, PHONOPHOBIA (LITERALLY HATRED OF LIGHT, HATRED OF SOUND) The exaggerated, almost intolerable sensitivity to these which frequently occur in the course of a migraine (see pages 26–27).

PLETHORA Congestion.

PRODROME (LITERALLY, "RUNNING BEFORE") The early or inaugural features of a migraine which often serve as a warning of an impending attack.

PROSOPAGNOSIA A specific inability to recognize *faces*—and also facial and bodily *expressions.* This may give rise to disorientation, and even depersonalization, derealization, and so on.

PSEUDOMIGRAINE Term often used for the occurrence of migraine, or migraine-like symptoms, in consequence of an anatomical abnormality in the brain (a tumor, a malformation, an aneurysm, etc.). *These are rare.* Pseudomigraines may also be called symptomatic migraines—to distinguish them from idiopathic attacks which have no such structural abnormality underlying them.

PSYCHOPHYSIOLOGICAL A highfalutin word for the simplest and deepest mystery in the world—the relation of "soul" and "body," and specifically, their going together in health and disease. Migraine is here portrayed as a most common and striking *psychophysiological reaction*, involving changes of attitude and mood inseparable from all the physical changes (see *Psychosomatic; Neuropsychological*).

PSYCHOSOMATIC Physical responses to mental or emotional stimuli, for example, the occurrence of ulcers, asthma—and, of course, migraine—when these can be related to heightened emotion or stress.

PTOSIS   Drooping of an eyelid.

SCINTILLATION   The sort of twinkling which is very characteristic of many of the visual phenomena of migraine—especially the crescentic expanding scotomata—the twinkling of phosphenes—and of cinematic vision.

SCOTOMA (LITERALLY, DARKNESS OR SHADOW)   Dramatic disturbances in vision and the visual field, taking the form of strange and often twinkling brilliances (scintillating scotomata), or strange blindnesses and absences of vision. Without doubt scotomata, of one sort or another, are the most common feature of migraine other than headache and, possibly, commoner than headache itself (see chapter 3).

SPECTRUM   A luminous scotoma in the visual field, colored and arched like a rainbow (see chapter 3).

SPLANCHNIC   Involuntary tissues and activities of the viscera: often engorged, and increased, in the early portions of a migraine—as with vascular (and glandular) appearance and activity.

STERNUTATORY   Provocative of sneezinglike snuff. Useful on occasion in terminating a migraine.

STIGMATA   Stigmata are sings or marks of disease—or, indeed, of anything else (such as the stigmata of grace—or disgrace). The term carries a signification over and above the purely medical terms "pathognomonic" and "diagnostic," indicating that the sufferer is "marked" and singled out. One might say that over and above the medical problems of having a disorder stand the problems of being *stigmatized* by it. Epileptics may be most cruelly (and unjustly) stigmatized; migraineurs, mercifully, are much less so.

SYNAESTHESIA   A "fusion" between normally distinct senses, so that sounds, for example, may be "seen," felt, and tasted (wonderfully described in *The Mind of a Mnemonist* by Luria). Probably a primitive state—may be normal in early infancy.

SYNCOPE   A brief loss or interruption of consciousness—a blackout.

SYNDROME   literally, like "concurrence" or "concourse," a *running-together*). A key word and key concept in our understanding of migraine, or of any other medical or "organic" condition. A syndrome is an *association*, but not just a random or mechanical one (like a junk shop). It is an organic association of features which *naturally* go together, and which therefore form a sort of composite or unity. Thus we may speak of migraine syndromes, Parkinsonian syndromes, personality syndromes, as well as others. We may perceive a syndrome, or that something *is* a syndrome, long before we are able to dissect it: and classical medicine (or *nosology*) is a natural history of such syndromes —as biology is a natural history and classification of organic beings.

SYMPATHETIC/PARASYMPATHETIC   These are the two great divisions of the *autonomic* (or vegetative) nervous system (see also *Autonomic*). Actions of the sympathetic system "tone up" the organism—increasing muscular tone, blood flow to muscles, heart action, blood pressure, wakefulness, energy, and affect other functions, thus preparing the organism for work, or fight-flight (sometimes called *ergotropic*). The parasympathetic system, by contrast, is concerned with consolidation, conservation, rest—and, when active (after meals, during sleep, and in the latter part of a migraine) *reduces* energy, vigilance, heart rate, muscle tone, and so on, while increasing the activity of the viscera and glands (sometimes called *trophotropic*). There is normally a fine "tuning" or balance between these two systems—but this is grossly disturbed in a migraine.

SYMPATHOTONIC/VAGOTONIC (*SEE SYMPATHETIC/PARASYMPATHETIC, AUTONOMIC, ETC.*) Old terms, once widely used, indicating a preponderant tendency to overstimulation of the sympathetic system (which would be shown as irritability, rage, tension, etc.), or of the opposite parasympathetic or vagal system (which would be shown as weakness, collapse, withdrawal, etc.). Such abnormal sensitivities, and lack of autonomic balance, have been considered as characteristic, or common, in migraineurs.

SYMPATHY (LITERALLY "FEELING TOGETHER" OR "SUFFERING TOGETHER") Often used with regard to various *organs*, in the older views of migraine, for example, the stomach suffering in sympathy with the head (see pages 3–4).

TACHYCARDIA, BRADYCARDIA Exceptionally rapid or exceptionally slow heart beat, respectively.

TINNITUS A high-pitched ringing sound, which may occur briefly in a migraine, sometimes accompanied by distortions in hearing, partial deafness, or vertigo. Tinnitus is the auditory equivalent of scintillations or phosphenes in sight, as formication and paresthesia are their equivalents in touch.

TRANSUDATION A passage of fluid from one compartment of the body, or one tissue, to another. Passage *out*, that is, on to, the surface of an organ or the skin, is *exudation*.

TROPHIC The *nutritive* functions of nerves and blood are called "trophic." If they are inadequate, we see dystrophy, or atrophy. Such changes are rare, and usually transient, in migraine, and occur in relation to extremities, such as skin, nails, hair.

TURBINATES Bony structures in the nostrils, resembling little scrolls or turbans.

UNCINATE SEIZURES Epileptic seizures (or migraines) arising in the *uncus*, deep in the brain. Such attacks are characterized by strange smells, a strange feeling of "having been there before" (*déjà vu*), sometimes vivid recollections of childhood, and occasionally speech disturbances.

URTICARIA Hives.

VASOVAGAL Having reference to the vagus nerve, and its relation to the tone of blood vessels. This is suddenly diminished in a so-called vasovagal attack (or faint).

VERTIGO A sensation of spinning—very sickening and intolerable—with an acute loss of orientation and balance.

Bibliography

ABERCROMBIE, J. (1829). *Local Affections of Nerves*. Churchill, London.

AIRY, G. B. (1865). "The Astronomer Royal on Hemiopsy." *Philosophical Magazine* 30:19–21.

AIRY, HUBERT. (1870). "On a Transient Form of Hemianopsia." *Phil. Trans. R. Soc. London* 160:247–270.

ALAJOUANINE, T., (1963). "Dostoievski's Epilepsy." *Brain* 86:209–21.

ALEXANDER, F. (1948). "Fundamental Concepts of Psychosomatic Research," pp. 3–13, in *Studies in Psychosomatic Medicine: an approach to the causes and treatment of vegetative disorders*. The Ronald Press, New York.

ALEXANDER, F., and FRENCH, T. M. (1948). *Studies in Psychosomatic Medicine: an Approach to the Causes and Treatment of Vegetative Disorders*. The Ronald Press, New York.

ALEXANDER, FRANS. (1950). *Psychosomatic Medicine: its Principles and Applications*. W. W. Norton & Co., New York.

ALVAREZ, W. C. (1945). "Was There Sick Headache in 3000 BC?" *Gastroenterology* 5:524.

———. (1959). "Some Characteristics of the Migrainous Woman." *N.Y. State J. Med.* 59:2176.

———. (1960). "The Migraine Scotoma as Studied in 618 Persons." *Amer. J. Ophth* 49:489.

ANDERSON, P. G. (1975). "Ergotamine Headache." 15:118–121.

ARETAEUS. (1856). *The Extant Works of Aretaeus the Cappadocian*. (Francis Adams's translation: printed for the Sydenham Society.) Wertheimer & Co., London.

ARING, C. D. (1972). "The Migrainous Scintillating Scotoma." *J.A.M.A.* 220:519–522.

BALYEAT, R. M. (1933). *Migraine: Diagnosis and Treatment*. J. B. Lippincott Co., Philadelphia & London.

BARKLEY, G. L., TEPLEY, N., SIMKINS, R., MORAN, J., and WELCH, K. M. (1990). "Neuromagnetic Fields in Migraine: Preliminary Findings." *Cephalalgia* 10 (no. 4):171–176.

BARRIE, M. A., FOX, W. R., WEATHERALL, M. and WILKINSON, M. I. P. (1968). "Analysis of Symptoms of Patients with Headache and their Response to Treatment with Ergot Derivatives." *Quart. J. Med.* 37:319. (See also leading article on this subject in *Brit. Med. J.* of 4 January 1969.)

BEAUMONT, G. E. (1952). *Medicine.* (6th ed.) J. & A. Churchill, London.

BICKERSTAFF, E. R. (1961). "Basilar Artery Migraine." *Lancet* 1:15.

———. (1961). "Impairment of Consciousness in Migraine." *Lancet* 2:1057.

BLAU, J. N. ed. (1987). *Migraine: Clinical, Therapeutic, Conceptual and Research Aspects.* London, Chapman and Hall Medical.

BLAU, J. N. and WHITTY, C. W. M. (1955). "Familial Hemiplegic Migraine." *Lancet* 2:1115.

BLEULER, E. (1958). *Dementia Praecox, or the Group of Schizophrenias.* International Universities Press, New York.

BOISMONT, A. BRIERRE DE. (1853). *Hallucinations: Or, the Rational History of Apparitions, Visions, Dreams, Ecstasy, Magnetism and Somnambulism.* Lindsay & Blakiston, Philadelphia.

BRADLEY, W. G., HUDGSON, P., FOSTER, J. B. and NEWELL, D. J. (1968). "Double-blind Controlled Trial of a Micronized Preparation of Flumedroxone (Demigran) in Prophylaxis of Migraine." *Brit. Med. J.* 2:531.

BRADSHAW, P. and PARSONS, M. (1963). "Hemiplegic Migraine: a Clinical Study." *Quart. J. Med.* 34:65.

BREWSTER, D. (1865). "On Hemiopsy, or Half-Vision," reprinted in *Trans. Roy. Soc. Edinburgh* 24:15–18, 1867.

BRUYN, G. W. (1968). "Complicated Migraine," in *Handbook of Clinical Neurology*, ed. P. J. Vinken and G. W. Bruyn. Amsterdam: Elsevier Science Publishing Co.

———. (1986). "Migraine Equivalents," in *Handbook of Clinical Neurology*, 48:155–171, ed. by F. C. Rose. Amsterdam: Elsevier.

BURN, J. H. (1963). *The Autonomic Nervous System.* Blackwell, Oxford.

CANNON, W. B. (1920). *Bodily Changes in Pain, Hunger, Fear, and Rage.* (2nd ed.) D. Appleton & Co., New York.

CAPLAN, L., CHEDRU, F., LHERMITTE, F., and MAYMAN, C. (1981). "Transient Global Amnesia and Migraine." *Neurology* 31:1167–1170.

CHARCOT, J.-M. (1892). *Clinique des Maladies du Systeme Nerveux*, pp. 71–89. Paris, Babe et Cie.

COHN, R. (1949). *Clinical Electroencephalography.* McGraw-Hill Book Co. Inc., New York.

CRITCHLEY, MACDONALD. (1936). "Prognosis in Migraine." *Lancet* 1:35.

———. (1963). "What is Migraine?" *J. Coll. Gen. Pract.* 6 (supp. 4):5.

———. (1964). "The Malady of Anne, Countess of Conway: a case for commentary," pp. 91–97, in *The Black Hole and Other Essays.* Pitman Medical Publ. Co., London, 1964.

———. (1966). "Migraine: From Cappadocia to Queen Square," in *Background to Migraine.* Heinemann, London.

CROWELL, G. F., et al. (1984). "The Transient Global Amnesia-Migraine Connection." *Archives of Neurology.* 41:75–79.

DARWIN, CHARLES. (1890). *The Expression of the Emotions in Man and Animals.* (2nd ed.) Murray, London.

DAVIES, PAUL. (1989). *The Cosmic Blueprint: New Discoveries in Nature's Ability to Order the Universe.* Simon and Schuster, New York.

DEUTSCH, F. (1959). *On the Mysterious Leap from the Mind to the Body.* International Universities Press, New York.

DEXTER, J. D., and RILEY, T. L. (1975). "Studies in Nocturnal Migraine." *Headache* 15:51–62.

DIAMOND, SEYMOUR, and DALESSIO, DONALD J. (1982). *The Practicing Physician's Approach to Headache* (3rd ed.) Williams & Wilkins, Baltimore.

DOW, D. J. and WHITTY, C. W. M. (1947). "Electroencephalographic Changes in Migraine." *Lancet* 2:52.

DUNNING, H. S. (1942). "Intracranial and Extracranial Vascular Accidents in Migraine." *Arch. Neurol. Psychiatr.* 48:396.

EDELMAN, G. M. (1990). *The Remembered Present: A Biological Theory of Consciousness.* New York, Basic Books.

EKBOM, K. A. (1987). "Treatment of Cluster Headache: Episodic and Chronic," in *Migraine,* ed. J. N. Blau, pp. 433–448. London, Chapman and Hall Medical.

ELKIND, A. H., FRIEDMAN, A. P., BACHMAN, A., SIEGELMAN, S. S., and SACKS, O. W. (1968). "Silent Retroperitoneal Fibrosis Associated with Methysergide Therapy." *Journal of the American Medical Association* 206:1041–1044.

ELLERTSON, B., et al. (1987). "Psychophysiological Response Patterns in Migraine Before and After Temperature Biofeedback." *Cephalalgia* 7:109–124.

ENGEL, G. L., FERRIS, E. B. and ROMANO, J. (1945). "Focal Electroencephalographic Changes during the Scotomas of Migraine." *Amer. J. Med. Sc.* 209:650.

ERMENTROUT, G. B., and COWEN, J. D. (1979). "A Mathematical Theory of Visual Hallucination Patterns." *Biological Cybernetics* 34:137–150.

FARQUHAR, H. G. (1956). "Abdominal Migraine in Children." *Brit. Med. J.* 1:1062.

FEIGENBAUM, MITCHELL J. (1980). "Universal Behavior in Non-Linear Systems." *Los Alamos Science* 1:4–27.

FITZ-HUGH, T. JR. (1940). "Praecordial Migraine: an Important Form of 'Angina Innocens.'" *New Int Clinics* 1 (series 3):143.

FLATAU, E. (1912). *Die Migräne.* Monogr. Gesamtgeb., Neurol. Psychiat., Heft II. Berlin, Spring.

FOUCAULT, M. (1965). *Madness and Civilization.* Random House, New York.

FREUD, SIGMUND. (1952) [1920]. *A General Introduction to Psychoanalysis.* Reprinted by Washington Square Press, New York.

FRIEDMAN, A. P., HARTER, D. H. and MERRITT, H. H. (1961). "Ophthalmoplegic Migraine." *Trans. Amer. Neur. Ass.* 86:169.

FROMM-REICHMANN, F. (1937). "Contributions to the Psychogenesis of Migraine." *Psychoanal. Rev.* 24:26.

FULLER, G. N., and GALE, M. V. (1988). "Migraine Aura as Artistic Inspiration," *British Medical Journal* 297:1670–1672, December 24, 1988.

FURMANSKI, A. R. (1952). "Dynamic Concepts of Migraine: A Character Study of One Hundred Patients." *Arch. Neurol. Psychiat.* 67:23.

GARDENER, J. W., MOUNTAIN, G. E. and HINES, E. A. (1940). "The Relationship of Migraine to Hypertension Headache." *Amer. J. Med. Sc.* 200:50.

GARRETT, ELIZABETH. (1870). "Sur la Migraine," doctoral thesis, Paris. (This thesis has been translated into English by Marcia Wilkinson.)

GELLHORN, ERNST. (1967). *Principles of Autonomic-Somatic Integration.* University of Minnesota Press, Minneapolis.

GIBBS, E. L. and GIBBS, F. A. (1951). "Electroencephalographic Evidence of Thalamic and Hypothalamic Epilepsy." *Neurology* 1:136.

GIBBS, F. A., and GIBBS, E. L. (1941). *Atlas of Electroencephalography.* Lew A. Commings Co., Cambridge, Mass. Reprinted by Addison-Wesley Press Inc., Cambridge, Mass., 1950.

GILLES DE LA TOURETTE, G. (1898). *Leçons de Clinique Thérapeutique sur les Maladies du Système Nerveux.* Bailliere, Paris.

GILLES DE LA TOURETTE, G., and BLOCQ, P. (1887). "Sur le Traitment de la Migraine Ophtalmique Accompagnée." *Prog. Med.,* 2me ser. 5:476–477.

GOODELL, H., LEWONTIN, R. and WOLFF, H. G. (1954). "The Familial Occurrence of Migraine Headache: a Study of Heredity." *Ass. Research Nerv. Ment. Dis.* 33:346.

GOODMAN, L. S., and GILMAN, A. (1955). *The Pharmacological Basis of Therapeutics.* (2nd ed.) Macmillan, New York.

GOWERS, W. R., SIR. (1964) [1881]. *Epilepsy and Other Chronic Convulsive Diseases: their Causes, Symptoms, and Treatment.* Dover Publications Reprint, New York.

———. (1988). *A Manual of Diseases of the Nervous System.* Vol. 2: 776–795. J. & A. Churchill, London.

———. (1895). "Subjective Visual Sensations." *Trans. Ophthalmol. Soc. U.K.* 15:20–44.

———. (1904). *Subjective Sensations of Sight and Sound: Abiotrophy, and Other Lectures.* P. Blakiston's Son & Co., Philadelphia.

———. (1907). *The Borderland of Epilepsy: Faints, Vagal Attacks, Vertigo, Migraine, Sleep Symptoms, and their Treatment.* P. Blakiston's Son & Co., Philadelphia.

GRAHAM, J. R. (1952). "The Natural History of Migraine: Some Observations and a Hypothesis." *Trans. Amer. Clin. & Climat. Ass.* 64:61.

GREENE, R. (1963). "Migraine—the Menstrual Aspect." *J. Coll. Gen. Pract.* 6 (supp. 4):15.

GREPPI, E. (1955). "Migraine Ground." *Int. Archiv. Allergy App. Immun.* 7:305.

GRIMES, E. (1931). "The Migraine Instability." *Med. J. Rec.* 134:417.

GRODDECK, GEORGE. (1949). *The Book of the It.* (Authorised translation of *Das Buch vom Es,* 1923.) Random House, New York.

HACHINSKI, V. C., PORCHAWKA, J., and STEELE, J. C. (1973). "Visual Symptoms in the Migraine Syndrome," *Neurology* 23:570–579.

HEBB, D. O. (1954). "The Problem of Consciousness and Introspection" in *Brain Mechanisms and Consciousness*, edited by J. F. Delafresnaye. Charles C. Thomas, Springfield, Ill.

————. (1968). "Concerning Imagery," *Psychological Review* 75:466–477.

HEBERDEN, WILLIAM. (1802). *Commentaries on the History and Cure of Diseases*. T. Payne, London.

HERSCHEL, J. F. W. (1858). "On Sensorial Vision," reprinted in *Familiar Lectures on Scientific Subjects*. London: Alexander Strahan, 1866.

HEYCK, H. (1956). *Neue Beiträge für klinik und Pathogenese der Migräne*. Theime, Stuttgart.

————. (1964). *Der Kopfschmerz* (3rd ed.) Stuttgart.

HORTON, B. T. (1956). "Histaminic Cephalgia: Differential Diagnosis and Treatment." *Proc. Mayo Clinic* 31:325.

HUBEL, D. H., and WIESEL, T. N. (1963). "Shape and Arrangement of Columns in Cat's Striate Cortex." *J. Physiology* (London) 165:559–568.

JACKSON, J. HUGHLINGS. (1931). *Selected Writings of John Hughlings Jackson*. Edited by James Taylor. Hodder & Stoughton, London.

JANET, P. (1921). "A Case of Sleep lasting Five Years, with Loss of Sense of Reality." *Arch. Neurol. & Psychiat.* 6:467.

JARCHO, SAUL. (1968). "Migraine in Astronomers and 'Natural Philosophers.'" *Bulletin of the New York Academy of Sciences*, v. 44, no. 7:886–891.

JOHNSON, E. S., KADAM, N. P., HYLANDS, D. M., and HYLANDS, P. J. (1985). "Efficacy of Feverfew as Prophylactic Treatment of Migraine." *British Medical Journal* 291:569–573.

JONES, ERNEST. (1949). *On the Nightmare*. Hogarth Press, London.

KEELER, M. H. (1968). "Marihuana-induced Hallucinations," *Diseases of the Nervous System* 29:314–315.

————. (1970). "Kluver's Mechanisms of Hallucination as Illustrated by the Paintings of Max Ernst," in *Origin and Mechanisms of Hallucination*, ed. W. Keup. Plenum Press, New York.

KIMBALL, R. W., FRIEDMAN, A. P. and VALLEJO, E. (1960). "Effect of Serotonin in Migraine Patients." *Neurology* 10:107.

KLEE, A. (1968). *A Clinical Study of Migraine with Particular Reference to the Most Severe Cases*. Munksgaard, Copenhagen.

————. (1975). "Perceptual Disorders in Migraine," in *Modern Topics in Medicine*, ed. J. Pearce, pp. 45–51. London, Heinemann.

KLUVER, HEINRICH (1928 and 1942). *Mescal and Mechanisms of Hallucination*, republished as a single volume, 1966. Chicago, University of Chicago Press.

KONORSKI, JERZY. (1967). *Integrative Activity of the Brain: an Interdisciplinary Approach*. University of Chicago Press, Chicago.

KUNKLE, E. C. (1959). "Acetylcholine in the Mechanism of Headache of the Migraine Type." *Arch. Neurol. Psychiat.* 81:135.

LANCE, JAMES W. (1982). *Mechanisms and Management of Headache* (4th ed.) Butterworth Scientific, London & Boston.

————. (1986). *Migraine and Other Headaches*. Scribner's, New York.

————. (1990). "A Concept of Migraine and the Search for the Ideal Headache Drug." *Headache* 30:17.

LANCE, J. W. and ANTHONY, M. (1960). "Some Clinical Aspects of Migraine." *Arch. Neurol.* 15:356.

LANCE, J. W., ANTHONY, M. and HINTERBERGER, H. (1967). "The Control of Cranial Arteries by Humoral Mechanisms and its Relation to the Migraine Syndrome." *Headache* 7:93.

LASHLEY, K. S. (1931). "Mass Action in Cerebral Function." *Science* 73:245–254.

———. (1941). "Patterns of Cerebral Integration indicated by Scotomas of Migraine." *Arch. Neurol. Psychiat.* 46:331.

LAURITZEN, M. (1987). "Cortical Spreading Depression as a Putative Migraine Mechanism." *TINS* 10:8–13.

LEÃO, A. (1944). "Spreading Depression of Activity in the Cerebral Cortex." *Neurophysiol.* 7:359.

LEES, F. and WATKINS, S. M. (1963). "Loss of Consciousness in Migraine". *Lancet* 2:647.

LENNOX, W. G. (1941). *Science and Seizures: New Light on Epilepsy and Migraine.* Harper & Bros., New York.

LENNOX, W. G., and LENNOX, M. A. (1960). *Epilepsy and Related Disorders.* (2 volumes.) Little, Brown & Co., Boston.

LEROY, R. (1922). "The Syndrome of Lilliputian Hallucinations." *J. Nerv. & Ment. Dis.* 56:325.

———. (1926). "The Affective State in Lilliputian Hallucinations." *J. Ment. Sci.* 72:179–186.

LIPPMAN, C. W. (1952). "Certain Hallucinations Peculiar to Migraine," *J. Nervous and Mental Disease* 116:346–351.

———. (1953). "Hallucinations of Physical Duality in Migraine." *J. Nerv. & Ment. Dis.* 117:345.

LIVEING, EDWARD. (1873). *On Megrim, Sick-Headache, and Some Allied Disorders: A Contribution to the Pathology of Nerve-Storms.* Churchill, London.

LURIA, A. P. (1966). *Higher Cortical Functions in Man.* (Translated by Basil Haigh.) Basic Books, New York.

MANDELBROT, BENOIT. (1982). *The Fractal Geometry of Nature.* San Francisco, Freeman.

MASTERS, R. E. L., and HOUSTON, J. (1967). *The Varieties of Psychedelic Experience.* Dell, New York.

———. (1968). *Psychedelic Art.* Grove Press, New York.

MILES, P. W. (1958). "Scintillating Scotoma: Clinical and Anatomical Significance of Pattern, Size, and Movement." *J.A.M.A.* 167:1810.

MILLER, J. *The Body in Question.* In preparation.

MILLER, W. R. (1936). "Psychogenic Factors in Polyuria of Schizophrenia." *J. Nerv. & Ment. Dis.* 84:418.

MILNER, P. M. (1958). "Note on a Possible Correspondence between the Scotomas of Migraine and the Spreading Depression of Leão." *Electroenceph. Clin. Neurophysiol.* 10:705.

MINGAZZINI, G. (1926). "Klinischer Beitrag zum Studium der cephalalgischen und hemikranischen Psykosen." *Z. ges. Neurol. Psychiatr.* 101:428.

MOBIUS. (1894). *Die Migräne.* Wien.

MOERSCH, F. P. (1924). "Psychic Manifestations in Migraine." *Amer. J. Psychiat.* 3:697–716.

MOREAU DE TOURS, JACQUES JOSEPH. (1973). *Hashish and Mental Illness.* Raven Press, New York. (Translation of 1845 original "Du Haschisch et de l'alienation mentale, etudes psychologique," Masson, Paris.)

MULLER, STEFAN C., PLESSER, THEO, and HESS, BENNO. (1989). "Structural Elements of Dynamical Chemical Patterns," *Leonardo* 22:3–10.

OLESEN, Jes. (1991). "Cerebral and Extracranial Circulatory Disturbances in Migraine: Pathophysiological Implications." *Cerebrovascular and Brain Metabolism Reviews* 3:1–28. New York, Raven Press.

OLESEN, J., LARSEN, B., and LAURITZEN, M. (1981). "Focal Hyperemia Followed by Spreading Oligemia and Impaired Activation of rCBF in Classical Migraine," *Annals of Neurology* 9:344.

OSTER, G. (1970). "Phosphenes," *Scientific American* 222:83–87.

PAVLOV, I. P. (1928–41). *Lectures on Conditioned Reflexes.* (Translated by W. Horsley Gantt.) International Publishers, New York.

PENFIELD, W. (1958). *The Excitable Cortex in Conscious Man.* Charles C. Thomas, Springfield.

PENFIELD, W. and PEROT, P. (1963). "The Brain's Record of Auditory and Visual Experience—a Final Summary and Discussion." *Brain* 86:595.

PENFIELD, W., and RASMUSSEN, T. (1950). *The Cerebral Cortex of Man.* The Macmillan Co., New York.

PETERS, J. C. (1853). *A Treatise on Headache.* William Radde, New York.

PIORRY, P. (1831). "Memoire sur une des Affections Désignées sous le Nom de Migraine ou Hémicranie." *J. Univ. hebd. Méd Chir,* prat. 2(1831):5–18; *J. Méd Chir.,* prat. Paris, 2e éd. Tome II (1936):33–34; *Traité Méd.,* prat. Tome VIII (1850):75.

PLANT, GORDON T. (1986). "The Fortification Spectra of Migraine," *British Medical Journal* 293:1613–1617, December 20, 1986.

PRIGOGINE, ILYA. (1980). *From Being to Becoming.* W. H. Freeman, San Francisco.

PRIGOGINE, ILYA, and STENGERS, ISABELLE. (1984). *Order Out of Chaos.* Bantam Books, New York.

RANSON, R., IGARASHI, H., MACGREGOR, E. A., and WILKINSON, M. (1991). "The Similarities and Differences of Migraine with Aura and Migraine without Aura: A Preliminary Study," *Cephalalgia* 11 (no. 4):189–192, September 1991.

RASCOL, A., CAMBIER, J., GUIRAUD, B., MANELFE, C., DAVID, J., and CLANET, M. (1979). "Accidents Ischemique Cerebraux au Cours de Crises Migraineuses," *Rev. Neurol* (Paris) 135:867.

RASKIN, NEIL HUGH. (1988). *Headache* (2nd ed.) Churchill Livingstone, New York.

———. (1990). "Conclusions." *Headache* 30:24.

RICHARDS, W. (1971). "The Fortification Illusions of Migraine," *Scientific American* 224:88–96.

ROSE, E. CLIFFORD, and GAWEL, M. (1979). *Migraine: The Facts.* Oxford University Press, Oxford.

RIEFF, P. (1959). *Freud: The Mind of the Moralist.* Doubleday & Co., New York.
SACKS, OLIVER. (1992). "The Last Hippie." *New York Review of Books* 39, no.
    6:58–62.
————. (1987). *A Leg to Stand On.* Harper & Row, New York.
————. (1987). *The Man Who Mistook His Wife for a Hat and Other Clinical
    Tales.* Harper & Row, New York.
SCHREIBER, A. O., and CALVERT, P. C. (1986). "Migrainous Olfactory Halluci-
    nations." *Headache* 26:513–514.
SELBY, G., and LANCE, J. W. (1960). "Observations on 500 cases of Migraine
    and Allied Vascular Headache." *J. Neurol. Neurosurg. Psychiat.* 23:23.
SELYE, H. (1946). "The General Adaptation Syndrome and Diseases of Adapta-
    tion." *J. Clinic. Endocrinol.* 6:117.
SICUTERI, F. (1959). "Prophylactic and Therapeutic Properties of Methyl Lyser-
    gic Acid Butanolamide in Migraine." *Int. Arch. Allergy* 15:300.
SIEGEL, RALPH. (1990). "Chaos and the Single Neuron in Area VI of the Cat."
    Abstracts Soc. Neuroscience 16:230.
SIEGEL, RONALD K. (1977). "Hallucinations." *Scientific American* 237 (no.
    4):132–140, October 1977.
SIEGEL, RONALD K., and JARVIK, MURRAY E. (1975). "Drug-Induced Hallucina-
    tions in Animals and Man," in *Hallucinations,* ed. R. K. Siegel and L. J. West.
    John Wiley & Sons, New York.
SINGER, CHARLES. (1958). "The Visions of Hildegard of Bingen," in *From Magic
    to Science.* Dover, New York.
STRAUSS, H. and SELINSKY, H. (1941). "EEG Findings in Patients with Migrain-
    ous Syndrome." *Trans. Amer. Neurol. Ass.* 67:205.
SYMON, D. N. K., and RUSSELL, G. (1986). "Abdominal Migraine: A Childhood
    Syndrome Defined." *Cephalalgia* 6:223–228.
SYMONDS, C. (1952). "Migrainous Variations." *Trans. Med. Soc. London*
    67:237. Reprinted in Symonds, *Studies in Neurology.* London, Oxford Uni-
    versity Press, 1970.
THOMPSON, D'ARCY W. (1942). *On Growth and Form.* Cambridge, Cambridge
    University Press.
TISSOT, SIMON ANDRÉ. 1770). *An Essay on the Disorders of People of Fashion.*
    (Translated by F. B. Lee.) S. Bladon, London. See also the last volume of *Traité
    des nerfs et leurs maladies,* of which 83 pages are devoted to the subject of
    migraine. Paris, 1778–1790.
TOURRAINE, G. A. and DRAPER, G. (1934). "The Migrainous Patient: A Consti-
    tutional Study." *J. Nerv. & Ment. Dis.* 80:1.
TURING, A. M. (1952). "The Chemical Basis of Morphogenesis." *Philos. Trans.
    Roy. Soc.* B237:37.
VAHLQUIST, B. and HACKZELL, G. (1949). "Migraine of Early Onset." *Acta
    Paediatrica* 38:622.
WEIR MITCHELL, S. (1887) "Neuralgic Headache with Apparitions of Unusual
    Character." *Amer. J. Med. Science* 93–94; 415–419.
WEISS, E., and ENGLISH, O. S. (1957). *Psychosomatic Medicine: A Clinical Study
    of Psychophysiological Reactions.* W. B. Saunders Co., Philadelphia & Lon-
    don.

WELCH, K. M. A. (1987). "Migraine: A Biobehavioral Disorder." *Archives of Neurology* 44:323–327.

WHITEHOUSE, D., PAPPAS, J. A., ESCALA, P. H. and LIVINGSTON, S. (1967). "Electroencephalographic Changes in Children with Migraine." *New Eng. J. Med.* 276:23.

WHITTY, C. W. M. (1953). "Familial Hemiplegic Migraine." *J. Neurol. Neurosurg. Psychiat.* 16:172.

———. (1971). "Migraine Variants." *British Medical Journal* 1:38–40.

WHYTT, ROBERT. (1768). *Diseases commonly called Nervous, Hypochondriac, or Hysteric.* Becket, Pond, & Balfour, Edinburgh.

WILKINSON, M., and BLAU, J. N. (1985). "Are Classical and Common Migraine Different Entities?" *Headache* 25:211–212.

WILLIS, THOMAS. (1684). *De Morb. Convuls.* (Amstel, 1670), *De Anima Brutorum* (Oxon, 1672). First English translation (Pordage) in *Dr. Willis' practice of Physick, Being the Whole Works of that Renowned and Famous Physician.* London.

WILSON, S. A. K. (1940). *Neurology.* Vol. 2:1570. Butterworth's.

WOLFF, H. G. (1963). *Headache and other Head-Pain.* Oxford University Press, New York.

Further information and help can be obtained from:

The National Headache Foundation
5252 North Western Avenue
Chicago, IL 60625
U.S.A.
800–843–2256

The Migraine Foundation
120 Carlton Street, Suite 210
Toronto, Ontario M5A 4K2
Canada
800–663–3557

The Migraine Trust
45 Great Ormond Street
London WC1 3HD
England
071–278–2676

The British Migraine Association
178a High Road
Bayfleet, Weybridge
Surrey KT14 7ED
England
0932–352–468

Index

Dr. Oliver Sacks was born in London in 1933 to a medical family: both of his parents were physicians. He was educated in London, Oxford, California and New York. His first clinical experience was with the care of migraine patients—he feels his real education as a physician began here. His central interest is always the individual's experience of and struggle with neurological disorder. Dr. Sacks is Professor of Neurology at the Albert Einstein College of Medicine in New York, and the author of *A Leg to Stand On, The Man Who Mistook His Wife for a Hat, Seeing Voices*, and *Awakenings*, which has recently been adapted as a feature film.

Designer: U. C. Press Staff
Compositor: J. Jarrett Engineering, Inc.
Text: 10/13 Sabon
Display: Sabon
Printer: Edwards Brothers, Inc.
Binder: Edwards Brothers, Inc.